Modelling Degradation of Bioresorbable Polymeric Medical Devices

Related titles

Computational modelling of biomechanics and biotribology in the musculoskeletal system
(ISBN 978-0-85709-661-6)

Bio-tribocorrosion in biomaterials and medical implants
(ISBN 978-0-85709-540-4)

Durability and reliability of medical polymers
(ISBN 978-1-84569-929-1)

Woodhead Publishing Series in Biomaterials:
Number 83

Modelling Degradation of Bioresorbable Polymeric Medical Devices

Edited by

J. Pan

ELSEVIER

AMSTERDAM • BOSTON • CAMBRIDGE • HEIDELBERG
LONDON • NEW YORK • OXFORD • PARIS • SAN DIEGO
SAN FRANCISCO • SINGAPORE • SYDNEY • TOKYO
Woodhead Publishing is an imprint of Elsevier

WP
WOODHEAD
PUBLISHING

Woodhead Publishing is an imprint of Elsevier
80 High Street, Sawston, Cambridge, CB22 3HJ, UK
225 Wyman Street, Waltham, MA 02451, USA
Langford Lane, Kidlington, OX5 1GB, UK

British Library Cataloguing-in-Publication Data
A catalogue record for this book is available from the British Library

Library of Congress Control Number: 2014944394

ISBN 978-1-78242-016-3 (print)
ISBN 978-1-78242-025-5 (online)

For information on all Woodhead Publishing publications
visit our website at http://store.elsevier.com/

Contents

List of contributors

X. Chen University of Leicester, Leicester, UK

A. Gleadall University of Nottingham, Nottingham, UK

X. Han Loughborough University, Loughborough, UK

J. Pan University of Leicester, Leicester, UK

Woodhead Publishing Series in Biomaterials

1 **Sterilisation of tissues using ionising radiations**
Edited by J. F. Kennedy, G. O. Phillips and P. A. Williams
2 **Surfaces and interfaces for biomaterials**
Edited by P. Vadgama
3 **Molecular interfacial phenomena of polymers and biopolymers**
Edited by C. Chen
4 **Biomaterials, artificial organs and tissue engineering**
Edited by L. Hench and J. Jones
5 **Medical modelling**
R. Bibb
6 **Artificial cells, cell engineering and therapy**
Edited by S. Prakash
7 **Biomedical polymers**
Edited by M. Jenkins
8 **Tissue engineering using ceramics and polymers**
Edited by A. R. Boccaccini and J. Gough
9 **Bioceramics and their clinical applications**
Edited by T. Kokubo
10 **Dental biomaterials**
Edited by R. V. Curtis and T. F. Watson
11 **Joint replacement technology**
Edited by P. A. Revell
12 **Natural-based polymers for biomedical applications**
Edited by R. L. Reiss et al.
13 **Degradation rate of bioresorbable materials**
Edited by F. J. Buchanan
14 **Orthopaedic bone cements**
Edited by S. Deb
15 **Shape memory alloys for biomedical applications**
Edited by T. Yoneyama and S. Miyazaki
16 **Cellular response to biomaterials**
Edited by L. Di Silvio
17 **Biomaterials for treating skin loss**
Edited by D. P. Orgill and C. Blanco
18 **Biomaterials and tissue engineering in urology**
Edited by J. Denstedt and A. Atala

41 **Wear of orthopaedic implants and artificial joints**
Edited by S. Affatato
42 **Biomaterials in plastic surgery: Breast implants**
Edited by W. Peters, H. Brandon, K. L. Jerina, C. Wolf and V. L. Young
43 **MEMS for biomedical applications**
Edited by S. Bhansali and A. Vasudev
44 **Durability and reliability of medical polymers**
Edited by M. Jenkins and A. Stamboulis
45 **Biosensors for medical applications**
Edited by S. Higson
46 **Sterilisation of biomaterials and medical devices**
Edited by S. Lerouge and A. Simmons
47 **The hip resurfacing handbook: A practical guide to the use and management of modern hip resurfacings**
Edited by K. De Smet, P. Campbell and C. Van Der Straeten
48 **Developments in tissue engineered and regenerative medicine products**
J. Basu and J. W. Ludlow
49 **Nanomedicine: Technologies and applications**
Edited by T. J. Webster
50 **Biocompatibility and performance of medical devices**
Edited by J.-P. Boutrand
51 **Medical robotics: Minimally invasive surgery**
Edited by P. Gomes
52 **Implantable sensor systems for medical applications**
Edited by A. Inmann and D. Hodgins
53 **Non-metallic biomaterials for tooth repair and replacement**
Edited by P. Vallittu
54 **Joining and assembly of medical materials and devices**
Edited by Y. (Norman) Zhou and M. D. Breyen
55 **Diamond-based materials for biomedical applications**
Edited by R.Narayan
56 **Nanomaterials in tissue engineering: Fabrication and applications**
Edited by A. K. Gaharwar, S. Sant, M. J. Hancock and S. A. Hacking
57 **Biomimetic biomaterials: Structure and applications**
Edited by A. J. Ruys
58 **Standardisation in cell and tissue engineering: Methods and protocols**
Edited by V. Salih
59 **Inhaler devices: Fundamentals, design and drug delivery**
Edited by P. Prokopovich
60 **Bio-tribocorrosion in biomaterials and medical implants**
Edited by Y. Yan
61 **Microfluidic devices for biomedical applications**
Edited by X.-J. James Li and Y. Zhou
62 **Decontamination in hospitals and healthcare**
Edited by J. T. Walker

63 **Biomedical imaging: Applications and advances**
Edited by P. Morris
64 **Characterization of biomaterials**
Edited by M. Jaffe, W. Hammond, P. Tolias and T. Arinzeh
65 **Biomaterials and medical tribology**
Edited by J. Paolo Davim
66 **Biomaterials for cancer therapeutics: Diagnosis, prevention and therapy**
Edited by K. Park
67 **New functional biomaterials for medicine and healthcare**
E.P. Ivanova, K.Bazaka and R. J. Crawford
68 **Porous silicon for biomedical applications**
Edited by H. A. Santos
69 **A practical approach to spinal trauma**
Edited by H. N. Bajaj and S. Katoch
70 **Rapid prototyping of biomaterials: Principles and applications**
Edited by R.Narayan
71 **Cardiac regeneration and repair Volume 1: Pathology and therapies**
Edited by R.-K. Li and R. D. Weisel
72 **Cardiac regeneration and repair Volume 2: Biomaterials and tissue engineering**
Edited by R.-K. Li and R. D. Weisel
73 **Semiconducting silicon nanowires for biomedical applications**
Edited by J.L. Coffer
74 **Silk biomaterials for tissue engineering and regenerative medicine**
Edited by S. Kundu
75 **Biomaterials for bone regeneration: Novel techniques and applications**
Edited by P.Dubruel and S. Van Vlierberghe
76 **Biomedical foams for tissue engineering applications**
Edited by P. Netti
77 **Precious metals for biomedical applications**
Edited by N. Baltzer and T. Copponnex
78 **Bone substitute biomaterials**
Edited by K. Mallick
79 **Regulatory affairs for biomaterials and medical devices**
Edited by S. F. Amato and R. Ezzell
80 **Joint replacement technology Second edition**
Edited by P. A. Revell
81 **Computational modelling of biomechanics and biotribology in the musculoskeletal system: Biomaterials and tissues**
Edited by Z. Jin
82 **Biophotonics for medical applications**
Edited by I. Meglinski
83 **Modelling degradation of bioresorbable polymeric medical devices**
Edited by J. Pan

84 **Perspectives in total hip arthroplasty: Advances in biomaterials and their tribological interactions**
S. Affatato
85 **Tissue engineering using ceramics and polymers Second edition**
Edited by A. R. Boccaccini and P. X. Ma
86 **Biomaterials and medical device-associated infections**
Edited by L. Barnes and I. R. Cooper
87 **Surgical techniques in total knee arthroplasty (TKA) and alternative procedures**
Edited by S. Affatato
88 **Lanthanide oxide nanoparticles for moleccular imaging and therapeutics**
Edited by G. H. Lee
89 **Surface modificationof magnesium and its alloys for biomedical applications Volume 1: Biological interactions, mechanical properties and testing**
Edited by T. S. N. Sankara Narayanan, I. S. Park and M. H. Lee
90 **Surface modification of magnesium and its alloys for biomedical applications Volume 2: Modification and coating techniques**
Edited by T. S. N. Sankara Narayanan, I. S. Park and M. H. Lee
91 **Medical modelling: The application of advanced design and rapid prototyping techniques in medicine Second Edition**
Edited by R. Bibb, D. Eggbeer and A. Paterson
92 **Switchable and responsive surfaces for biomedical applications**
Edited by Z. Zhang
93 **Biomedical textiles for orthopaedic and surgical applications: Fundmentals, applications and tissue engineering**
Edited by T. Blair

Part One

Fundamental methods of modelling degradation of bioresorbable polymeric medical devices

Introduction to computer modelling for the design of biodegradable medical devices

1

J. Pan
University of Leicester, Leicester, UK

1.1 Introduction

This book is for readers who use biodegradable polymers in medical applications and wish to use computer modelling to help their research or device development.

An implanted medical device that disappears after serving its function is extremely attractive. In October 2010 a heart patient was treated using a biodegradable and drug-eluting stent by Professor Anthony Gershlick at the University Hospitals of Leicester. This was the first case of using a biodegradable stent in the UK. The stent is made of a polylactide (PLA) and designed to restore blood flow by opening a narrowed artery and providing support while the opened area heals. The stent combines scaffolding and drug release for the artery – the narrowing can be treated with resolution of the patient's symptoms, and the released drug attenuates the response of injured tissue that is caused by the high pressure deployment of the stent. Once no longer required, the stent slowly dissolves over a period of 2 years through pathways in the Krebs cycle to carbon dioxide and water. A permanent implant is not left behind, allowing the artery to be more functionally normal. Similar concepts are being used or developed in a wide range of applications. Sutures made of biodegradable polymers have been successfully used in surgeries since the 1970s. Screws and plates made of similar polymers have been used to fix broken bones. Biodegradable wafers loaded with anticancer drugs have been placed into the cavity after cancer surgery to slowly release the drugs, helping to prevent the cancer from returning. Intensive research is being carried out worldwide in using porous foams made of biodegradable polymers as scaffolds for tissue regeneration. In all these applications, the biodegradable devices firstly provide some temporary functions, then degrade to let biology take over, and are eventually metabolised into carbon dioxide and water.

The degradation time of these devices varies from weeks to years depending on applications. Testing different design ideas for biodegradable devices requires long-term (up to 5 years) *in vitro* and *in vivo* experiments, and ultimately human clinical trials. Consequently, virtual testing using computer modelling is particularly helpful. Although experimental tests will play a dominant role in the foreseeable future, any use of computer modelling in the early design stage can significantly accelerate device development.

Modelling Degradation of Bioresorbable Polymeric Medical Devices. http://dx.doi.org/10.1533/9781782420255.1.3

The most important feature of biodegradable devices is that they ‘disappear’ after serving their functions. Consequently, the focus of this book is on degradation rate. Modelling polymer degradation is also a precondition for calculating drug release rate from degrading devices such as drug-eluting coronary stents and tissue engineering scaffolds. Broadly speaking, the degradation rate of a polymeric device is affected by

1. type and properties of the raw polymer,
2. manufacturing and sterilisation conditions,
3. *in vivo* environment of the device, and
4. shape and size of the device.

Each of these factors can be further subdivided, and the degradation rate depends on a long list of variables. There is significant uncertainty when relating the degradation rate of a device back to these factors. In particular, the *in vivo* nature of device degradation is not yet fully understood. Currently, it is not possible to set up a computer model for a device and predict its degradation rate taking into account all of these variables.

The immediate aim of this book is therefore rather modest and limited to the shape and size design of devices. A mathematical framework is presented which uses ‘material data’ accumulated from existing polymers and devices and calculates the degradation rate of a device that is made of the same polymer under similar manufacturing conditions but of a different design. This type of computer modelling has matured in engineering for ‘degradation’ problems. For example, the approach is routinely used to calculate fatigue and creep damage of engineering components for design modifications. For biodegradable devices, this modest level of computer modelling is already a leap forward from the trial-and-error approach that is currently practised.

The research literature and ongoing research are, however, far more ambitious. The ultimate goal of computer modelling is to predict the degradation rate taking all the variables as input. This means performing polymer design and component design together, as well as manipulating the manufacturing process, all in a computer model. For biodegradable devices, the task is more challenging than engineering applications because of the interaction between the device and tissue. This book aims to introduce the first step and stimulate further research. Costache *et al.* (2010) have provided a review on computational methods for the development of polymeric biomaterials.

The book is also limited to devices that degrade through bulk degradation rather than surface erosion. Bulk degradation is the dominating mechanism for applications except for drug delivery devices which often degrade through surface erosion. Conservative licensing means only a few polymers have been commonly used. Typical examples are polyesters such as PLA, polyglycolide (PGA) and polycaprolactone (PCL). These polyesters are used either alone or to make copolymers or polymer blends to achieve different degradation rates and mechanical and functional properties. In the rest of the book, the term ‘biodegradable polymers’ is used to refer to this group of polymers.

The book assumes basic knowledge on biodegradable polymers. There are many books available, such as that edited by Ratner *et al.* (2013), which provide comprehensive coverage on biodegradable polymers. In particular, a book edited by Buchanan (2008) provides in-depth coverage on degradation mechanisms of biodegradable materials.

1.2 General modelling techniques useful in studying device degradation

In order to set out the background for degradation models presented in the following chapters, this section provides an overview of three computer modelling techniques, namely molecular dynamics, Monte Carlo method and finite element method. These techniques have been developed and widely used in other disciplines and are very useful in studying polymer and device degradation. The scope and limitations of these techniques are introduced. Full details of molecular dynamic models and Monte Carlo models can be found in Leach (2001). Full details on the finite element method can be found in Davies (2011).

1.2.1 Molecular dynamic models

In molecular dynamic models, polymer chains are modelled atom by atom. Forces on each atom exerted by its surrounding atoms are calculated according to the nature of the chemical bond and the distance between the atom and the surrounding atoms. Different mathematical relations are used for different type of bonds, with unique sets of parameters for each atomic species. The variables in the model are the locations of the atoms. At any instant of time, the accelerations of the atoms are calculated according to Newton's law and their velocities and positions are updated using a small timestep. Repeating the procedure provides the trajectories of all the atoms. Figure 1.1 shows an example of molecular models for a semi-crystalline polymer.

Biodegradation of a polymeric device is the cleavage of polymer chains caused by the hydrolysis reaction between water molecules and polymer chains. In theory, the chain cleavage event can be directly modelled using molecular dynamics by mixing water molecules with polymer chains. The input for such a model is the number of water molecules and the chemical composition and structure of the polymer chains. In the computer simulation, water molecules would react with the polymer chains, eventually breaking their backbone. The degradation rate could therefore be obtained from the simulation. This would allow polymer design at the molecular level for a targeted degradation rate. Such a calculation is, however, not yet possible. This is because the time scale that a molecular dynamic simulation can reach is typically a few nano-seconds while the actual time taken by a chain cleavage event is many weeks or months. Molecular dynamics follows the motion of all the atoms, including their thermal vibration which requires extremely small timesteps and hence a huge number of repeated calculations. Most of these details are irrelevant to the chain cleavage but difficult to be filtered out in the modelling method.

A more subtle issue is that the interaction between atoms is often a 'group behaviour' while the simplistic inter-atomic force depends only on the pair of atoms under

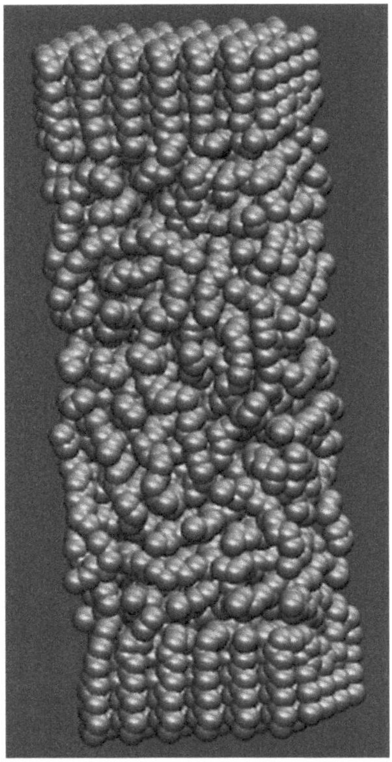

Figure 1.1 A molecular model for semi-crystalline polymer. (*Source*: from Ding *et al.*, 2012).

consideration. This group behaviour is governed by quantum mechanics. Direct solution of the governing equations (e.g. the density function theory) of quantum mechanics is only possible for a small group of atoms. The inter-atomic forces in the literature may or may not reflect the reality for a long-term event such as polymer chain cleavage even if the computing time is not an issue.

Despite its limitations, molecular models in its current state can be helpful for understanding the biodegradation of polymers. For example, it can be used to calculate the change in potential energy of a polymer chain during chain cleavage. Figure 1.2 shows the results obtained by Karst and Yang (2006). In such calculations, one is interested in comparing the states of the polymer chains before and after a cleavage event, rather than the actual cleavage process. The chain cleavage is artificially introduced instead of being computed. This reduction in the potential energy is the driving force for the chain cleavage. The calculated change in energy can be used to rank the degradation rates of different polymers, copolymers or polymer blends.

Molecular models have been used to understand the change in Young's modulus caused by polymer chain scissions (Ding *et al.*, 2012). Chapter 9 provides some

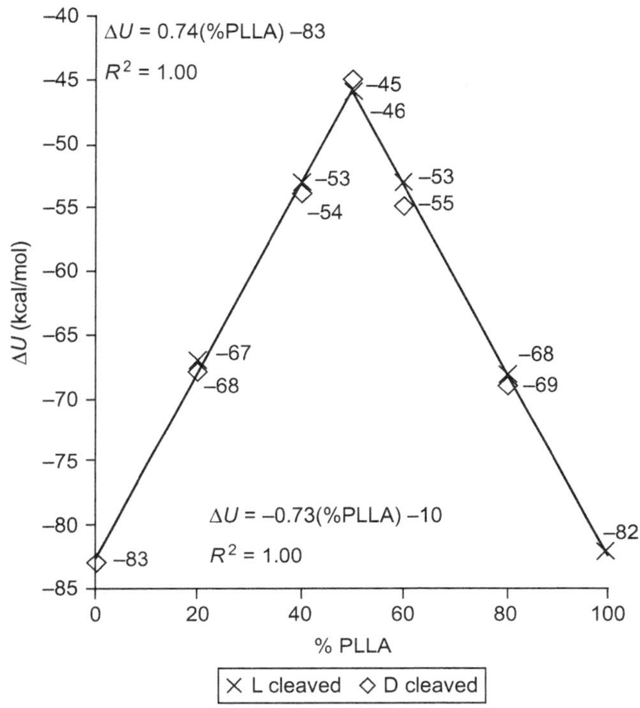

Figure 1.2 Change in potential energy (ΔU) for hydrolysis of various blends of poly(L-lactic acid) (PLLA) and poly(D-lactic acid) (PDLA) graphed by % PLLA in the blend and by whether a PLLA (L-cleaved) or PDLA (D-cleaved) was cleaved, from Karst and Yang (2006).

further details for such studies. It is also possible to use molecular dynamics to study interactions between biomaterials and proteins.

1.2.2 Monte Carlo models

In a Monte Carlo model, the random elements of the degradation process are directly executed by computer. For example, the exact location of a chain cleavage is random. If one wishes to find out the evolution of molecular weight distribution as more and more polymer chains are cleaved, an analogical experiment could be to get a few hundreds of long strings and cut them randomly using scissors. Measuring the lengths of all the strings after certain number of scissions gives the new distribution of the string length. This experiment can be performed numerically in a computer for tens of thousands of polymer chains in a split of a second. The Monte Carlo simulation does not relate the molecular weight change to real time. A scission rate can be imposed to the simulation which is known as kinetic Monte Carlo method (Gillespie, 1976). Figure 1.3 presents an example (Gleadall and Pan, 2013) where the Monte Carlo simulation is compared with experimental data of Tsuji (2002). Chapter 10 provides further details on this topic.

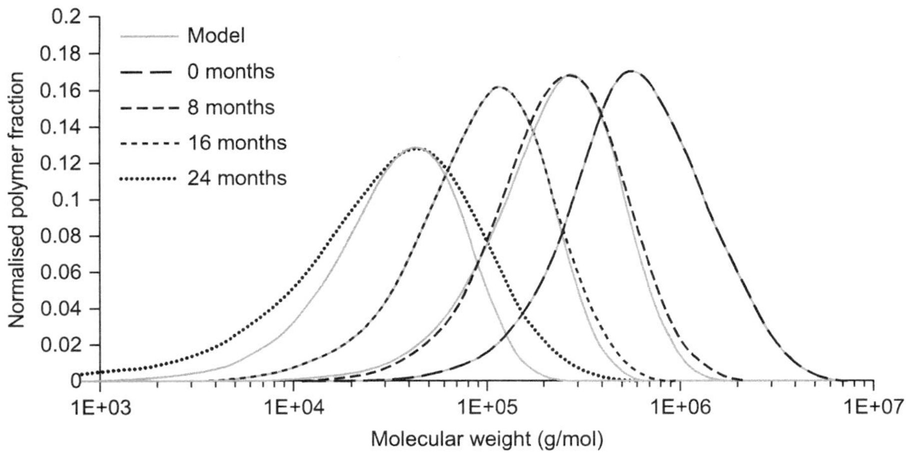

Figure 1.3 Comparison between Monte Carlo simulations (grey lines) for molecular weight distribution and experimental data (dashed lines) of Tsuji (2002) for a PDLA at different times of degradation, from Gleadall and Pan (2013).

Monte Carlo method can also be used to simulate diffusion of small oligomers in a polymer matrix. In fact, the method was first invented to simulate neutron diffusion in fissionable materials (Metropolis, 1987). To understand how this is done, one can consider the simpler problem of simulating the path along which a football rolls down a hill. From a given location, a computer simulation can make multiple attempts to move the ball by a small distance in several random directions. The changes in the height of the ball location can be calculated for all the attempts. The attempt (direction) that makes the largest drop in height is accepted. Repeating the procedure many times provides the trajectory of the football. In the diffusion problem, the driving force for the migration of an oligomer is the change in its chemical potential. Difficulty arises when one uses this method to directly simulate oligomer diffusion in a device, which is many orders of magnitude larger than a single oligomer and may have a huge number of oligomers. To make the computing possible, the Monte Carlo model has to be 'coarse-grained', i.e. a large number of oligomers are lumped together. This could destroy the underlying physics in the model. The Monte Carlo method is at its best when used to study the diffusion coefficient in a small representative unit of the polymer. The diffusion of oligomers out of a device is better treated macroscopically using continuum models, which is the topic of Chapter 6.

1.2.3 Finite element method

The finite element method can model the change of physical or chemical variables, the concentration of a chemical species for example, over space and time in a device. The most powerful aspect of the method is that it can deal with devices of any shape, no matter whether this is a screw with a helical thread, a scaffold with random pores, or a coronary stent of any complicated design.

The degradation of a device made of a polyester such as PLA or PGA is not uniform inside the device. The average molecular weight of the polymer chains varies with location as well as time. This is because the carboxylic end groups of the polymer chains have a high degree of acid dissociation. As shown in Figure. 1.3, chain scission produces more and more short chains, making the local environment more and more acidic. Near the surface of a device, the short chains can diffuse into the surrounding medium, which reduces the local acidity and slows down the chain scission. At the core of the device, the short chains cannot leave as quickly, which leads to a high local acidity and faster chain scission. This makes the degradation of a device heterogeneous (Grizzi *et al.*, 1995).

The mathematical equations that govern the heterogeneous degradation are presented in Chapter 6. A key variable in the equations is the concentration of the short chains. These short chains diffuse from where their concentration is high to where it is low. This principle can be combined with the requirement for matter conservation and written into a mathematical equation. Before the computer age, such equations were very difficult to solve for real devices. It is almost impossible to find an analytical function to describe how the concentration varies with space and time in a device of sophisticated shape. The finite element method overcomes this difficulty by using two key ideas:

1. Divide the device into many small elements and use concentrations at the vertexes of an element to control the concentration field inside the element.

Plate I (a) in the colour section between pages 130 and 131 shows a finite element model for a single representative unit of a scaffold. It is very easy to use the irregular tetrahedral elements to model devices of sophisticated shapes. The vertexes of the elements are named as 'nodes'. The tetrahedral elements share a common set of concentrations at the nodes. The distribution of concentration inside an element is less important if the elements are sufficiently small. This is like controlling the shape of a fishing net by holding all the knots. Instead of trying to find a mathematical function to describe the concentration in the entire device, the finite element method finds discrete values of the concentration at the nodes.

2. Rewrite the local equations into a global principle

If a fishing net is loosely hung over two supporting lines, it will form a shape between the lines. The physics of the shape can be described by balancing the tensions of the strings and the gravity at each knot. However, balancing force is a principle local to each knot, which is difficult to use because each knot is different. Alternatively and equivalently, the positions of all the knots make the potential energy of the entire net minimum. This is a global principle and much easier to use. The total potential energy of the net can be written in terms of the positions of all the knots. The requirement of making the potential energy minimum then helps to find these positions.

Similarly, it is difficult to apply the principle that 'short chains diffuse from where concentration is high to where it is low' to the tetrahedral elements shown in Plate I (a). This is because the elements are of irregular shape and size and connected irregularly with each other. The finite element method resolves this difficulty by using a global principle. Moving the short chains from one place to another requires energy. A biodegradable device is a system made of polymer chains, short chains and water. Just as the shape of the fishing net is formed to minimise its potential energy, short chains diffuse out of a device to reduce the total free energy of the system. We therefore have the following global principle:

rate of free energy reduction = rate of energy consumption by diffusion

Both sides of the equation can be expressed in terms of the rates of change in the concentration at all the finite element nodes. The global principle therefore leads to a set of governing equations for the rates of concentration at all the finite element nodes. These equations can be numerically integrated, giving the variation of the concentration with time at all the nodes. Plate I (b) shows the distribution of average molecular weight after a period of degradation. Further details of the finite element analysis can be found in Chapter 7.

All local mathematical equations can be rewritten into a global principle, although many of the principles do not make an explicit sense such as minimising the potential energy. The finite element method can therefore be conveniently used to model intercoupling and multi-physics problems.

A limitation of the traditional finite element method is that it is difficult to deal with breaking up and fragmentation of devices which occur in the later stage of biodegradation. However, recent progress in computational mechanics, for example the development of a so-called Materials Point Method, may help to resolve this issue in the near future. Figure 1.4 shows an example of computer simulated fragmentation of a ceramic coating (Li *et al.,* 2012). The approach can be applied to device fragmentation during biodegradation.

For the design of biodegradable devices, the finite element method can already be used to

1. Optimise the shape and size of a device to achieve required deformation behaviour and failure load.
2. Calculate load sharing between a device and its supporting tissue as a device degrades.
3. Calculate drug release profile from a device.
4. Calculate molecular weight and degree of crystallinity as functions of time and location. The calculation also provides profile of monomer/pH release from a degrading device.

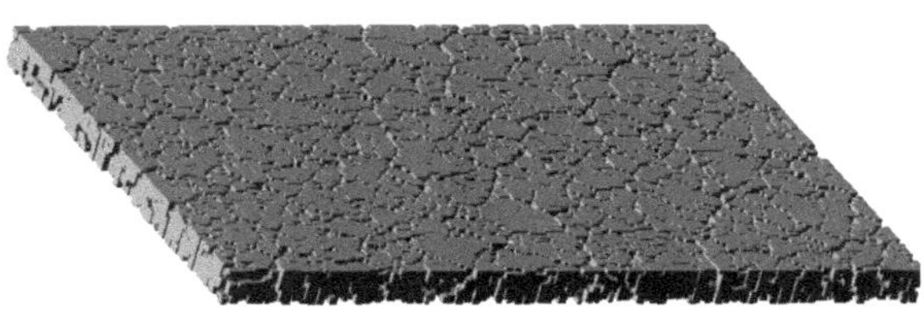

Figure 1.4 Computer simulated fragmentation of a ceramic coating on a solid substrate using the material point method, from Li *et al.* (2012). The method can be adapted to model device fragmentation during later stage of degradation.

1.3 The degradation pathway and models presented in this book

Biodegradation of implanted devices is a two-phase process: chemical hydrolysis of the polymer backbone and active metabolism of the degradation products. During the first phase, water penetrates the biodegradable device, attacking the ester bonds and converting the long polymer chains into shorter water-soluble oligomers. This is known as the hydrolysis reaction. In the second phase, enzymes released from white blood cells attack these fragments turning them into natural monomeric acids found in the body, such as lactic acid. These acids enter the citric acid cycle and are excreted as water and carbon dioxide. The device loses all its functions by the end of the first phase, and the models presented in this book are limited to this phase.

The hydrolysis of polyester molecules produces shorter chains (oligomers) with acid and alcohol end groups. These acid end groups have a high degree of dissociation and therefore give rise to an acidic environment, which significantly accelerates the hydrolysis rate. The hydrolysis reaction is therefore autocatalytic. If some small and water-soluble oligomers can diffuse away, then the acidity of the local environment is changed. The interplay between oligomer diffusion and the hydrolysis reaction is therefore a central issue that the model must consider. Furthermore, the oligomers diffuse in a degrading polymer, which has increasing porosity, crystallinity and water content as degradation progresses. The variation of the effective diffusion coefficient with respect to these factors has to be considered.

Most of the polyesters are semi-crystalline polymers, although their copolymers are often intrinsically amorphous. The crystalline phase is difficult for water to penetrate and hydrolyse. The degree of crystallinity can increase significantly during biodegradation in both initially amorphous and semi-crystalline polymers. This is because the cleavage of the polymer chains provides extra mobility to the chains and leads to further crystallisation. The model has to consider the interplay between the hydrolysis reaction and crystallisation.

In this book this sequence of events and their various underlying processes is described by a set of mathematical equations from which all the characteristic parameters of a degrading device can be calculated using numerical methods. Simplicity is a major driver for the approach taken here, which can be traced back to the work by Joshi and Himmelstein (1991). On the other hand, the work by Perale *et al.* (2009) is a good example for a different approach that could have been taken.

Part One of the book introduces the mathematical equations step by step with increasing complexity. The six chapters in Part One follow a natural logic flow. It is useful to point out that Section 6.6 provides an overview on the conditions in which the different models can be used. The mathematical models involve a large number of equations, variables and parameters. Some variable or parameter can take a subtly different meaning in a different context. A complete set of equations with the definitions of all the variables and parameters are always summarised after some new issues or factors are introduced in each chapter. Consequently, readers do not have to go back to the previous chapters to look for an equation or a definition for a symbol. This approach means that Part One contains some repeating materials which is worthy for the purpose of clarity and readability. Part Two of the book presents advanced and separate topics. Each chapter in Part Two is independent.

1.4 Challenges and unresolved issues

There are many challenges in using biodegradable polymers for medical applications. For example, the polymeric screws and plates are not yet strong enough for many orthopaedic fixations. When they degrade, an acidic environment is often generated, which may lead to local inflammation. The biodegradable stents are a little chunky and cannot dilate to a very large extent. Large dilation is needed for applications such as treating new-born babies with a congenital heart disease. The current generation of polymeric coronary stents degrades too slowly, in a couple of years against the ideal scenario of 6 months or so. In tissue engineering, many researchers are working on various scaffolds to generate the tissue they want from stem cells. The biggest challenge is how to insure angiogenesis in a timely fashion within the scaffold construct. For mathematical modelling to play a major role in resolving these issues, progress is required in two directions:

1. Integrating material design, device design and processing control – this will open up the design space significantly, even working with existing polymers and their composites. New polymers and their composites can also be purposely designed for existing or new applications. Multi-scale and multi-physics modelling is needed to achieve this goal, which is a major research theme in materials modelling.
2. Modelling tissue response to, and interaction with, degrading materials – this is perhaps the most challenging task in computer modelling. Sengers *et al.* (2007) provided a comprehensive review in the context of tissue engineering.

These challenges and unresolved issues provide the ideal opportunity for further research. Nevertheless, the existing modelling techniques can already help to accelerate device design. The difficulty is to break the discipline barrier between computer modelling and biomaterial science – a task this book attempts to achieve.

Acknowledgements

Most of the research work presented in this book was carried out by previous and current PhD students at the University of Leicester including Xinpu Chen, Lifeng Ding, Andrew Gleadall, Xiaoxiao Han and Ying Wang. Many colleagues from Leicester and other institutions also contributed to this work including Helen Atkinson, Fraser Buchanan, Ruth Cameron, Ruslan Davidchalk, David Farrar, Simon Gill, Ruoyu Huang, Wenguang Jiang, Minna Kellomäki, Marc-Anton Kruft, Csaba Sinka, Wenjuan Niu and Neil Weir. Their individual contributions are referenced where appropriate in the following chapters. Ismael Morenogomez read the original version of Chapter 5 and suggested a number of corrections.

The papers published by these authors, however, reflected a step-by-step development and gradual maturing of the mathematical models. The book is, therefore, not simply a collection of the previously published work but an attempt to re-present the complete mathematical framework in a consistent manner.

References

Buchanan FJ (2008) *Degradation Rate of Bioresorbable Materials*, Woodhead Publishing Limited, Cambridge, UK.

Costache AD, Ghosh J, Knight DD and Kohn J (2010) Computational methods for the development of polymeric biomaterials. *Advanced Engineering Materials*, **12** (1–2):B3–B17.

Davies AJ (2011) *The Finite Element Method: An Introduction with Partial Differential Equations*, second edition, Oxford University Press, Oxford, UK.

Ding L, Davidchalk R and Pan J (2012) A molecular dynamics study of Young's modulus change of semi-crystalline polymers during degradation by chain scissions. *Journal of the Mechanical Behaviour of Biomedical Materials*, **5**:224–230.

Gillespie DT (1976) A general method for numerically simulating the stochastic time evolution of coupled chemical reactions. *Journal of Computational Physics*, **22**:403–434.

Gleadall A and Pan J (2013) Computer simulation of polymer chain scission in biodegradable polymers. *Journal of Biotechnology & Biomaterials*, **3**:154.

Grizzi I, Garreau H, Li S and Vert M (1995) Hydrolytic degradation of devices based on poly [DL-lactic acid] size dependence. *Biomaterials*, **16**:305–311.

Joshi A and Himmelstein KJ (1991) Dynamics of controlled release from bioerodible matrices. *Journal of Controlled Release*, **15**:95–104.

Karst D and Yang Y (2006) Molecular modeling study of the resistance of PLA to hydrolysis based on the blending of PLLA and PDLA. *Polymer*, **47**:4845–4850.

Leach AR (2001) *Molecular Modelling – Principle and Applications*, second edition, Prentice Hall, Person Education Ltd. Harlow England.

Li F, Pan J and Cocks ACF (2012) A new numerical scheme for computer simulation of multiple cracking in ceramic films during constrained sintering. *Modelling and Simulation in Materials Science and Engineering*, **20**:035008 (16p).

Metropolis N (1987) The beginnings of the Monte Carlo method. *Los Alamos Science*, special issue, **15**:125–130.

Perale G, Arosio P, Moscatelli D, Barri V, Müller M, Maccagnan S and Masi M (2009) A new model of resorbable device degradation and drug release: transient 1-dimension diffusional model. *Journal of Controlled Release*, **136**:196–205.

Ratner BD, Hoffman AS, Schoen FJ and Lemons JE (2013) *Biomaterials Science: An Introduction to Materials in Medicine*, third edition, Academic Press Limited, London, UK.

Sengers B, Taylor M, Please C and Oreffo R (2007) Computational modeling of cell spreading and tissue regeneration in porous scaffolds. *Biomaterials*, **28**:1926–1940.

Tsuji H (2002) Autocatalytic hydrolysis of amorphous-made polylactides: effects of L-lactide content, tacticity, and enantiomeric polymer blending. *Polymer*, **43**:1789–1796.

Modelling degradation of amorphous biodegradable polyesters: basic model

2

J. Pan, X. Chen
University of Leicester, Leicester, UK

2.1 Introduction

It is convenient to start the discussion of degradation models with amorphous polymers. A typical application of amorphous polymers in medical devices is the drug-carrying layer of coronary stents. Calculating the degradation rate of the polymer is the first step to predict drug-release profile from a stent. Furthermore, all semi-crystalline polymers contain an amorphous phase. It is therefore logical to focus attention on amorphous polymers first. Semi-crystalline polymers are considered in Chapter 4.

A degrading polymer is considered as being made of three constituents – long chains, short chains and water molecules as schematically illustrated in Figure 2.1. The short chains are defined as monomers and oligomers whose degrees of polymerisation (number of ester units) are less than an upper limit. All the other chains are considered as 'long' ones. Polymer degradation is the cleavage of the long chains, reducing their average length (molecular weight) and producing short chains.

In reality the polymer chains always have a distribution of molecular weights. Figure 2.1 shows an example of molecular weight distributions of a degrading polymer at different times. As the polymer degrades, the chains cleave almost randomly and the distribution curve shifts from the right to the left. The distinction between 'long' and 'short' chains seems arbitrary after a first glance at Figure 2.2. However, chains that are shorter than about 8 units of polymerisation are water soluble and can diffuse out of a device, while longer chains cannot. These short chains play an important and distinctive role in the degradation process, which will be discussed step by step in this book. As degradation proceeds, the long chains gradually become short ones. The modelling focuses on this transition rather than following the evolution of the molecular weight distribution. *Avoiding the complexity of chain length distribution and separating the chains into two distinctive groups of 'long' and 'short' ones is a central simplification and assumption in all the models presented in this book.* The simplification was first introduced by Wang *et al.* (2008) and Han and Pan (2009). An exception is Chapter 10, where the evolution of chain distribution is explicitly modelled.

For devices that degrade through bulk degradation, water molecules diffuse into a device much faster than the rate of its degradation. As a rule of thumb, water

Modelling Degradation of Bioresorbable Polymeric Medical Devices. http://dx.doi.org/10.1533/9781782420255.1.15

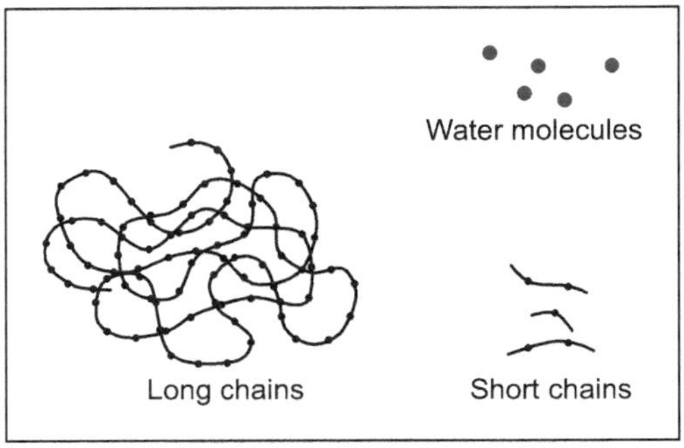

Figure 2.1 Schematic illustration of the three constituents of a degrading polymer.

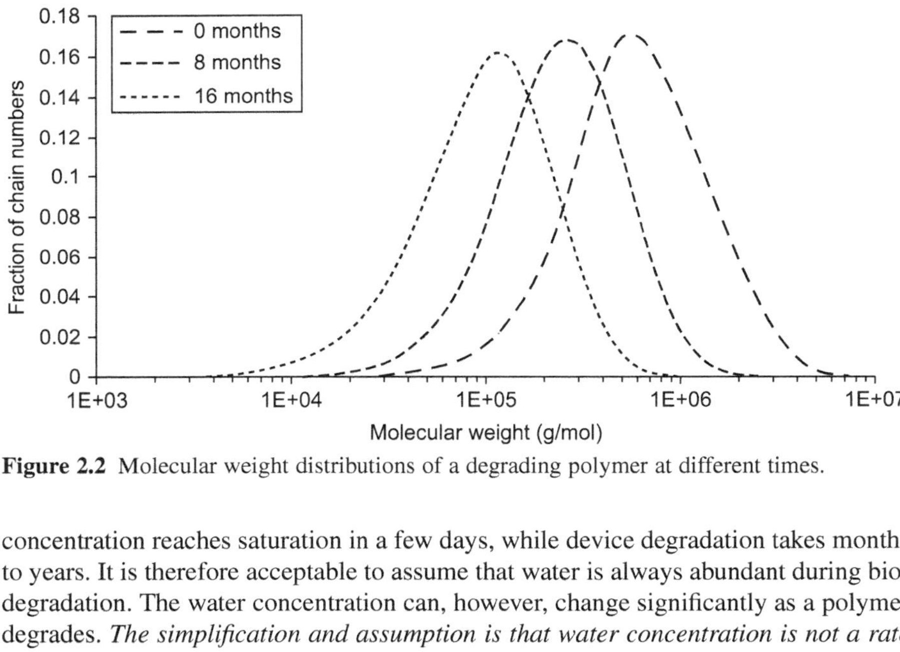

Figure 2.2 Molecular weight distributions of a degrading polymer at different times.

concentration reaches saturation in a few days, while device degradation takes months to years. It is therefore acceptable to assume that water is always abundant during biodegradation. The water concentration can, however, change significantly as a polymer degrades. *The simplification and assumption is that water concentration is not a rate limiting factor for degradation and hence there is no need to follow the change in water concentration in a mathematical model* (Wang *et al.*, 2008; Han and Pan, 2009).

The long chains are characterised by their number-averaged molecular weight, which is denoted as M_n. As a polymer degrades, M_n reduces with time which is a typical measurement in a degradation experiment. The total number of ester units of all the long chains per unit volume is denoted as C_e. This is an important variable, because it is the ester bonds that water molecules attack during degradation. As more and more short chains are produced, C_e gradually decreases, reducing the number of ester bonds available for water molecules to attack.

The average degree of polymerisation of all the short chains is denoted as m. For simplicity, m is assumed to remain constant during degradation. The total number of

Table 2.1 Calculations of M_n, C_e, m and C_{ol}

Chain number	1	2	3	4	5		
Long chains	100	200	700	1000	2000	$M_n = 800\ M_{unit}$	$C_e = 4000$
Short chains	2	4	6	–	–	$m = 4$	$C_{ol} = 12$

M_{unit} – molecular weight of one ester unit.

ester units of all the short chains per unit volume is denoted as C_{ol}. This is another important variable in the degradation. As the long chains are turning into short ones, C_{ol} increases at the expense of C_e. However, diffusion of the short chains out of the device reduces C_{ol}. The diffusion process also leads to a non-uniform distribution of C_{ol} in a device, taking higher values at the core of the device and lower values near its surface. If polymerisation is incomplete during the manufacturing process, then a significant number of residual monomers and oligomers may exist at the beginning of the degradation, i.e. we may have $C_{ol} > 0$ at $t = 0$.

To illustrate the definitions of M_n, C_e, m and C_{ol}, Table 2.1 presents a hypothetical polymer consisting of five long chains and three short chains in a unit volume. For each chain, the number in the table represents its total number of ester units. The number-averaged molecular weight for the long chains is calculated by

$$M_n = M_{unit} \times \frac{(100 + 200 + 700 + 1000 + 2000)}{5} = 800 M_{unit}$$

in which M_{unit} is the molecular weight of one ester unit. The concentration of ester bonds of the long chains is calculated by

$$C_e = 100 + 200 + 700 + 1000 + 2000 = 4000$$

The average degree of polymerisation of the short chains is calculated by

$$m = \frac{(2 + 4 + 6)}{3} = 4$$

The concentration of ester bonds of the short chains is calculated by

$$C_{ol} = 2 + 4 + 6 = 12$$

In practice the number concentrations of C_e and C_{ol} are very large values. It is therefore more convenient to use molar concentration (mol/m^3) in actual calculations.

2.2 Hydrolysis rate equation

Considering three examples of polyesters the ester bonds are the weak links when exposing to water. Hydrolysis reaction between ester bonds and water molecules cleaves the polymer chains. Figure 2.3 shows the chain scission process using poly(lactide) (PLA) as an example. After the cleavage, the two loose ends terminate as a hydroxyl alcohol group (R′–OH) and a carboxylic acid end group (R–COOH). Here R and R′ denote the remainders of the polymer chain. The reaction can be catalysed by H^+ that may exist in the material. In fact, the carboxylic end groups have a high degree of acid dissociation. Thus the reaction promotes itself once it starts, i.e. the reaction is autocatalytic. The actual steps of the autocatalytic reaction are complex and subject to debate.

In order to write a general equation for practical polymers including co-polymers and polymer blends, details of the chemical structure are ignored and all the ester bonds are treated as equal. The hydrolysis reaction is phenomenologically described as

$$\text{ESTER BONDS} + H_2O \xrightarrow{H^+} R{-}COOH + R'{-}OH \qquad [2.1]$$

Using R_s to represent the total number of chain scissions per unit volume of the material, the changing rate of R_s can be written (Wang *et al.*, 2008; Han and Pan, 2009):

$$\frac{dR_s}{dt} = k_1 C_e + k_2' C_e C_{H^+} \qquad [2.2]$$

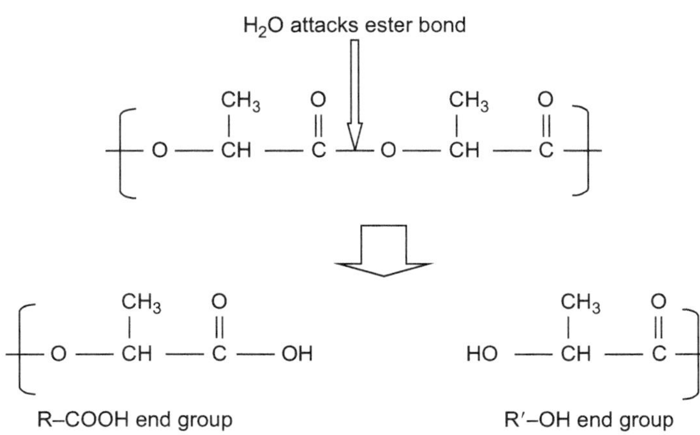

Figure 2.3 Scission of a PLA chain producing a carboxylic acid end group (R–COOH) and a hydroxyl alcohol end group (R′–OH).

in which C_e is the concentration of ester bonds of the polymers and C_{H^+} is the concentration of H^+. The first term on the right hand side reflects that part of the hydrolysis reaction may occur without the catalyst H^+. The second term represents autocatalytic hydrolysis reaction. k_1 and k_2' are the corresponding reaction constants. The concentration of water molecules does not appear in the equation because it is assumed that they are always abundant despite the fact that the water concentration can change significantly during degradation.

The acid disassociation of the carboxylic end groups can be expressed as

$$\mathrm{R{-}COOH} \Leftrightarrow \mathrm{R{-}COO^-} + \mathrm{H^+} \quad [2.3]$$

This reaction is fast and reversible, and can be treated as being always at equilibrium with an equilibrium expression of

$$K_a = \frac{C_{\mathrm{H^+}} C_{\mathrm{COO^-}}}{C_{\mathrm{COOH}}} \quad [2.4]$$

in which C_X represents concentration of the subscript species X and K_a represents the equilibrium constant. K_a is known at given temperatures. For example, PLA and poly(glycolide) (PGA) have $K_a = 1.349 \times 10^{-4}$ ($p\mathrm{K_a}$= 3.87) at 37°C. The charge balance requires that $C_{\mathrm{H^+}} = C_{\mathrm{COO^-}}$ and Equation [2.4] leads to

$$C_{\mathrm{H^+}} = \left[K_a C_{\mathrm{COOH}}\right]^{1/2} \quad [2.5]$$

Substituting Equation [2.5] into Equation [2.2] gives the following expression for scission rate

$$\frac{dR_s}{dt} = k_1 C_e + k_2 C_e \left[C_{\mathrm{COOH}}\right]^{1/2} \quad [2.6]$$

in which a new reaction constant has been introduced: $k_2 = k_2'\left[K_a\right]^{1/2}$.

2.3 Production of short chains

Scissions of polymer chains produce short chains. If all the scissions occur at ester bonds next to the polymer chain ends, then each chain scission creates a monomer. This is known as end scission, as illustrated in Figure 2.4a. Using R_{ol} to represent the number of ester units of the short chains per unit volume, we have

$$R_{ol} = R_s. \quad [2.7]$$

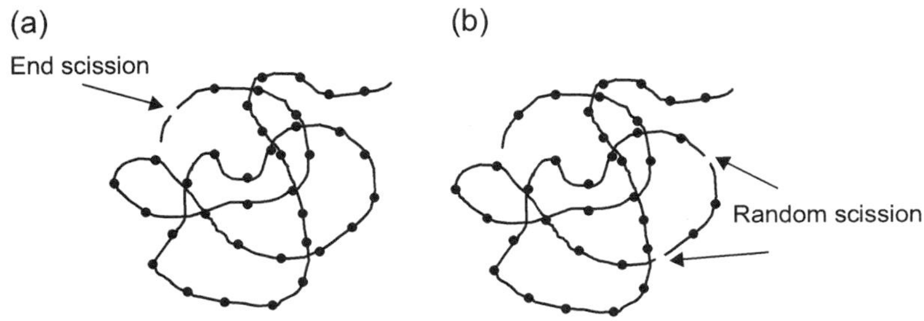

Figure 2.4 (a) End and (b) random scissions of polymer chains, dots represent ester bonds.

On the other hand, if the chain scissions occur randomly along the polymer chains, as illustrated in Figure 2.4b, then there is a small chance that two scissions work together to produce a short chain, or one scission occurs a few units away from the chain end. Using statistical analysis, Flory (1953) obtained

$$\frac{R_{ol}}{C_{e0}} = \sum_{i=1}^{q} i\left(\frac{R_s}{C_{e0}}\right)^2\left(1-\frac{R_s}{C_{e0}}\right)^{i-1} \approx \frac{1}{2}\left(q+q^2\right)\left(\frac{R_s}{C_{e0}}\right)^2 \quad [2.8]$$

in which q is the upper limit for the number of ester units of all the short chains and C_{e0} is the initial concentration of ester bonds of the polymer. The approximation in Equation [2.8] is accurate if R_s is much smaller than C_{e0}.

To compare the effects of end and random scission, let us consider a hypothetical polymer which has a typical degree of polymerisation (number of ester units) of 1000 and assume ten scissions occurred on each chain. If all the scissions occur at the chain ends, the degree of polymerisation will be reduced to 990 and the amount of short chains will be increased to $R_{ol} = (10/1000)C_{e0} = 10^{-2}C_{e0}$. Alternatively, if all the scissions occur randomly, the degree of polymerisation will be reduced to about 100, at which the polymer would have lost all its useful properties. Using $R_s / C_{e0} = 10/1000 = 0.01$ and $q = 8$ in Equation [2.8] gives $R_{ol} = 3.6\times10^{-3}C_{e0}$. This simple calculation demonstrates two important points:

1. random scission is much more efficient in reducing molecular weight than end scission; and
2. end scission is more efficient in generating short chains than random scission.

Pure end scission cannot explain the observed molecular weight reduction because it is too slow for end scission to reduce the average molecular weight. On the other hand, pure random scission cannot always explain the observed weight loss because too few short chains would be available to diffuse out of the device. Gleadall *et al.* (2014) studied the existing data in the literature and concluded that the degradation of common biodegradable polymers is typically a combination of random and end scissions. The chain ends are more susceptible to cleavage, which produces most of the monomers responsible for weight loss. However, it is the random scission that dominates the reduction in molecular weight. Section 3.5 provides a full discussion on these issues.

In general, the production of short chains can be empirically related to chain scission using (Han *et al.*, 2010)

$$\frac{R_{ol}}{C_{e0}} = \alpha\left(\frac{R_s}{C_{e0}}\right)^{\beta} \qquad [2.9]$$

in which α and β are empirical parameters. If the relative ratio between the rates of end and random scissions is known, then Monte Carlo simulation can be used to calculate the short chain production. The values of α and β can be obtained by fitting Equation [2.9] with the Monte Carlo results. This is the topic of Chapter 10. In practice this ratio is generally unknown, and the use of co-polymers and polymer blends further complicates the simulation. Consequently, α and β have to be treated as empirical parameters in general.

2.4 Master equation for chain scission

Using C_{chain0} to represent the number of polymer chains per unit volume at the beginning of the degradation, each scission produces a –COOH end group and we have

$$C_{\text{COOH}} = C_{\text{chain0}} + R_s \qquad [2.10]$$

Similarly, using C_{e0} to represent the initial concentration of ester bonds of the long chains, the short chains are produced at the expense of C_{e0}. Using Equation [2.9] gives

$$C_e = C_{e0} - R_{ol} = C_{e0}\left[1 - \alpha\left(\frac{R_s}{C_{e0}}\right)^{\beta}\right] \qquad [2.11]$$

Submitting Equations [2.10] and [2.11] into Equation [2.6] gives

$$\frac{dR_s}{dt} = C_e\left\{k_1 + k_2\left[C_{\text{COOH}}\right]^{1/2}\right\} = C_{e0}\left[1 - \alpha\left(\frac{R_s}{C_{e0}}\right)^{\beta}\right]\left\{k_1 + k_2\left[C_{\text{chain0}} + R_s\right]^{1/2}\right\} \qquad [2.12]$$

It is sometime convenient to use a normalised form of the above equation. Defining

$$\overline{R}_s = \frac{R_s}{C_{e0}} \qquad [2.13]$$

$$\overline{k}_2 = C_{e0}^{0.5} k_2 \qquad [2.14]$$

Equation [2.12] can then be rewritten as

$$\frac{d\overline{R}_s}{dt} = \left(1 - \alpha \overline{R}_s^{\beta}\right)\left[k_1 + \overline{k}_2 \left(N_{\text{dp0}}^{-1} + \overline{R}_s\right)^{1/2}\right] \qquad [2.15]$$

in which N_{dp0} is the initial degree of polymerisation given by

$$N_{\text{dp0}} = \frac{C_{e0}}{C_{\text{chain0}}} \qquad [2.16]$$

The number-averaged molecular weight M_n is the total weight of the polymer chains divided by the total number of chains, i.e. we have

$$M_n = \frac{C_{e0} M_{\text{unit}}}{C_{\text{chain0}} + R_s} \qquad [2.17]$$

in which M_{unit} represents the molecular weight of a repeating unit of the polymer chain. Using M_{n0} to represent the initial molecular weight of a polymer, Equation [2.17] can be rewritten in a normalised form

$$\overline{M}_n = \frac{M_n}{M_{n0}} = \frac{1}{1 + N_{\text{dp0}} \overline{R}_s} \qquad [2.18]$$

When measuring the molecular weight, using gel permeation chromatography (GPC) for example, the short chains are too small to be detected. Furthermore, the short chains do not contribute to the mechanical properties of a polymer, and including them in the number-averaged calculation distorts the true state of the polymer. It is therefore often necessary to exclude short chains from the calculation. Recalling that R_{ol} represents the total number of ester units of all the short chains, and m represents the average degree of polymerisation of the short chains, the number of short chains is given by R_{ol}/m. Averaged molecular weight excluding the short chains is then calculated as

$$M_n = \frac{\left(C_{e0} - R_{ol}\right) M_{\text{unit}}}{C_{\text{chain0}} + R_s - R_{ol}/m} \qquad [2.19]$$

which can be normalised by M_{n0} as

$$\bar{M}_n = \frac{M_n}{M_{n0}} = \frac{1 - \alpha \bar{R}_s^{\beta}}{1 + N_{\mathrm{dp0}} \left(\bar{R}_s - (\alpha / m) \bar{R}_s^{\beta} \right)} \quad [2.20]$$

2.5 Summary of equations and list of symbols

In summary, the normalised chain scission can be calculated by integrating the following master equation

$$\frac{d\bar{R}_s}{dt} = \left(1 - \alpha \bar{R}_s^{\beta}\right)\left[k_1 + \bar{k}_2 \left(N_{\mathrm{dp0}}^{-1} + \bar{R}_s\right)^n\right] \quad [2.15]$$

The averaged molecular weight is calculated using

$$\bar{M}_n = \frac{M_n}{M_{n0}} = \frac{1}{1 + N_{\mathrm{dp0}} \bar{R}_s} \quad [2.18]$$

If one wishes to exclude the short chains, then the averaged molecular weight is calculated using

$$\bar{M}_n = \frac{M_n}{M_{n0}} = \frac{1 - \alpha \bar{R}_s^{\beta}}{1 + N_{\mathrm{dp0}} \left(\bar{R}_s - (\alpha / m) \bar{R}_s^{\beta} \right)} \quad [2.20]$$

The definitions of all the symbols in the master equation are collected together here and grouped for convenience and clarity.

(I) Variables that change with time

- $\bar{R}_s = R_s / C_{eC}$ – total number of chain scissions per unit volume normalised by the initial number of ester units of all the chains per unit volume. Unit for all the concentrations: mol/m^3.
- $\bar{M}_n = M_n / M_{n0}$ – number-averaged molecular weight normalised by its initial value. Unit for molecular weight: g/mol.

(II) Parameter describing the initial condition of a polymer

- N_{dp0} – initial degree of polymerisation (DP). DP is defined as average number of ester units per polymer chain.

(III) Empirical parameters

- m – average DP of the short chains, dimensionless, typically set as 4–6.
- α, β – empirical parameters for short chain production, dimensionless.

(IV) Kinetic rate constants

- k_1 – hydrolysis rate constant for non-catalytic reaction; unit: 1/time.
- $\overline{k}_2 = C_{e0}^n k_2$ – hydrolysis rate constant for autocatalytic reaction; unit: 1/time.
- n – acid dissociation exponent of –COOH groups, which should be 0.5 but may be changed empirically to fit experimental data; dimensionless.

To restore the model to its dimensional format, one needs to know the initial average molecular weight M_{n0}. Usually the initial density ρ_0 and the molecular weight of a repeating unit M_{unit} are also known for a polymer. The initial values for the ester bond concentration C_{e0} and the DP N_{dp0} can be calculated as

$$C_{e0} = \frac{\rho_0}{M_{\text{unit}}} \qquad [2.21]$$

and

$$N_{\text{dp0}} = \frac{M_{n0}}{M_{\text{unit}}} \qquad [2.22]$$

2.6 Analytical solutions of the master equation

It is possible to simplify the master equation in some limiting conditions and to obtain analytical solutions.

2.6.1 *Solution for early stage degradation by non-catalytic hydrolysis*

In many studies we are only interested in the early stage of the polymer degradation. In this case the total amount of ester units of the short chains, R_{ol}, is much smaller than the ester bond concentration, C_{e0}, which means $\alpha \overline{R}_s^{\beta} \ll 1$. Furthermore, if the hydrolysis is non-catalytic, i.e. $\overline{k}_2 = 0$, then Equation [2.15] is reduced to

$$\frac{d\overline{R}_s}{dt} = k_1 \qquad [2.23]$$

which gives

$$\overline{R}_s = k_1 t \qquad [2.24]$$

Using Equation [2.24] in Equation [2.18] gives

$$M_n = \frac{M_{n0}}{1 + k_1 N_{\mathrm{dp}0} t} \qquad [2.25]$$

which can be rewritten as

$$\frac{1}{M_n} = \frac{1}{M_{n0}} + \frac{1}{M_{\mathrm{unit}}} k_1 t \qquad [2.26]$$

2.6.2 Solution for early stage degradation by autocatalytic hydrolysis

If we assume $\alpha \bar{R}_s^{\beta} << 1$ and that the hydrolysis is entirely autocatalytic, i.e. $k_1 = 0$, then Equation [2.15] is reduced to

$$\frac{d\bar{R}_s}{dt} = \bar{k}_2 \left(N_{\mathrm{dp}0}^{-1} + \bar{R}_s \right)^{1/2} \qquad [2.27]$$

which can be integrated to give

$$\bar{R}_s = \left[N_{\mathrm{dp}0}^{-1/2} + \frac{1}{2} \bar{k}_2 t \right]^2 - N_{\mathrm{dp}0}^{-1} \qquad [2.28]$$

Using Equation [2.28] in [2.18] gives

$$M_n = \frac{M_{n0}}{\left(1 + (1/2) N_{\mathrm{dp}0}^{1/2} \bar{k}_2 t \right)^2} \qquad [2.29]$$

which can be rewritten as

$$\left(\frac{1}{M_n} \right)^{1/2} = \left(\frac{1}{M_{n0}} \right)^{1/2} + \frac{1}{2} \left(\frac{1}{M_{\mathrm{unit}}} \right)^{1/2} \bar{k}_2 t \qquad [2.30]$$

In the literature, Equations [2.26] and [2.30] are often used to determine if a polymer degrades by autocatalytic hydrolysis reaction. In a degradation experiment, M_n is measured as a function of time. Using the measured data, $1/M_n$ and $(1/M_n)^{1/2}$ are plotted against time t. If $1/M_n$ versus time forms a straight line, then it is concluded that the hydrolysis is non-catalytic and k_1 can be calculated from the gradient of the line. On the other hand, if $(1/M_n)^{1/2}$ versus time forms a straight line, it is then concluded that the hydrolysis is autocatalytic and k_2 can be calculated from the gradient of the line. It is, however, often found that the two equations can only fit the very early stage of the measured experimental data.

2.7 Numerical solution of the master equation

In general, the master Equation [2.15] can only be integrated numerically. This is in fact very straightforward. Various commercial software can be used to integrate the equation. Alternatively, users can write a simple computer code to perform this integration. In this section, a numerical procedure and its corresponding computer code are provided.

2.7.1 A numerical scheme

For any known set of parameters of α,β, k_1, $\overline{k}_2$ and $N_{\mathrm{dp}0}$, the right hand side of Equation [2.15] is a simple function of $\overline{R}_s$, i.e. we can write

$$\frac{d\overline{R}_s}{dt} = f\left(\overline{R}_s\right) \tag{2.31}$$

in which

$$f\left(\overline{R}_s\right) = \left(1 - \alpha\overline{R}_s^{\beta}\right)\left[k_1 + \overline{k}_2\left(N_{\mathrm{dp}0}^{-1} + \overline{R}_s\right)^{1/2}\right] \tag{2.32}$$

We also know that at $t = 0$, $\overline{R}_s = 0$, which is the initial condition for the master equation. Using the definition of differentiation, we have

$$\frac{d\overline{R}_s}{dt} \approx \frac{\overline{R}_s\left(t+\Delta t\right) - \overline{R}\left(t\right)_s}{\Delta t} \approx f\left(\overline{R}_s\right) \tag{2.33}$$

in which Δt is a small time length. Consequently, we can write

$$\overline{R}_s\left(t+\Delta t\right) = \overline{R}_s\left(t\right) + \Delta t \times f\left(\overline{R}_s\right) \tag{2.34}$$

The following numerical scheme can therefore be used to calculate $\overline{R}_s$ as a function of time t

1. Input m, α,β, $N_{\mathrm{dp}0}$, k_1 and $\overline{k}_2$
2. Set Δt (see explanation below)

3. $t = 0$, $\bar{R}_s = 0$
4. Calculate $f\left(\bar{R}_s\right)$
5. $t = t + \Delta t$
6. $\bar{R}_s = \bar{R}_s + \Delta t \times f\left(\bar{R}_s\right)$
7. Calculate $\bar{M}_n$ using either Equation [2.18] or [2.20]
8. Output t, $\bar{R}_s$, $\bar{M}_n$
9. If $\bar{M}_n$ is close to zero then stop, otherwise go back to Step 4 and repeat the above procedure using the current value of $\bar{R}_s$.

For the numerical solution to be correct, Δt has to be sufficiently small. Although there are guidelines for the choice of Δt in numerical analysis, they strongly depend on the nature of $f\left(\bar{R}_s\right)$. In practice, a trial-and-error approach works better. One can start with a guessed value of Δt (say 1 day) and perform the numerical calculation. Then reduce Δt (say by half) and repeat the calculation. If the repeated analysis gives a different result (of $\bar{R}_s$ at a time t), then the guessed value of Δt is not small enough. One should continue to reduce Δt until further reduction does not lead to any change in the numerical result. At this point the numerical solution has converged to the correct one.

Figure 2.5 provides an example of the numerical solution for M_n / M_{n0} versus time using $m = 4$, $\alpha = 0.4$, $\beta = 1$, $N_{\mathrm{dp0}} = 1000$, $k_1 = 5\times10^{-4}$ / week and $k_2 = 5\times10^{-3}$ / week. The dashed line in the figure was calculated using the computer programme provided in Section 2.7.3. In the numerical integration we have used $\bar{R}_{s,\max} = 0.1$ and $N = 10^5$

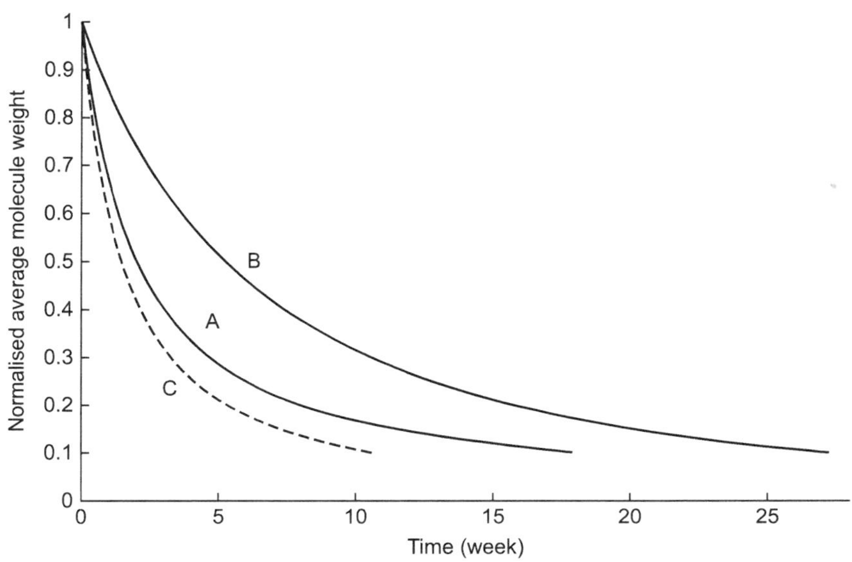

Figure 2.5 Normalised molecular weight as function of time obtained using (A) Equation [2.25] (B) Equation [2.29] and (C) numerical integration of Equation [2.15].

to ensure convergence (see Section 2.7.2). Equation [2.25] with $k_1 = 5\times10^{-4}$ / week (case A) and Equation [2.29] with $\bar{k}_2 = 5\times10^{-3}$ / week (case B) are also plotted in the figure.

2.7.2 Structure of a C++ programme for the numerical calculation

A computer programme is provided in Section 2.7.3 which is short enough for a reader to type in and try the numerical integration. Figure 2.6 shows the flow chart of the programme. It starts by inputting all the parameters and setting the initial conditions. A while loop is then used to perform the repeated calculations. The calculation

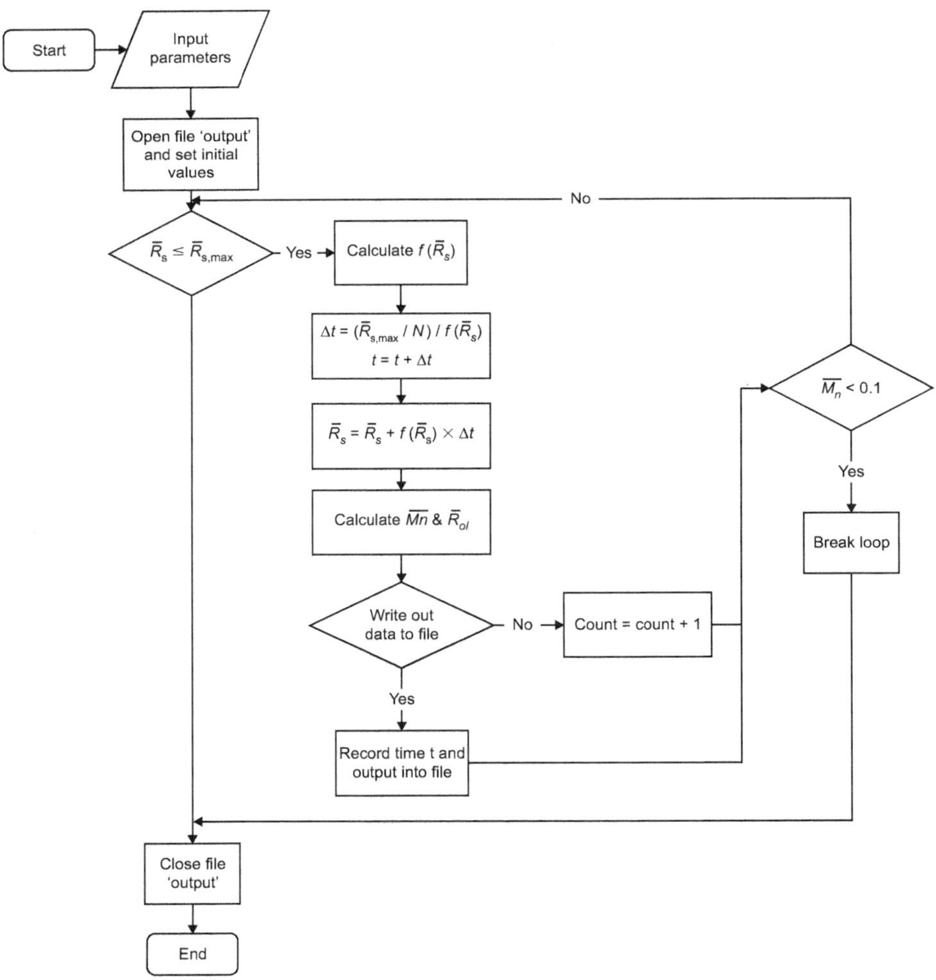

Figure 2.6 Flow chart of a C++ programme for the numerical integration.

continues until either $\bar{R}_s$ has gone beyond a maximum value, $\bar{R}_{s,\max}$ which is set by the user, or $\bar{M}_n$ has become less than 0.1. In the loop $f(\bar{R}_s)$ is calculated using Equation [2.32] by calling a separate function, $\bar{R}_s$ is defined by Equation [2.34] and $\bar{M}_n$ is calculated using Equation [2.18] by calling two separate functions. The time step Δt is set by requiring

$$\Delta t \times \frac{d\bar{R}_s}{dt} \times N = \Delta t \times f(\bar{R}_s) \times N = \bar{R}_{s,\max} \qquad [2.35]$$

which means $\bar{R}_{s,\max}$ is reached by approximately N time steps. N is an empirical number set by the user and has to be large enough to ensure convergence. It is normal that $N = 10^4 \sim 10^5$ has to be used. Because of the large number of time steps, it is unnecessary to write out data at every time step. The programme writes out 5000 data points at maximum throughout the calculation. This is achieved by using an output index 'count' and the condition 'if (count == read_data)' in the programme. The variable names used in the programme are listed as following:

(I) Input parameters

1. m – average DP of short chains
2. n – acid dissociation exponent of –COOH groups
3. alpha, beta – (α, β) empirical parameters for short chain production
4. $Ndp0$ – (N_{dp0}) initial DP
5. $k1$, $k2\_bar$ – $(k_1, \bar{k}_2)$ hydrolysis rate constants for non-catalytic and autocatalytic reaction respectively
6. Rs_bar_MAX - $(\bar{R}_{s,\max})$ maximum value of $\bar{R}_s$ beyond that the calculation stops
7. N – number of time steps to reach $\bar{R}_{s,\max}$
8. Ce0 – (C_{e0}) initial value for the ester bond concentration
9. Cchain0 – (C_{chain0}) initial value for the number of polymer chains

(II) Output parameters

1. t – time
2. Rs_bar – $(\bar{R}_s)$ normalised number of chain scissions per unit volume
3. Rol_bar – $\bar{R}_{ol}$ normalised number of ester units of short chains per unit volume
4. Mn_bar – $\bar{M}_n$ normalised number-averaged molecule weight

(III) Working variables

1. $function\_of\_Rs\_bar$ – function for calculating $f\left(\bar{R}_s\right)$
2. $calculate\_Mn\_bar$ – function for calculating $\bar{M}_n$
3. $delta\_t$ – Δt length of time step
4. $count$ – output index, initially set as 0 and reset as zero after each writing out of data

2.7.3 The C++ programme

```
#include <stdio.h> #include <math.h> #include <stdlib.h>     //(call C++ libraries)
double function_of_Rs_bar(double, double, double, double, double, double, double);
```

double calculate_Mn_bar(double, double);
//(give function prototype of two subroutines function_of _Rs_bar and calculate_Mn_bar, which will be used afterwards to calculate $f(\bar{R}_s)$ and $\overline{M_n}$ respectively)

```
int main ()      //(set main function)
{  double t=0.0, delta_t=0.0;     //(arguments)
   double k1, k2_bar, n, alpha, beta, m, Rs_bar_Max, Ce0, Cchain0;
   int N;
    printf("Input initial m value: "); scanf("%lf", &m);
    printf("Input Rs_bar_Max: "); scanf("%lf", &Rs_bar_Max);
    printf("Input number N: "); scanf("%d", &N);
    printf("Input parameters, n: "); scanf("%lf", &n);
    printf("Input parameters, alpha: "); scanf("%lf", &alpha);
    printf("Input parameters, bata: "); scanf("%lf", &beta);
    printf("Input parameters, k1: "); scanf("%lf", &k1);
    printf("Input parameters, k2_bar: "); scanf("%lf", &k2_bar);
    printf("Input parameters, Ce0: "); scanf("%lf", &Ce0);
    printf("Input parameters, Cchain0: "); scanf("%lf", &Cchain0);
       double Ndp0;
       int read_data;
       Ndp0=Ce0/Cchain0;          //(calculate Ndp0.)
       read_data=N/5000;          //(select maximum 5000 sets of data)
     FILE *output; output = fopen("output.txt", "w");     //(open file "output")
    double Rs_bar=0.0, Rol_bar=0.0, Mn_bar=1.0;     //(set initial value for outputs)
         int count=0;                    //(set initial value of count.)
      double f _Rs_bar =0.0;          //(use to call function_of_Rs_bar later)
      fprintf(output, "  t   \tRs_bar    \tMn_bar    \tRol_bar\n");    //(print out the title
      of outputs in file)
    while (Rs_bar<=Rs_bar_Max)        //(set up a while loop to do the reporting
    calculation)
   {   if (t==0) fprintf(output, "%.8lf    \t%.8lf    \t%.8lf    \t%.8lf\n",    t, Rs_bar,
   Mn_bar, Rol_bar);
   //(print out initial output values in file)
        if (count == read_data) //(write data to file)
        {  fprintf(output, "%.8lf \t%.8lf \t%.8lf \t%.8lf\n", t, Rs_bar, Mn_bar,
        Rol_bar);
        count = 0;   }
        else { count = count+1; }
        f _Rs_bar= function_of_Rs_bar(alpha, beta, k1, k2_bar, Ndp0, Rs_bar, n);
        //(call subroutine function_of_Rs_bar)
        delta_t = (Rs_bar_Max/N)/f_Rs_bar;     //(calculate delta_t)
        t = t+delta_t;       //(update time t)
        Rs_bar=Rs_bar+f_of_Rs_bar*delta_t;       //(calculate Rs_bar using equation
        (2.34))
        Rol_bar=alpha*pow(Rs_bar, beta);        //(calculate Rol_bar using equation
        (2.9))
```

```
        Mn_bar=calculate_Mn_bar(Ndp0, Rs_bar);        //(call subroutine) calculate_
        Mn_bar to calculate Mn_bar
        if (Mn_bar<0.1) break;      }
    fclose(output);         //(close file "output")
    system ("pause");       }

    double function_of_Rs_bar(double alpha, double beta, double k1, double k2_bar,
    double Ndp0, double Rs_bar, double n)
    {
        return (1-alpha*pow(Rs_bar, beta))*(k1+k2_bar*pow((1/Ndp0+Rs_bar),n));
    }       //(a subroutine to calculate f(R̄s) use equation (2.15))
    double calculate_Mn_bar(double Ndp0, double Rs_bar)
    {
        return 1/(1+Ndp0*Rs_bar);
    }       //(a subroutine to calculate M̄n use equation (2.18))
```

2.8 Concluding remarks

Equations [2.26] and [2.30] have been widely used in the literature to interpret degradation data for their simplicity. The validity of these equations is often limited to the very early stage of the degradation. For amorphous polymers, the master Equation [2.15] is more generally valid. However, short chain diffusion is ignored, which is the topic of the following chapters.

References

Flory PJ (1953) *Principles of Polymer Chemistry*. Ithaca and London, Cornell University Press.

Gleadall A, Pan J, Kruft MA and Kellomäki M (2014) Degradation mechanisms of bioresorbable polyesters, part 1: effects of random scission, end scission and autocatalysis. *Acta Biomaterialia*, **10**:2223–2232.

Han X and Pan J (2009) A model for simultaneous degradation and crystallisation in biodegradable polymers. *Biomaterials*, **30**:423–430.

Han X, Pan J, Buchannan F, Weir N and Farrar D (2010) Analysis of degradation data of bioresorbable polymers obtained at elevated and physiological temperatures using mathematical models. *Acta Biomaterialia*, **6**:3882–3889.

Wang Y, Pan J, Han X, Sinka IC and Ding L (2008) A phenomenological model for the degradation of biodegradable polymers. *Biomaterials*, **29**:3393–3401.

Modelling degradation of amorphous biodegradable polyesters: advanced model

3

J. Pan, X. Chen
University of Leicester, Leicester, UK

3.1 Introduction

The master Equation [2.15] presented in Chapter 2 cannot deal with short chain diffusion. The diffusion of short chains into the surrounding tissue reduces the concentration of carboxylic end groups inside a device and hence slows its degradation rate. Furthermore, the small chains near the surface of a device can diffuse out more quickly than those at the core. Consequently, the core degrades faster than the surface shell and a thick device degrades faster than a thin one. Grizzi *et al.* (1995) were the first to point out that short chain diffusion is responsible for the heterogeneous degradation and size effect observed in their experiments. It is therefore important to build the effect of short chain diffusion into the rate equation for chain scission. Both the long and short chains terminate with carboxylic end groups, but only those on the short chains can diffuse out. This chapter presents a rate equation for chain scission in which the carboxylic end groups on long and short chains are separated. A full treatment of short chain diffusion is the topic of Chapter 6. In this chapter when solving the equation it is assumed that the short chain diffusion can be ignored. The validity of this assumption can be found in Section 6.6.

A related issue is that carboxylic end groups on the short and long chains may have different capacities as catalysts for the hydrolysis reaction. Those on the long polymer chains have limited mobility, and may not fully contribute to the hydrolysis reaction. It is also possible to cap the chain ends during polymer processing with different function groups to tailor the degradation rate. Separating the two groups in the master equation provides the flexibility for switching off the catalytic effect of carboxylic end groups on the long chains.

This chapter also further elaborates the different roles played by end and random scissions on the degradation process, which was briefly mentioned in Section 2.3.

Modelling Degradation of Bioresorbable Polymeric Medical Devices. http://dx.doi.org/10.1533/9781782420255.1.33

3.2 Partition of carboxylic end groups on long and short chains

This section provides a rate equation for polymer chain scission in which the effect of carboxylic end groups of the long and short chains is separated using a set of partitioning parameters.

3.2.1 Rate equation for chain scission

The carboxylic end groups are divided into two types:

1. those of the long chains, which are not water soluble and cannot diffuse out of the device, represented by $C_{\mathrm{COOH}}^{\mathrm{long}}$
2. those of the short chains, which are water soluble and can diffuse, represented by $C_{\mathrm{COOH}}^{\mathrm{short}}$.

Let us reconsider the hydrolysis rate equation

$$\frac{dR_s}{dt} = k_1 C_e + k_2' C_e C_{\mathrm{H^+}} \qquad [2.2]$$

and the expression for the concentration of H^+

$$C_{\mathrm{H^+}} = \left[K_a C_{\mathrm{COOH}}\right]^{1/2} \qquad [2.5]$$

Splitting the two types of carboxylic end groups, Equation [2.5] is rewritten as

$$C_{\mathrm{H^+}} = \left[K_a \left(\chi_1 C_{\mathrm{COOH}}^{\mathrm{long}} + \chi_2 C_{\mathrm{COOH}}^{\mathrm{short}}\right)\right]^{1/2} \qquad [3.1]$$

in which χ_1 and χ_2 are two partitioning parameters which take values between zero and one. For example, Equation [3.1] is reduced to Equation [2.5] by setting $\chi_1 = \chi_2 = 1$; and the contribution from the long chains can be switched off by setting $\chi_1 = 0$ and $\chi_2 = 1$.

The number of carboxylic end groups on the long chains increases with chain scission and decreases with the production of short chains, which can be expressed as

$$C_{\mathrm{COOH}}^{\mathrm{long}} = C_{\mathrm{chain0}} + R_s - \frac{R_{ol}}{m} \qquad [3.2]$$

in which C_{chain0} is the concentration of long chain at the beginning of the degradation, R_{ol} is the number of ester units of all the short chains that have been generated, by

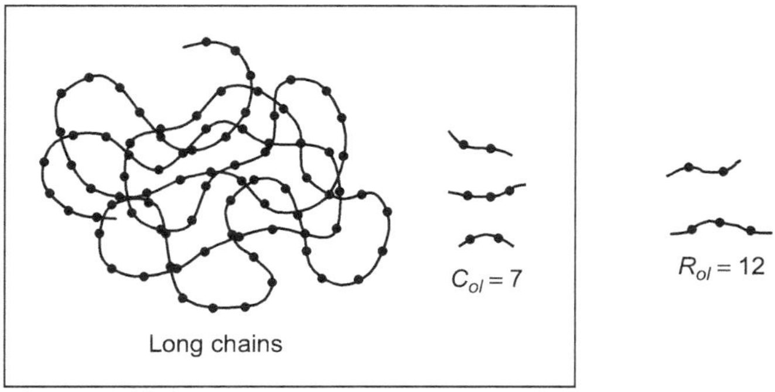

Figure 3.1 Current and accumulated short chains. Two short chains have left the polymer while three remain inside. Dots represent ester bonds.

chain scission and m is the average number of ester units of the short chains. R_{ol} is related to R_s through Equation [2.9], using which Equation [3.2] can be rewritten as

$$C_{\mathrm{COOH}}^{\mathrm{long}} = C_{\mathrm{chain0}} + R_s - C_{e0}\frac{\alpha}{m}\left(\frac{R_s}{C_{e0}}\right)^{\beta} \qquad [3.3]$$

Because the short chains may diffuse out of a device, at any given time the concentration of the short chains in a polymer can be different from R_{ol}. The number of ester units of short chains that are currently in the polymer is denoted as C_{ol}. The difference between R_{ol} and C_{ol} is schematically illustrated in Figure 3.1. If polymerisation during the manufacturing of a device is incomplete, then the material may contain a significant amount of residual short chains. This means C_{ol} may have a non-zero initial value, referred to as C_{ol0}, at the beginning of the degradation. On the other hand R_{ol} counts for only the short chains that are generated by chain scission and is always zero at the beginning of degradation.

The number of carboxylic end groups on the short chains inside the polymer is given by

$$C_{\mathrm{COOH}}^{\mathrm{short}} = \frac{C_{ol}}{m} \qquad [3.4]$$

Combining Equations [2.2], [3.1], [3.3] and [3.4] gives

$$\frac{dR_s}{dt} = k_1 C_e + k_2 C_e\left[\chi_1\left(C_{\mathrm{chain0}} + R_s - C_{e0}\frac{\alpha}{m}\left(\frac{R_s}{C_{e0}}\right)^{\beta}\right) + \chi_2\frac{C_{ol}}{m}\right]^n \qquad [3.5]$$

in which n is the acid dissociation exponent, which should be 0.5 but can take other empirical values, and $k_2 = k_2'\left[K_a\right]^n$.

3.2.2 Master equation without short chain diffusion

A full treatment of diffusion of the short chains is provided in Chapter 6. In the remaining part of this chapter, it is assumed that the diffusion is prohibited. In this case all the short chains produced by chain scissions remain in the material and we have:

$$C_{ol} = C_{ol0} + R_{ol} = C_{ol0} + \alpha C_{e0}\left(\frac{R_s}{C_{e0}}\right)^{\beta} \quad [3.6]$$

Using Equation [3.6] and $C_e = C_{e0} - R_{ol}$ in Equation [3.5] leads to the following master equation for chain scission

$$\frac{d\bar{R}_s}{dt} = \left(1-\alpha\bar{R}_s^{\beta}\right)\left\{k_1 + \bar{k}_2\left[\bar{C}_0 + \chi_1\bar{R}_s + \left(\chi_2 - \chi_1\right)\frac{\alpha}{m}\bar{R}_s^{\beta}\right]^n\right\} \quad [3.7]$$

The averaged molecular weight is calculated using

$$\bar{M}_n = \frac{M_n}{M_{n0}} = \frac{1}{1+N_{\text{dp0}}\bar{R}_s} \quad [2.18]$$

If one wishes to exclude the short chains, then the averaged molecular weight is calculated using

$$\bar{M}_n = \frac{M_n}{M_{n0}} = \frac{1-\alpha\bar{R}_s^{\beta}}{1+N_{\text{dp0}}\left(\bar{R}_s - (\alpha/m)\bar{R}_s^{\beta}\right)} \quad [2.20]$$

The definitions of all the symbols in the master equation are listed here for the convenience of readers.

1. Variables that change with time
   - $\bar{R}_s = R_s / C_{e0}$ – total number of chain scissions per unit volume normalised by the initial number of ester units of all the chains per unit volume. Unit for all the concentrations: mol/m^3.
   - $\bar{M}_n = M_n / M_{n0}$ – number-averaged molecular weight normalised by its initial value. Unit for molecular weights: g/mol.
2. Parameter describing initial conditions of a polymer
   - N_{dp0} – initial degree of polymerisation (DP). DP is defined as the average number of ester units per polymer chain.
   - $\bar{C}_0$ – normalised initial concentration of –COOH end groups

$$\overline{C}_0 = \frac{1}{C_{e0}}\left(\chi_1 C_{\text{chain}0} + \chi_2 \frac{C_{ol0}}{m}\right) \qquad [3.8]$$

in which $C_{\text{chain}0}$ is the initial number of long chains per unit volume, C_{ol0} is the initial total number of ester units of short chains per unit volume and C_{e0} is the initial number of ester units per unit volume.

3. Empirical parameters
   - m – average DP of the short chains, dimensionless, typically set as 4–6.
   - α, β – empirical parameters for short chain production, dimensionless.
   - χ_1, χ_1 – partitioning parameters for the long and short chains to act as catalyst, dimensionless.
4. Kinetic constants
   - k_1 – hydrolysis rate constant for non-catalytic reaction; unit: 1/time.
   - $\bar{k}_2 = C_{e0}^n k_2$ – hydrolysis rate constant for autocatalytic reaction; unit: 1/time.
   - n – acid disassociation exponent of –COOH groups which should be 0.5 but may be changed empirically to fit experimental data; dimensionless.

3.3 Analytical solutions to the master equation

Under various restrictive conditions, it is possible to obtain analytical solutions to the master Equation [3.7]. These analytical solutions are provided here without derivation.

3.3.1 Early stage degradation ($\alpha \overline{R}_s^{\beta} \ll 1$), pure autocatalytic hydrolysis ($k_1 = 0$), either $\beta = 1$ or $\chi_2 = \chi_1 = 1$, and $n = 1$

In this case Equation [3.7] can be simplified as

$$\frac{d\overline{R}_s}{dt} = \bar{k}_2\left[\overline{C}_0 + A\overline{R}_s\right] \qquad [3.9]$$

where

$$A = \chi_1 + (\chi_2 - \chi_1)\frac{\alpha}{m} \qquad [3.10]$$

Equation [3.9] can be integrated to give

$$\overline{R}_s = \frac{1}{A}\overline{C}_0\left(e^{A\bar{k}_2 t} - 1\right) \qquad [3.11]$$

In the case that no separation is made between carboxylic end groups on the long and short chains ($\chi_2 = \chi_1 = 1$), Equation [3.11] leads to

$$\ln\left(M_n\right) = \ln\left(M_{n0}\right) - k_2' C_{e0} K_a t \tag{3.12}$$

which is used in some literature.

3.3.2 Early stage degradation ($\alpha \bar{R}_s^\beta << 1$), pure autocatalytic hydrolysis ($k_1 = 0$), either $\beta = 1$ or $\chi_2 = \chi_1 = 1$, and $n \neq 1$

In this case Equation [3.7] can be simplified as

$$\frac{d\bar{R}_s}{dt} = \bar{k}_2 \left[\bar{C}_0 + A\bar{R}_s\right]^n \tag{3.13}$$

where

$$A = \chi_1 + \left(\chi_2 - \chi_1\right)\frac{\alpha}{m} \tag{3.10}$$

Equation [3.13] can be integrated to give

$$\bar{R}_s = \frac{1}{A}\left[\left(\bar{C}_0\right)^{1-n} + A(1-n)\bar{k}_2 t\right]^{1/1-n} - \frac{\bar{C}_0}{A} \tag{3.14}$$

If $\chi_2 = \chi_1 = 1$, and $n = 0.5$, then the above solution is reduced to Equation [2.28].

3.3.3 Early stage degradation ($\alpha \bar{R}_s^\beta << 1$), pure autocatalytic hydrolysis ($k_1 = 0$), only the short chains act as catalyst ($\chi_1 = 0$ and $\chi_2 = 1$), no residual oligomers at the beginning of the degradation ($\bar{C}_0 = 0$) and $n\beta \neq 1$

In this case the master Equation [3.7] is reduced to

$$\frac{d\bar{R}_s}{dt} = \bar{k}_2 \left[\frac{\alpha}{m}\bar{R}_s^\beta\right]^n \tag{3.15}$$

which can be integrated to give

$$\bar{R}_s = \left[(1 - n\beta)\bar{k}_2 \left(\frac{\alpha}{m} \right)^n t \right]^{1/(1-n\beta)} \qquad [3.16]$$

It can be concluded that $n\beta < 1$ otherwise the function is not defined.

3.3.4 Non-catalytic hydrolysis ($\bar{k}_2 = 0$) without the assumption of early stage degradation and $\beta = 1$

The master Equation [3.7] is reduced to

$$\frac{d\bar{R}_s}{dt} = k_1 \left(1 - \alpha \bar{R}_s \right) \qquad [3.17]$$

and its solution is

$$\bar{R}_s = \frac{1}{\alpha}\left(1 - e^{-\alpha k_1 t} \right) \qquad [3.18]$$

3.3.5 Non-catalytic hydrolysis ($\bar{k}_2 = 0$) without the assumption of early stage degradation and $\beta = 2$

The master Equation [3.7] is reduced to

$$\frac{d\bar{R}_s}{dt} = k_1 \left(1 - \alpha \bar{R}_s^2 \right) \qquad [3.19]$$

and its solution is

$$\bar{R}_s = \frac{1}{\sqrt{\alpha}} \frac{e^{2\sqrt{\alpha} k_1 t} - 1}{e^{2\sqrt{\alpha} k_1 t} + 1} \qquad [3.20]$$

3.3.6 Pure autocatalytic hydrolysis ($k_1 = 0$) without the assumption of early stage degradation, $\beta = 1$ and $n = 0.5$

The master Equation [3.7] is reduced to

$$\frac{d\bar{R}_s}{dt} = \bar{k}_2\left(1-\alpha\bar{R}_s\right)\left[\bar{C}_0 + A\bar{R}_s\right]^{0.5} \quad [3.21]$$

and its solution is

$$\bar{R}_s = \frac{H^2}{A\alpha}\frac{(1+Ge^{-\sqrt{\alpha H\bar{k}_2 t}})^2}{(1-Ge^{-\sqrt{\alpha H\bar{k}_2 t}})^2} - \frac{\bar{C}_0}{A} \quad [3.22]$$

in which

$$A = \chi_1 + (\chi_2 - \chi_1)\frac{\alpha}{m},\ H = \sqrt{(\bar{C}_0\alpha + A)}\ \text{and}\ G = \frac{\sqrt{\alpha\bar{C}_0} - H}{\sqrt{\alpha\bar{C}_0} + H} \quad [3.23]$$

3.4 Numerical solution and a parametric study of the model

In general, the master Equation [3.7] has to be integrated numerically. In fact, the numerical scheme and computer programme presented in Section 2.7 can be directly used for the integration by replacing the expression for function *f* with

$$f(\bar{R}_s) = \left(1-\alpha\bar{R}_s^{\beta}\right)\left\{k_1 + \bar{k}_2\left[\bar{C}_0 + \chi_1\bar{R}_s + (\chi_2 - \chi_1)\frac{\alpha}{m}\bar{R}_s^{\beta}\right]^n\right\} \quad [3.24]$$

As a demonstration example, Figure 3.2 shows the comparison between the analytical solution of Equation [3.22] and its corresponding numerical solution. The following parameters are used: $m = 4$, $\chi_1 = 0$, $\chi_2 = 1$, $\alpha = 0.4$, $\beta = 1$, $N_{dp0} = 1000$, $\bar{C}_0 = 0$, $k_1 = 0$ and $\bar{k}_2 = 1$/week. This set of parameters leads to $A = 0.1$, $H = 0.316$ and $G = -1$. The numerical method makes it possible to study how the different parameters affect the model prediction. This is sometimes called a parametric study.

3.4.1 Effect of $\bar{k}_2 / k_1$

The ratio of $\bar{k}_2 / k_1$ reflects the relative rate of autocatalytic hydrolysis with respect to non-catalytic hydrolysis. Figure 3.3 shows the calculated molecular weight as a function of time using a range of different parameters. Curve A in the figure represents in fact 6 different curves all overlapping with each other. This groups of curves shares a common ratio of $\bar{k}_2 / k_1 = 1$. The numerical calculation therefore shows that for this ratio of $\bar{k}_2 / k_1$, changing the values of χ_1, χ_2, α, β and n has no effect on the calculated

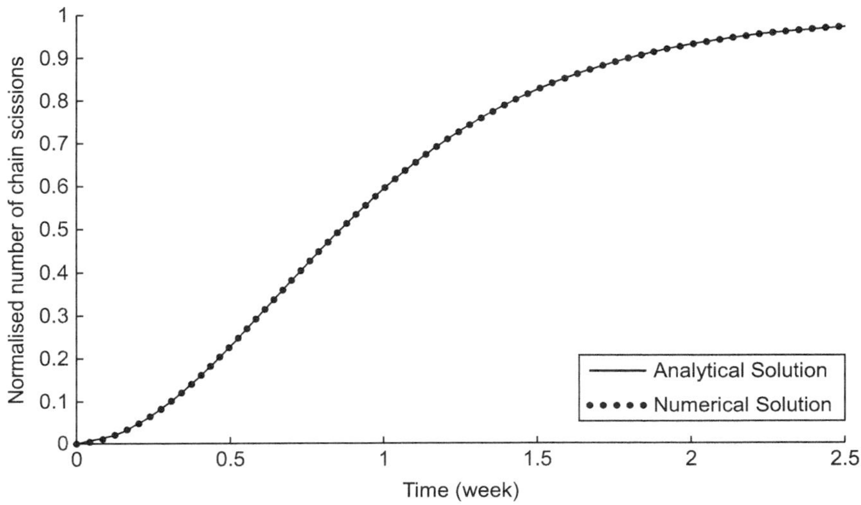

Figure 3.2 Comparison between analytical solution of Equation [3.22] and its corresponding numerical solution.

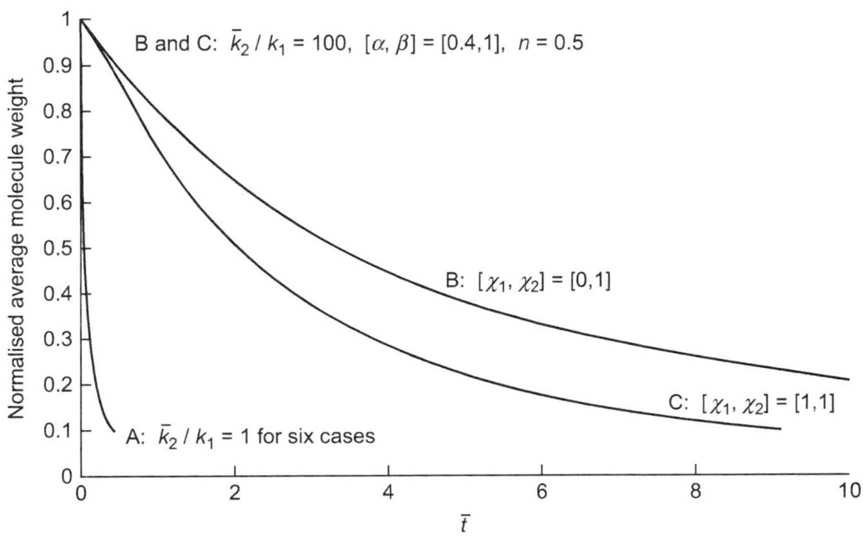

Figure 3.3 Average molecular weight as functions of time calculated using different parameters. Curve A represents a set of six curves which overlap each other using $\bar{k}_2 / k_1 = 1$, $[\alpha, \beta] = [0.4, 1]$, $[28, 2]$; $n = [0.1, 0.5]$ and $[\chi_1, \chi_2] = [0, 1]$, $[1, 1]$. Curves B and C are for $\bar{k}_2 / k_1 = 100$.

molecular weight as a function of time. This is because these parameters are all related to autocatalytic hydrolysis, i.e. the second term in Equation [2.2]. The numerical analysis suggests that when $\bar{k}_2 / k_1$ approaches unity, the autocatalytic term can be ignored. Curves B and C in Figure 3.3 were obtained using a common ratio of $\bar{k}_2 / k_1 = 100$ and two different sets of values of χ_1, χ_2, α, β and n. It can be observed at this ratio of $\bar{k}_2 / k_1$, changing the values of these parameters has a major effect on the results. This suggests that at this ratio of $\bar{k}_2 / k_1$, the autocatalytic term in Equation [2.2] dominates the hydrolysis reaction. This issue is further discussed in Section 6.6.2. In all the cases, following parameters were used: $m = 4$, $\bar{C}_0 = 0$ and $N_{\mathrm{dp0}} = 2307$.

3.4.2 Effect of α and β

These two parameters control the number of short chains produced by chain scission according to Equation [2.9]:

$$\frac{R_{ol}}{C_{e0}} = \alpha\left(\frac{R_s}{C_{e0}}\right)^{\beta} \qquad [2.9]$$

To demonstrate this, Figure 3.4 shows the calculated molecular weight as functions of time using two sets of parameters: case A uses $\alpha = 28$, $\beta = 2$, $k_1 = 5\times10^{-4}$ / week and $\bar{k}_2 = 0.01$ / week, while case B uses $\alpha = 0.4$, $\beta = 1$, $k_1 = 1\times10^{-6}$ / week and $\bar{k}_2 = 0.01$ / week. A common set of the remaining parameters, $m = 4$, $\bar{C}_0 = 0$,

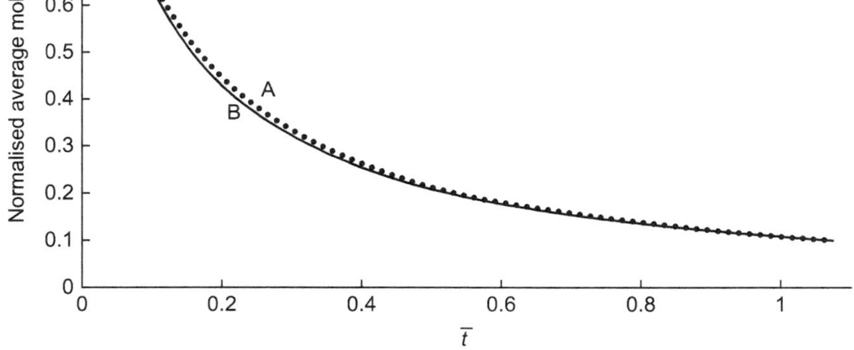

Figure 3.4 Calculated average molecular weight as functions of time for two different set of parameters.

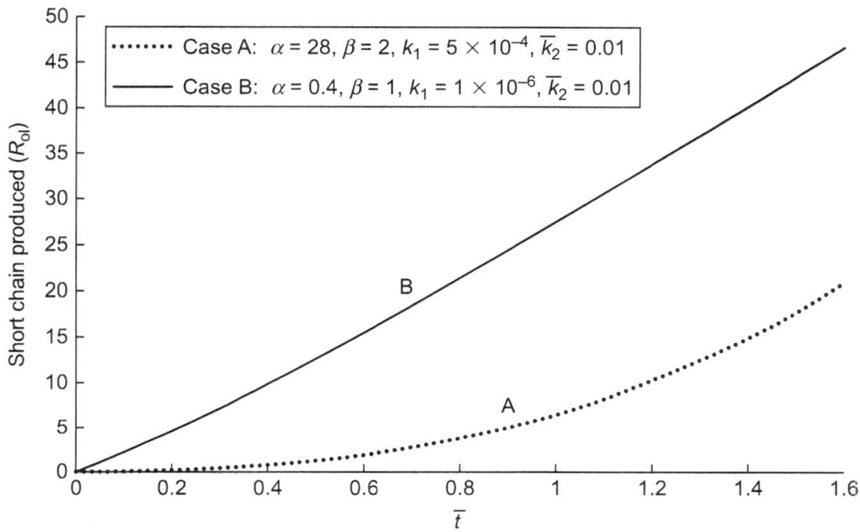

Figure 3.5 Calculated number of ester units of all the short chains produced by chain scission as functions of time for two different sets of parameters.

$N_{dp0} = 2307, \chi_1 = 0$, $\chi_2 = 1$ and $n = 0.5$, was used. The ratios of $\overline{k}_2 / k_1$ in the two cases are big enough for the hydrolysis reaction to be autocatalytic. Consequently, α and β have a significant effect on the results, which is, however, missing from Figure 3.4. The roles played by α and β become clear in Figure 3.5, which shows the calculated number of short chains produced as functions of time for the two cases. It is apparent that the short chain production is very different between the two cases. It can therefore be concluded that one cannot uniquely determine the values of α, β, k_1 and $\overline{k}_2$ from the data of average molecular weight as function of time alone. The information about short chain production (the very left end of the molecular weight distributions as shown in Figure 2.2) has to be available in order to determine the values for α and β.

3.4.3 Effect of χ_1 and χ_2

χ_1 and χ_2 are introduced into the model to partition the long and short chains. Their effect can be demonstrated by taking account of short chain diffusion in the model, which is the topic of Chapter 6. It is, however, useful to show this effect here together with the discussion on other model parameters. Figure 3.6 shows the calculated molecular weight as functions of time using two different sets of parameters: for case A $\chi_1 = 0$, $\chi_2 = 1$, $k_1 = 5\times10^{-5}$ / week and $\overline{k}_2 = 5\times10^{-4}$ / week, and for case B $\chi_1 = 1$, $\chi_2 = 1$, $k_1 = 1.2\times10^{-4}$ / week and $\overline{k}_2 = 2\times10^{-5}$ / week. A common set of the remaining parameters, $m = 4$, $\overline{C}_0 = 0$, $N_{dp0} = 2307$, $\alpha = 0.4$, $\beta = 1$ and $n = 0.5$, were used for both cases. The coefficient for short chain diffusion in non-degraded polymer was set

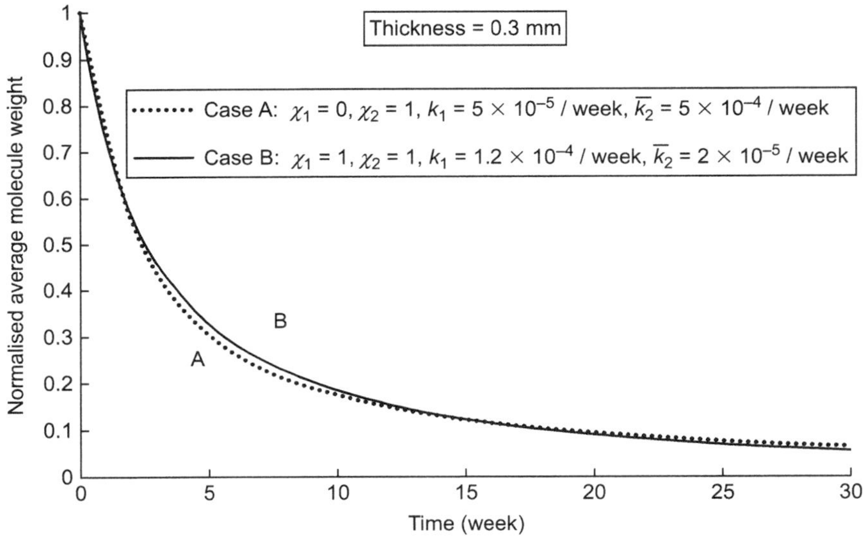

Figure 3.6 Calculated average molecular weight as functions of time for two different sets of parameters showing they give same prediction for samples with a thickness of 0.3 mm.

as $D_{\text{polymer}} = 3.3\times10^{-14}\text{m}^2/\text{week}$ for both cases (see Section 6.4.1). It can be observed from Figure 3.6 that the two sets of parameters give almost identical molecular weights as functions of time. These were, however, calculated using a sample thickness of 0.3 mm. Figure 3.7 shows the calculated results using the same sets of parameters but for a sample thickness of 2 mm. Different molecular weights as functions of time can be observed. This demonstrates that in order to uniquely determine the values for χ_1 and χ_2, one has to obtain experimental data using samples of different thicknesses.

3.4.4 Effect of $\overline{C}_0$

$\overline{C}_0$ is defined by Equation [3.8] and reflects the number of chain ends in the polymer at the beginning of the degradation. Acid disassociation of the –COOH end groups leads to an increasing level of H^+ and accelerates the degradation rate. If a large number of residual monomers exist, then $\overline{C}_0$ can play a significant role in the degradation behaviour. Because the –COOH end groups are only relevant if the hydrolysis is autocatalytic, let us focus on the case of pure autocatalytic hydrolysis by setting $k_1 = 0$ and $\overline{k}_2 = 1$. Figure 3.8 shows the calculated molecular weight as functions of time for five different values of $\overline{C}_0$. The calculation used a common set of parameters: $m = 4$, $N_{\text{dp}0} = 2307$, $\alpha = 0.4$, $\beta = 1$ and $n = 0.5$. If all the chain ends can act as catalysts, then $\overline{C}_0 = C_{\text{chain}0} / C_{e0}$, which is case D shown in Figure 3.8. Here $C_{\text{chain}0}$ is the initial concentration of chain ends and C_{e0} is the initial concentration of ester units of all the polymer chains. Case A assumes an extremely small value of $\overline{C}_0 = 10^{-10} C_{\text{chain}0} / C_{e0}$. Cases B and C represent some moderate values of

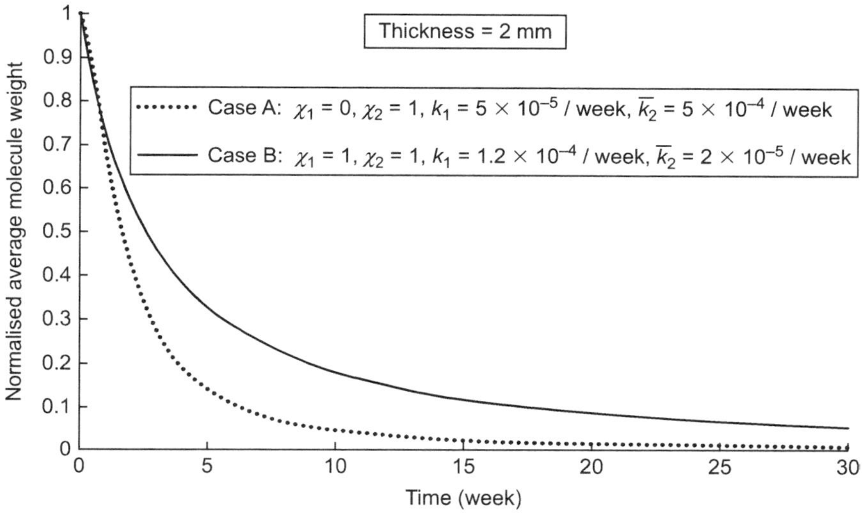

Figure 3.7 Calculated average molecular weight as functions of time for two different sets of parameters identical to those used in Figure 3.6 showing they give different predictions for samples with a thickness of 2 mm.

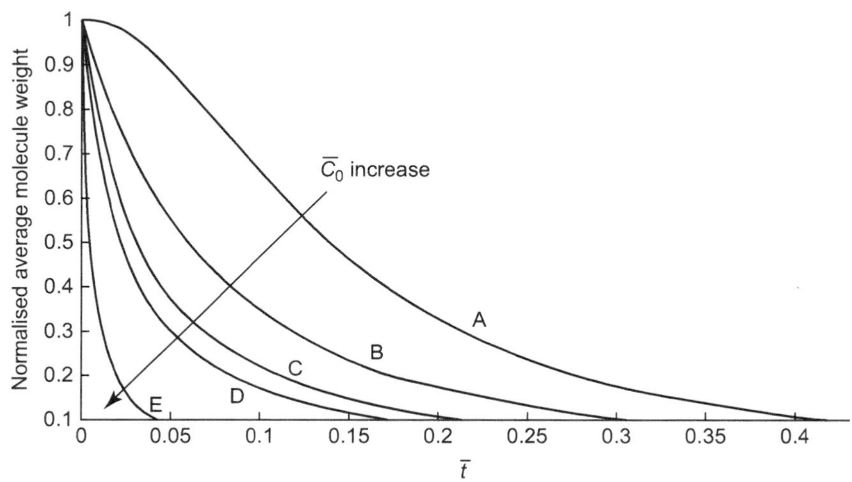

Figure 3.8 Effect of $\overline{C}_0$ on the degradation behaviour for pure autocatalytic hydrolysis (A) $\overline{C}_0 = 10^{-10} C_{\text{chain}0} / C_{e0}$, (B) $\overline{C}_0 = 0.1 C_{\text{chain}0} / C_{e0}$, (C) $\overline{C}_0 = 0.5 C_{\text{chain}0} / C_{e0}$, (D) $\overline{C}_0 = C_{\text{chain}0} / C_{e0}$ and (E) $\overline{C}_0 = 0.01$. $k_1 = 0$ and $\overline{k}_2 = 1$.

$\overline{C}_0 = 0.1 C_{\text{chain}0} / C_{e0}$ and $\overline{C}_0 = 0.5 C_{\text{chain}0} / C_{e0}$, respectively. Case E represents a very large value of $\overline{C}_0 = 0.01$, which means 1% of the ester units act as catalysts for the hydrolysis reaction. It is very clear that an increasing value of $\overline{C}_0$ changes both the shape of the curve and the rate of the degradation.

3.5 Separation of end scission from random scission

It is often claimed that biodegradable polymers degrade through random scissions of the polymer chains. However the ester bonds next to chain ends may hydrolyse faster than those inside the chains, which is known as end scission. To account for the effect of end scission, Gleadall *et al.* (2014) used separate equations for random scission rate, dR_{rs} / dt, and end scission rate, dR_{es} / dt, respectively, such that

$$\frac{dR_{rs}}{dt} = k_{r1}C_e + k'_{r2}C_eC_{H^+} \qquad [3.25]$$

and

$$\frac{dR_{es}}{dt} = k_{e1}C_{\text{end}} + k'_{e2}C_{\text{end}}C_{H^+} \qquad [3.26]$$

where C_e, C_{end} and C_{H^+} represent the concentrations of ester bonds, chain ends and H^+ respectively, and k_{r1}, k'_{r2}, k_{e1} and k'_{e2} represent the corresponding reaction constants. C_e should exclude ester bonds next to the chain ends, but this difference can be ignored because C_e is much larger than C_{end}. Only random scission produces new ends for the long chains, which leads to

$$C_{\text{end}} = 2\left(C_{\text{chain}0} + R_{rs}\right) \qquad [3.27]$$

in which $C_{\text{chain}0}$ is the number of long chains per unit volume at the beginning of the degradation.

In the master Equation [3.7], monomers and oligomers have been treated together as short chains. Here the concentrations of monomers and oligomers are followed separately. In principle, both end and random scissions produce monomers. However, the monomer production rate by random scission is much smaller than that by end scission. Using R_m to represent the concentration of monomers, it is assumed that only end scissions produce monomers, and we have

$$R_m = R_{es} \qquad [3.28]$$

Following Equation [2.8] in Section 2.3, oligomer production R_{ol} by random scission can be related to the total number of scissions R_{rs} through

$$R_{ol} = \alpha C_{e0}\left(\frac{R_{rs}}{C_{e0}}\right)^2 \qquad [3.29]$$

in which α depends on q, the upper limit to the number of ester units, and is taken as 28 here. Both end and random scissions reduce the long chains through the production of monomers and oligomers, which can be expressed as

$$C_e = C_{e0} - R_{ol} - R_m \tag{3.30}$$

The number of long chains increases with random scission and decreases with oligomer production. The concentration of –COOH end groups on the long chains is given by

$$C_{\text{COOH}}^{\text{long}} = C_{\text{chain0}} + R_{rs} - \frac{R_{ol}}{m} \tag{3.31}$$

The concentration of –COOH end groups on the short chains is given by

$$C_{\text{COOH}}^{\text{short}} = (C_{m0} + R_m) + \frac{1}{m}(C_{ol0} + R_{ol}) \tag{3.32}$$

in which C_{m0} and C_{ol0} represent the concentrations of residual monomers and oligomers at the beginning of the degradation, respectively. The concentration of C_{H^+} can then be calculated using Equation [3.1].

Combining Equations [3.1] and [3.25]–[3.32] leads to the following rate equations for random and end scissions in the normalised form:

$$\frac{d\bar{R}_{rs}}{dt} = \left[1 - \bar{R}_{es} - \alpha \bar{R}_{rs}^{\beta}\right]\left\{k_{r1} + \bar{k}_{r2}\left[\bar{C}_0 + \chi_1 \bar{R}_{rs} + \chi_2 \bar{R}_{es} + (\chi_2 - \chi_1)\frac{\alpha}{m}\bar{R}_{rs}^{\beta}\right]^n\right\} \tag{3.33}$$

and

$$\frac{d\bar{R}_{es}}{dt} = 2\left[\bar{C}_{\text{chain0}} + \bar{R}_{rs}\right]\left\{k_{e1} + \bar{k}_{e2}\left[\bar{C}_0 + \chi_1 \bar{R}_{rs} + \chi_2 \bar{R}_{es} + (\chi_2 - \chi_1)\frac{\alpha}{m}\bar{R}_{rs}^{\beta}\right]^n\right\} \tag{3.34}$$

where $\bar{R}_{rs} = R_{rs} / C_{e0}$, $\bar{R}_{es} = R_{es} / C_{e0}$, $\bar{k}_{r2} = C_{e0}^n k_{r2}$, $\bar{k}_{e2} = C_{e0}^n k_{e2}$, $C_{\text{chain0}} = C_{\text{chain0}} / C_{e0}$ and

$$\bar{C}_0 = \frac{1}{C_{e0}}\left(\chi_1 C_{\text{chain0}} + \chi_2 C_{m0} + \chi_2 \frac{C_{ol0}}{m}\right) \tag{3.35}$$

The number-averaged molecular weight can be calculated by modifying Equations [2.18] and [2.20] slightly, such that

$$\bar{M}_n = \frac{M_n}{M_{n0}} = \frac{1}{1+N_{dp0}\left(\bar{R}_{rs}+\bar{R}_{es}\right)} \quad [3.36]$$

or, if one wishes to exclude the short chains, use

$$\bar{M}_n = \frac{M_n}{M_{n0}} = \frac{1-\alpha\bar{R}_{rs}^{\beta}-\bar{R}_{es}}{1+N_{dp0}\left(\bar{R}_{rs}-(\alpha/m)\bar{R}_{rs}^{\beta}\right)} \quad [3.37]$$

Equations [3.33] and [3.34] can be integrated using a numerical scheme similar to that presented in Section 2.7.

3.6 Contributions from random and end scissions to polymer degradation

As discussed in Section 2.3, chain scissions cannot be purely random because pure random scission cannot produce enough oligomers to account for the level of mass loss observed in the experiments. On the other hand, the chain scissions cannot only occur next to the chain ends either, because the molecular weight reduction would be too slow. A few cleavages in the middle of the long chains can reduce the average molecular weight much more than the same number of cleavages does at the chain ends. The separation of end scission from random scission in the rate equations makes it possible to demonstrate the different roles played by the two scission mechanisms in polymer degradation (Gleadall *et al.*, 2014).

Figures 3.9 and 3.10 show molecular weight ($\bar{M}_n$, solid lines) and the accumulation of short chains ($\bar{R}_m + \bar{R}_{ol}$, dashed lines) as functions of time for random and end scissions, respectively. These were obtained by integrating Equations [3.33] and [3.34] numerically. When calculating the molecular weight, the small chains were excluded. It was assumed that only –COOH groups of the short chains act as catalysts, i.e $\chi_1 = 0$ and $\chi_2 = 1$. A typical set of material data for poly(lactide) (PLA) of M_{unit} = 72 g mol^{-1}, N_{chain0} = 4.35 mol m^{-3} and C_{e0} = 17 300 mol m^{-3} (representing M_{n0} = 286 000 g mol^{-1}) was used. In both figures the degradation time is normalised by a characteristic time t_c, which is the time taken for the molecular weight to reduce to 10% of its initial value. Consequently, the absolute values of the reaction constants do not have an effect and only their relative values are important. To eliminate the effect of any residual short chains on this demonstration, the initial concentrations of residual oligomers and monomers were set at an extremely small value of 10^{-10} C_{e0}.

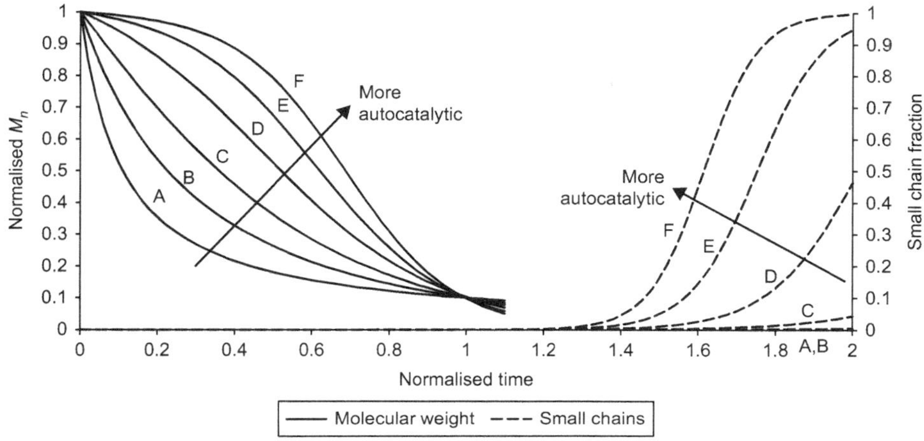

Figure 3.9 Random scission – molecular weight (solid lines) and accumulation of short chains (dashed lines) as functions of time. $\bar{k}_{r2}/k_{r1}$ = 0 (A), 5(B), 20 (C), 100 (D), 500 (E) and infinity(F). (*Source*: Taken from Gleadall *et al.*, 2014.)

In the case shown in Figure 3.9, k_{e1} and $\bar{k}_{e2}$ were set as zero to represent pure random scission. The ratio $\bar{k}_{r2}/k_{r1}$, reflecting the relative rate of autocatalytic hydrolysis to non-catalytic hydrolysis, was varied from 0 to infinity to cover a wide range of different polymers. It can be observed from Figure 3.9 that in all the cases the accumulation of short chains is insignificant until the molecular weight reaches a very small value. This means any measurable mass loss cannot be expected before the device breaks apart.

In the case shown in Figure 3.10, k_{r1} and $\bar{k}_{r2}$ were set as zero to reflect pure end scission. The relative rate of autocatalytic hydrolysis to non-catalytic hydrolysis, i.e. $\bar{k}_{e2}/k_{e1}$, was varied from zero to infinity to cover a wide range of different polymers. In strong contrast to Figure 3.9, the accumulation of short chains now occurs simultaneously with the reduction in molecular weight. This means significant mass loss can be expected if only end scission occurs.

To demonstrate that end scissions alone are too slow to reduce molecular weight, Figure 3.11 shows a fitting for the experimental data obtained by Beslikas *et al.* (2011) using the model prediction by Gleadall *et al.* (2014). The model also took account of chain cleavage-induced crystallisation and diffusion of the short chains, which will be discussed in later chapters of this book. Here we focus on the effect of random and end scissions. The best fit was achieved by $k_{r1} = k_{e1} = 0$ (i.e. fully autocatalytic hydrolysis) and of $\bar{k}_{e2}/\bar{k}_{r2} = 7500$, which indicates that end scission occurs much faster than random scission. This high relative rate of end scission is necessary to achieve the level of mass loss observed in the experiment. However, it is very interesting to examine the effect of the relatively small rate of random scission on the molecular weight reduction. The dashed lines in Figure 3.11 show the model prediction using the identical set of parameters, except that random scission is completely switched off. It can be observed that the molecular weight would remain almost constant if no

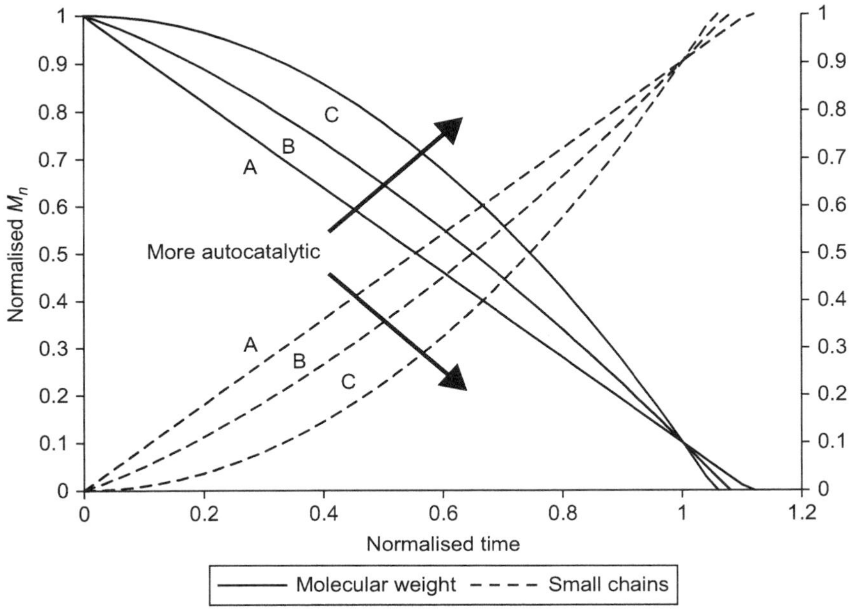

Figure 3.10 End scission – molecular weight (solid lines) and accumulation of short chains (dashed lines) as functions of time. $\bar{k}_{e2}/k_{e1}$ = 0 (A), 0.02 (B) and infinity (C). (*Source*: Taken from Gleadall *et al.*, 2014.)

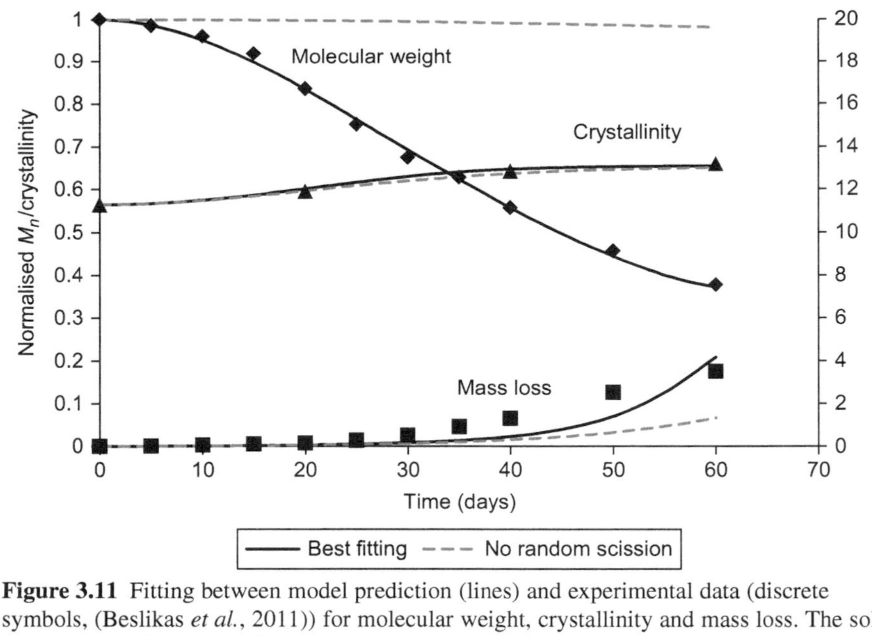

Figure 3.11 Fitting between model prediction (lines) and experimental data (discrete symbols, (Beslikas *et al.*, 2011)) for molecular weight, crystallinity and mass loss. The solid lines were obtained assuming fast end scission and much slower end scission. The dashed lines were obtained assuming pure end scission. (*Source*: Taken from Gleadall *et al.*, 2014.)

random scission had occurred. This clearly demonstrates that random scissions are critical in reducing molecular weight. It is clear that random and end scissions play different roles in the degradation of biodegradable polymers. Random scissions are largely responsible for the reduction in molecular weight, assuming that the small chains are not counted. End scissions are largely responsible for the production of short chains.

3.7 Concluding remarks

It is always possible to introduce more and more details in a mathematical model for polymer degradation. The model presented in Section 3.5 gives an example of introducing further details in contrast to that of Section 3.2. However a more detailed model also requires more parameters. The model in Section 3.5 is useful for understanding the underlying mechanims for polymer degradation. It is however over-complicated to be used in device design. Equations [3.5] or [3.7] in Section 3.5 has perhaps reached the right balance between complexity and practicality. The parametric study in Section 3.4 points to a potential experimental procedure to determine the parameters in the model.

References

Beslikas T, Gigis I, Goulios V, Christoforides J, Papageorgiou GZ and Bikiaris DN (2011) Crystallization study and comparative *in vitro-in vivo* hydrolysis of PLA reinforcement ligament. *International Journal of Molecular Sciences*, **12**:6597–6618.

Grizzi I, Garreau H, Li S and Vert M (1995) Hydrolytic degradation of devices based on poly [DL-lactic acid] size dependence. *Biomaterials*, **16**:305–311.

Gleadall A, Pan J, Kruft MA and Kellomäki M (2014) Degradation mechanisms of bioresorbable polyesters, part 1: effects of random scission, end scission and autocatalysis. *Acta Biomaterialia*, **10**:2233–2240.

Modelling degradation of semi-crystalline biodegradable polyesters

4

J. Pan
University of Leicester, Leicester, UK

4.1 Introduction

Some typical biodegradable polymers, such as poly(L-lactide) (PLLA) and poly(glycolide) (PGA), are partially crystalline (semi-crystalline). In these polymers part of the polymer chains line up or fold back and forth to form plates like crystallites. Unlike metals or ceramics, the polymer crystallites cannot grow much beyond a few nano metres. A single polymer chain can move in and out of many crystallites. A hierarchal structure is often formed: a group of lamellar crystallites are packed together. These groups then form large micron-sized spherulites. The crystalline phase is important in providing devices with the required mechanical properties. In degradation experiments of semi-crystalline polymers it has been widely observed that the degree of crystallinity increases significantly during degradation (Zong *et al.*, 1999; Tsuji and Ikada, 2000; Tsuji and Muramatsu, 2001). It has also been generally assumed that the crystallites are much harder to degrade than the amorphous phase (for example Zong *et al.* (1999)). During biodegradation, the hydrolysis reaction of the ester backbone leads to cleavage of the polymer chains. The chain cleavage occurs preferentially in the amorphous phase and provides extra mobility for the polymer chains to crystallise. Each chain cleavage effectively acts as a potential nucleation site for further crystallisation. This is known as chain cleavage-induced crystallisation and schematically shown in Figure 4.1.

The classical crystallisation theory due to Avrami (1939, 1940, 1941) has been shown to be generally valid for semi-crystalline polymers. The theory predicts that the volume of the crystalline phase per unit volume, known as degree of crystallinity and referred as X_c, depends exponentially on time:

$$X_c = 1 - e^{-(k_c t)^m} \qquad [4.1]$$

in which m is a constant, often referred to as the Avrami exponent, and k_c is a temperature dependent parameter reflecting the growth rate of a single crystal. This theory

Modelling Degradation of Bioresorbable Polymeric Medical Devices. http://dx.doi.org/10.1533/9781782420255.1.53

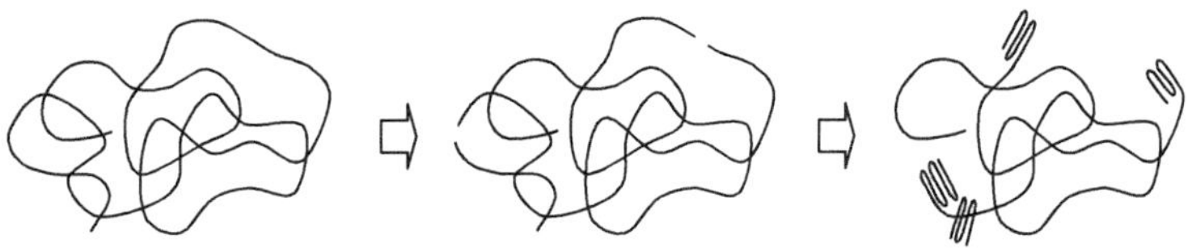

Figure 4.1 Cleavage-induced crystallisation of polymer chains.

does not directly apply to chain cleavage-induced crystallisation because it assumes that the nucleation sites for crystallites are pre-existent. It is therefore necessary to revisit the fundamentals of Avrami's theory and connect it with the rate equation for chain scission presented in Chapter 3. Before that, the rate equation has to be rewritten for polymers that contain a crystalline phase.

4.2 Rate equation for chain scission in semi-crystalline polymers

A degrading semi-crystalline polymer is considered as consisting of four species, as schematically shown in Figure 4.2:

1. amorphous long chains, which hydrolyse and can crystallise following cleavage; they are too large to diffuse out of a device
2. short chains, which are water soluble and can diffuse out of a device
3. crystallites, which are formed and grow but do not hydrolyse
4. water molecules, which are abundant.

Polymer degradation is a process that the long chains cleave, producing short chains and generating crystallites.

The rate Equation [3.5] for chain scission, as presented in Chapter 3, can be applied to the amorphous phase of a semi-crystalline polymer. Using superscript amp to represent the amorphous phase, the rate equation can be rewritten as:

$$\begin{aligned}\frac{dR_s^{\mathrm{amp}}}{dt} &= k_1 C_e^{\mathrm{amp}} + k_2' C_e^{\mathrm{amp}} C_{\mathrm{H^+}}^{\mathrm{amp}} \\ &= k_1 C_e^{\mathrm{amp}} + k_2 C_e^{\mathrm{amp}} \left[\chi_1 \left(C_{\mathrm{chain0}}^{\mathrm{amp}} + R_s^{\mathrm{amp}} - \frac{R_{ol}^{\mathrm{amp}}}{m} \right) + \chi_2 \frac{C_{ol}^{\mathrm{amp}}}{m} \right]^n\end{aligned} \quad [4.2]$$

in which k_1 and k_2' are reaction constants for non-catalytic and auto-catalytic hydrolyses, respectively, $k_2 = k_2'[K_a]^n$, χ_1 and χ_2 are parameters partitioning carboxylic end groups on the long and short chains, m is the average number of ester units of short chains, and n is the acid dissociation constant of the carboxylic end groups, which

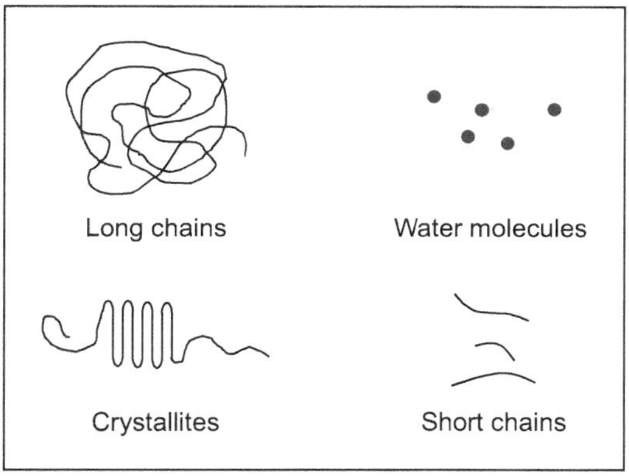

Figure 4.2 Schematic illustration of the four constitutes of a degrading semi-crystalline polymer.

should be 0.5 but could take other empirical values. The variables in Equation [4.2] are defined as:

R_s^{amp} – number of chain scissions per unit volume of the amorphous phase
C_e^{amp} – number of ester bonds of long chains in the amorphous phase per unit volume of the amorphous phase
$C_{\mathrm{H^+}}^{\mathrm{amp}}$ – number of cationic hydrogen (as catalyst) in the amorphous phase per unit volume of the amorphous phase
$C_{\mathrm{chain0}}^{\mathrm{amp}}$ – number of initial chain ends in the amorphous phase per unit volume of the amorphous phase
R_{ol}^{amp} – number of ester bonds of short chains which are produced by chain scissions per unit volume of the amorphous phase (excluding initial short chains and including those diffused out)
C_{ol}^{amp} – current number of ester bonds of short chains per unit volume of the amorphous phase (including initial short chains and excluding those diffused out).

For a detailed discussion on the difference between R_{ol}^{amp} and C_{ol}^{amp}, see Section 3.2.1.

All the concentrations in Equation [4.2] are defined over the volume of the amorphous phase. This volume decreases with time as the polymer continues to crystallise. It is more convenient to replace the variables by their counter parts, which are defined over the volume of the entire semi-crystalline polymer. For example, using R_s to represent number of chain scissions per unit volume of the semi-crystalline polymer, we have

$$R_s^{\mathrm{am}} = \frac{R_s}{1 - X_c} \qquad [4.3]$$

where X_c is the volume of crystalline phase per unit volume of the semi-crystalline polymer. Rearranging the above equation into $R_s = (1 - X_c) R_s^{\mathrm{am}}$ and differentiating both sides with respect to time gives

$$\frac{dR_s}{dt} = \left(1 - X_c\right)\frac{dR_s^{\text{am}}}{dt} - R_s^{\text{am}}\frac{dX_c}{dt} \qquad [4.4]$$

The second term on the left-hand side of Equation [4.4] needs to be dropped. This is because R_s is defined as the number of chain scissions that have ever occurred per unit volume of a polymer, i.e. it represents a historical record of chain scissions. Change in the crystalline volume does not alter this historical record and dX_c / dt does not have any effect on dR_s / dt. This definition of R_s is determined by the way in which R_s is used later in this section in order to calculate the extended degree of crystallinity and number-averaged molecular weight. In other words, it can be considered that R_s is defined through (Han and Pan, 2009)

$$\frac{dR_s}{dt} = \left(1 - X_c\right)\frac{dR_s^{\text{am}}}{dt} \qquad [4.5]$$

Applying transformation similarly to Equation [4.3] for all the other concentrations and using Equation [4.5], the rate Equation [4.2] can be rewritten as

$$\frac{dR_s}{dt} = k_1 C_e + k_2 C_e \left[\chi_1\left(C_{\text{chain0}} + R_s - \frac{R_{ol}}{m}\right) + \chi_2 \frac{C_{ol}}{m}\right]^n \left(\frac{1}{1 - X_c}\right)^n \qquad [4.6]$$

in which all the variables are now defined over the volume of the semi-crystalline polymer. For clarity, it is useful to repeat that C_{ol} represents the current concentration of short chains which can be changed by diffusion while R_{ol} represents a historical record of short chains produced by chain scission which cannot be changed by diffusion.

The issue of short chain diffusion will be dealt with in Chapter 6. In this chapter, we focus on situations where the short chain diffusion is very slow and can be ignored. In this case we have

$$C_{ol} = C_{ol0} + R_{ol} \qquad [4.7]$$

where C_{ol0} represents the residual concentration of short chains at the beginning of degradation. The empirical relation given by Equation [2.9] between short chain production and chain scission is used

$$\frac{R_{ol}}{C_{e0}} = \alpha\left(\frac{R_s}{C_{e0}}\right)^{\beta} \qquad [2.9]$$

in which C_{e0} represents the number of ester units of amorphous long chains per unit volume of the semi-crystalline polymer at the beginning of degradation. The reduction in the ester bond concentration of the long and amorphous chains comes from two parts: (i) short chain production, and (ii) crystallisation of the long chains, which can be expressed as

$$C_e = C_{e0} - R_{ol} - \omega(X_c - X_{c0}) \qquad [4.8]$$

in which ω is the number of ester units per unit volume of the crystalline phase and X_{c0} is the degree of crystallinity at the beginning of degradation. Using Equations [2.9], [4.7] and [4.8] in Equation [4.6] gives

$$\frac{d\bar{R}_s}{dt} = \left[1 - \alpha\bar{R}_s^{\beta} - \bar{\omega}(X_c - X_{c0})\right]\left\{k_1 + \bar{k}_2\left[\bar{C}_0 + \chi_1\bar{R}_s + (\chi_2 - \chi_1)\frac{\alpha}{m}\bar{R}_s^{\beta}\right]^n\left(\frac{1}{1-X_c}\right)^n\right\} \qquad [4.9]$$

in which the following normalisations have been used

$$\bar{R}_s = \frac{R_s}{C_{e0}} \qquad [4.10]$$

$$\bar{\omega} = \frac{\omega}{C_{e0}} \qquad [4.11]$$

$$\bar{k}_2 = C_{e0}^n k_2 \qquad [4.12]$$

and

$$\bar{C}_0 = \frac{1}{C_{e0}}\left(\chi_1 C_{\text{chain}0} + \chi_2\frac{C_{ol0}}{m}\right) \qquad [4.13]$$

It is helpful to compare the rate Equation [4.9] for semi-crystalline polymers with Equation [3.7] for amorphous polymers in Section 3.2.2. In the following two sections it will be shown that the degree of crystallinity X_c can be related to $\bar{R}_s$.

4.3 Actual and extended degrees of crystallinity

Avrami (1939, 1940, 1941) developed a classical theory for crystallisation which has been widely applied to different materials. In his theory Avrami introduced a concept of extended degree of crystallinity and established a relationship between the actual degree of crystallinity and the extended one. This relationship is central to the crystallisation theory and re-introduced here using a simple statistical argument.

The volume degree of crystallinity, X_c, is defined as the volume occupied by the crystalline phase per unit volume of a material. By definition X_c is less than or equal to unity. During crystallisation, crystals nucleate and grow. However, a crystal cannot grow freely for very long because at some stage it will impinge on surrounding crystals. The so-called extended volume degree of crystallinity, referred to as X_{ext} in this book, is defined as the imaginary volume occupied by the crystals assuming that they can grow freely (into each other) per unit volume of the material. Unlike X_c, the extended degree of crystallinity X_{ext} can be larger than unity. It is relatively easy to calculate X_{ext}. A relationship between X_{ext} and X_c is then needed in order to calculate the actual degree of crystallinity from the extended one.

Figure 4.3 shows schematically the growth of a new crystallite impinging on existing ones. The box shown in Figure 4.3a is a representative unit of the material. The grey area shown in Figure 4.3b indicates the overlapping part of the crystallite. To estimate the volume fraction of the overlapping section, let us perform a thought experiment: throwing the new crystal randomly into the box shown in Figure 4.3a and doing so repeatedly, there are some rare chances that the new crystal could overlap completely with existing crystals and some other chances that the new crystal falls into the 'free' space around the existing crystals. However, the most probable overlapping fraction is equal to the volume fraction of the existing crystal phase in the box, i.e. X_c. The total volume of the new crystallite is the extended volume which is referred to as dV_{ext}. The most probable volume of the overlapping part is then given by $X_c dV_{\text{ext}}$. By adding a new crystal randomly into the box, the most probable increase in the volume of the crystalline phase, indicated using the white part in Figure 4.3b, is given by

$$dV_c = dV_{\text{ext}} - X_c dV_{\text{ext}}. \qquad [4.14]$$

Dividing both sides by the volume of the box and rearranging the equation slightly give

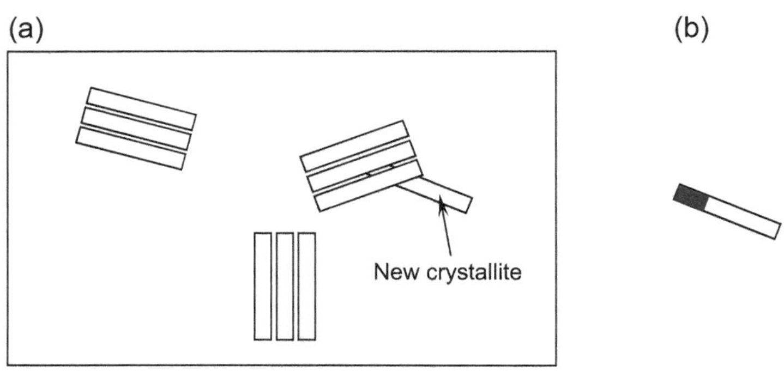

Figure 4.3 Impingement of crystal growth. (a) A representative unit of the material containing existing and new crystals and (b) a new crystal showing its extended and actual volumes.

$$\frac{dX_c}{dX_{\text{ext}}} = 1 - X_c \qquad [4.15]$$

which is the well-known relationship due to Avrami between the actual and extended degrees of crystallinity. It is purely based on the probability argument and does not involve any underlying mechanism for the crystal growth.

It is often necessary to modify Equation [4.15] empirically in order to fit experimental data. For example, the degree of crystallinity in polymers can never reach unity (fully crystalline), so a maximum limit to X_c can be introduced, $X_{c\max}$. An empirical impingement exponent λ is also frequently used in the literature such that

$$\frac{dX_c}{dX_{\text{ext}}} = \left[X_{c\max} - X_c\right]^{\lambda} \qquad [4.16]$$

If $\lambda = 1$, Equation [4.16] can be integrated to give

$$X_c = X_{c\max} - \left(X_{c\max} - X_{c0}\right)e^{-X_{\text{ext}}} \qquad [4.17]$$

in which X_{c0} is the degree of crystallinity at the beginning of degradation. If $\lambda \neq 1$ then Equation [4.16] can be integrated to give

$$X_c = X_{c\max} - \left[(\lambda - 1)X_{\text{ext}} + \left(X_{c\max} - X_{c0}\right)^{1-\lambda}\right]^{1/1-\lambda} \qquad [4.18]$$

In order to calculate X_c, one needs to calculate the extended volume of the polymer crystallites.

4.4 Extended degree of crystallinity of chain cleavage-induced crystallisation

It is relatively straightforward to calculate the extended degree of crystallinity X_{ext} because the calculation assumes that all the crystals grow freely into each other in the space. For crystallisation induced by chain cleavage, each broken chain acts as a potential nucleation site for crystallisation. The broken chains obtain some extra mobility and form new crystallites. This mobility is, however, very local and constrained by the surrounding chains. The crystallites cannot grow much larger than a few nanometres.

4.4.1 *Fast crystal growth*

If it can be assumed that the time taken by a crystallite to grow to its full size is much shorter than that taken by a chain scission, then the extended volume is simply the number of chain scissions times the average volume of the crystallites (Gleadall *et al.*, 2012). Not all chain scissions can lead to nucleation of crystallites. Using p to represent the probability for a newly broken chain to crystallise, and v_c to represent the average volume of the crystallites, then the extended degree of crystallinity is given by

$$X_{\text{ext}} = v_c \times (pR_s) = k_c \overline{R}_s \quad [4.19]$$

in which $\overline{R}_s = R_s / C_{e0}$ and a new dimensionless constant k_c is introduced for convenience such that

$$k_c = pv_c C_{e0} \quad [4.20]$$

Substituting Equation [4.19] in Equations [4.17] and [4.18] gives

$$X_c = X_{c\max} - (X_{c\max} - X_{c0}) e^{-k_c \overline{R}_s}, \text{for } \lambda = 1 \quad [4.21]$$

and

$$X_c = X_{c\max} - \left[(\lambda - 1) k_c \overline{R}_s + (X_{c\max} - X_{c0})^{1-\lambda} \right]^{1/1-\lambda}, \text{ for } \lambda \neq 1 \quad [4.22]$$

4.4.2 *Slow crystal growth*

If the rate of crystal growth is comparable to that of chain scission, then it becomes much less straightforward to calculate the extended degree of crystallinity (Han and Pan, 2009). For simplicity the actual shape of the crystallites is ignored, and r is used to represent the dimensions of a typical crystallite and r_c to represent the average dimension that all the crystallites can finally reach. It is further assumed that a crystallite, nucleated at time τ, grows with time t according to the following relation:

$$r = r_c \left(1 - e^{-(G/r_c)(t-\tau)}\right) \quad [4.23]$$

in which

$$G = \left.\frac{dr}{dt}\right|_{t=\tau} \quad [4.24]$$

This is essentially assuming that r firstly increases with time at an almost linear rate, G, and then slows down sharply as it reaches r_c. As an example, Figure 4.4

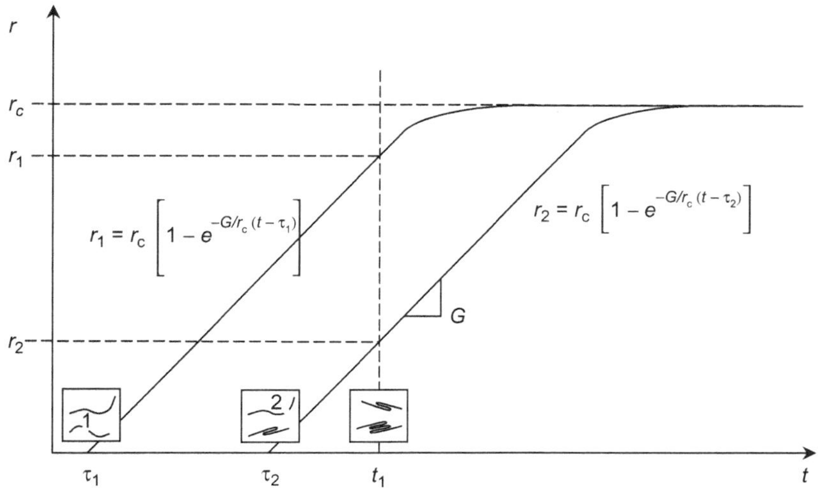

Figure 4.4 Growth of two crystallites nucleated at τ_1 and τ_2.

illustrates Equation [4.23] for two crystallites that are nucleated at τ_1 and τ_2, respectively. The vertical axis is the size of the crystallites, and the horizontal axis is the time. At any particular time t_1, the summation of the two crystallite volumes gives the extended volume of the crystalline phase.

In general, many crystallites of different sizes grow simultaneously as degradation proceeds. Each chain scission creates a potential site for a crystallite to nucleate. Considering a small time period $\Delta\tau$, the number of newly produced chain ends by chain scission over this period is $\Delta\tau \times \dot{R}_s(\tau)$. However, there is always a thermodynamic barrier, known as the activation energy, which a crystal has to overcome in order to grow from a nucleation site. To take the thermodynamic barrier into account, Avrami introduced a parameter ξ to represent the number fraction of nucleation sites that actually start to grow over a small period of time $\Delta\tau$. ξ has a unit of $1/t$ and is different from the probability p in Equation [4.19]. Using N to represent the concentration of nucleation sites, the number of nucleation sites per unit volume that actually start to grow at time τ is given by

$$\Delta N_{\text{grow}} = N(\tau) \times (\xi \times \Delta\tau) \quad [4.25]$$

To calculate $N(\tau)$, one can use

$$\frac{dN}{d\tau} = \frac{dR_s}{d\tau} - \frac{dN_{\text{grow}}}{d\tau} \quad [4.26]$$

i.e. over the time period $\Delta\tau$, the number of nucleation sites is increased by the number of chain scissions but decreased by those starting to grow.

However, some of the chain ends are swallowed by crystallites that are currently growing. The swallowing rate is given by the second term on the right-hand side of Equation [4.4], which was dropped in Section 4.2, i.e. we have

$$\frac{dN_{\text{swallow}}}{d\tau} = N^{\text{am}} \frac{dX_c}{d\tau} = \frac{N}{1-X_c} \frac{dX_c}{d\tau} \quad [4.27]$$

in which N^{am} represents the number of nucleation sites per unit volume of the amorphous phase. In conclusion the changing rate of the nucleation sites at time τ is given by

$$\frac{dN}{d\tau} = \frac{dR_s}{d\tau} - \frac{dN_{\text{grow}}}{d\tau} - \frac{dN_{\text{swallow}}}{d\tau} \quad [4.28]$$

Using Equation [4.25] for very small $\Delta\tau$ and Equation [4.27], Equation [4.28] can be rewritten as

$$\frac{dN}{d\tau} = \frac{dR_s}{d\tau} - \xi N - \frac{N}{1-X_c} \frac{dX_c}{d\tau} \quad [4.29]$$

which is the governing equation for the evolution of nucleation sites.

At degradation time t, the volume of a crystallite that was nucleated at time τ is referred to as $v(t-\tau)$. This volume can be related to the characteristic dimension r of the crystallite using a shape factor η such that

$$v(t-\tau) = \eta r^3 = \eta r_c^3 \left(1 - e^{-(G/r_c)(t-\tau)}\right)^3 \quad [4.30]$$

Recalling that $\Delta N_{\text{grow}}(\tau)$ is the number of nucleation sites per unit volume that actually start to grow at time τ, the increase in the extended degree of crystallinity over $\Delta\tau$ is given by

$$\Delta X_{\text{ext}} = v(t-\tau) \times \Delta N_{\text{grow}}(\tau) \quad [4.31]$$

Submitting Equations [4.25] and [4.30] into [4.31] gives

$$\Delta X_{\text{ext}} = \eta r_c^3 \left(1 - e^{-(G/r_c)(t-\tau)}\right)^3 \xi N(\tau) \Delta\tau = v_c \left(1 - e^{-(G/r_c)(t-\tau)}\right)^3 \xi N(\tau) \Delta\tau \quad [4.32]$$

where $v_c = \eta r_c^3$ represents the average volume of the crystallites. The extended degree of crystallinity is then the summation of all the incremental $\Delta X_{\text{ext}}(\tau)$ from the beginning of degradation to the current time t, i.e. we have

$$X_{\text{ext}}(t) = \int_0^t v_c \left(1 - e^{-(G/r_c)(t-\tau)}\right)^3 \xi N(\tau)\, d\tau \qquad [4.33]$$

4.5 Summary of governing equations for simultaneous chain scission and crystallisation

If diffusion of short chains is prohibited, the rate equation for chain scission of semi-crystalline polymers is given by

$$\frac{d\bar{R}_s}{dt} = \left[1 - \alpha\bar{R}_s^{\beta} - \bar{\omega}(X_c - X_{c0})\right]\left\{k_1 + \bar{k}_2\left[\bar{C}_0 + \chi_1\bar{R}_s + (\chi_2 - \chi_1)\frac{\alpha}{m}\bar{R}_s^{\beta}\right]^n\left(\frac{1}{1-X_c}\right)^n\right\} \qquad [4.9]$$

4.5.1 Assuming fast crystallisation relative to chain scission

If fast crystallisation is assumed, then the degree of crystallinity is given by

$$X_c = \begin{cases} X_{c\max} - (X_{c\max} - X_{c0})e^{-k_c\bar{R}_s} & \lambda = 1 \\ X_{c\max} - \left[(\lambda-1)k_c\bar{R}_s + (X_{c\max} - X_{c0})^{1-\lambda}\right]^{1/1-\lambda} & \lambda \neq 1 \end{cases} \qquad [4.21, 4.22]$$

By submitting Equations [4.21] or [4.22] into rate Equation [4.9], the left-hand side of Equation [4.9] is a function of $\bar{R}_s$. It can be expressed in the same format as Equation [2.31] as $d\bar{R}_s / dt = f(\bar{R}_s)$ and therefore can be integrated using the numerical scheme and corresponding computer programme presented in Section 2.7. The numerical solution provides $\bar{R}_s$ and X_c as functions of time.

Definitions for all the symbols in these equations are listed here for clarity and reader's convenience.

1. Variables that change with time
   - $\bar{R}_s = R_s / C_{eC}$ – total number of chain scissions normalised by the initial number of ester units of long chains in the amorphous phase, unit for all concentrations: mol/m^3.
   - X_c – volume degree of crystallinity, dimensionless.
2. Parameter describing initial conditions of the polymer
   - $\bar{C}_0$ – normalised initial concentration of –COOH end groups

$$\bar{C}_0 = \frac{1}{C_{e0}}\left(\chi_1 C_{\text{chain}0} + \chi_2 \frac{C_{ol0}}{m}\right)$$

in which $C_{\text{chain}0}$ is the initial number of long chains in the amorphous phase per unit volume, C_{ol0} is the initial total number of ester units of short chains per unit volume and C_{e0} is the initial number of ester units of the long chains in the amorphous phase per unit volume.

- X_{c0} – initial degree of crystallinity, dimensionless.
- $\bar{\omega} = \omega / C_{e0}$ – number of ester units per unit volume of the crystalline phase normalised by number ester units per unit volume of the amorphous phase.

3. Empirical parameters
   - m – average degree of polymerisation of the short chains, dimensionless, typically set as 4–6.
   - α, β – empirical parameters for short chain production, dimensionless.
   - χ_1, χ_1 – partitioning parameters for the long and short chains to act as catalyst, dimensionless.
   - λ – impingement exponent for crystal growth, dimensionless.
4. Kinetic constants
   - k_1 – hydrolysis rate constant for non-catalytic reaction, unit: 1/week.
   - $\bar{k}_2 = C_{e0}^n k_2$ – hydrolysis rate constant for autocatalytic reaction, unit:1/week.
   - n – acid dissociation exponent of the –COOH groups, usually taken as 0.5.
   - $k_c = p v_c C_{e0}$ in which p is the probability for a cleaved chain to form a crystallite and v_c is the average volume of the crystallites; dimensionless.
   - $X_{c\max}$ – maximum degree of crystallinity; dimensionless.

4.5.2 Without the assumption of fast crystallisation

If it cannot be assumed that crystallisation occurs much faster than chain scission, then the following set of equations should be used to calculate

1. concentration of nucleation sites

$$\frac{dN}{dt} = \frac{dR_s}{dt} - \xi N - \frac{N}{1 - X_c}\frac{dX_c}{dt} \qquad [4.29]$$

2. extended degree of crystallinity

$$X_{\text{ext}}(t) = \int_0^t v_c \left(1 - e^{-\bar{G}(t-\tau)}\right)^3 \xi N(\tau)\, d\tau \qquad [4.33]$$

3. degree of crystallinity

$$\frac{dX_c}{dX_{\text{ext}}} = \left[X_{c\max} - X_c\right]^{\lambda} \qquad [4.16]$$

The set of Equations [4.9], [4.16], [4.29] and [4.33] can be numerically integrated. Because these are a combination of differential and integration equations, their integration is less straightforward than using the method presented in Section 2.7. However, they pose no difficulty for a modern numerical method.

Definitions for the extra symbols in Equations [4.16], [4.29] and [4.33] are listed here.

1. Variables that change with time
   - N – number of nucleation sites per unit volume, unit: $1/m^3$.
   - X_{ext} – extended degree of crystallinity, dimensionless.
2. Parameter describing conditions of the polymer
   - v_c – average volume of the crystallites, unit: m^3.
3. Kinetic parameters
   - $\underline{\xi}$ – number fraction of nucleation sites that start to grow per unit time, unit: 1/week.
   - $\bar{G} = G / r_c$ – growth rate of crystallite normalised by the average size of the crystallites, unit: 1/week.

4.6 Calculation of number-averaged molecular weight

The average molecular weight can be calculated by either counting all the polymer chains or disregarding the short chains. The distinction between 'long' and 'short' chains is that the short ones are water soluble and can diffuse while the long ones cannot.

4.6.1 Counting all the long and short chains

If all the chains are counted in the calculation of the average molecular weight, then the number-averaged molecular weight of a semi-crystalline polymer is the total weight of all the chains in both amorphous and crystalline phases divided by the total number of polymer chains. If diffusion of short chains is prohibited, then the total weight remains as a constant. The total number of chains increases by the total number of chain scissions. The molecular weight can therefore be calculated as

$$M_n = \frac{\left(C_{e0} + \omega X_{c0}\right) M_{\text{unit}}}{N_{\text{chain0}} + R_s} \qquad [4.34]$$

The definitions of the various symbols in Equation [4.34] are listed below:

- C_{e0} – initial number of ester units of the long chains in the amorphous phase per unit volume of the semi-crystalline polymer
- X_{c0} – initial volume degree of crystallinity
- ω – number of ester units per unit volume of the crystalline phase
- M_{unit} – weight of a repeating unit of the polymer chain
- N_{chain0} – initial number of all the polymer chains per unit volume
- R_s – number of chain scissions per unit volume

The initial molecular weight is given by

$$M_{n0} = \frac{\left(C_{e0} + \omega X_{c0}\right) M_{\text{unit}}}{N_{\text{chain0}}} \quad [4.35]$$

Equation [4.34] can be written into a normalised format as

$$\bar{M}_n = \frac{M_n}{M_{n0}} = \frac{1}{1 + \left(C_{e0}/N_{\text{chian0}}\right)\bar{R}_s} \quad [4.36]$$

which is similar to Equation [2.18] for amorphous polymers, except that C_{e0} here is the initial number of ester units of long chains of *the amorphous phase* per unit volume and N_{chian0} is the number of polymer chains of the *entire polymer* including the crystalline phase. $C_{e0} / N_{\text{chain0}}$ is therefore no longer the degree of polymerisation of the polymer.

4.6.2 Discounting the short chains

If the short chains are not counted when calculating the average molecular weight, then the total number of ester units of the long chains reduces due to production of the short chains. The total weight of the long chains is given by $\left(C_{e0} + \omega X_{c0} - R_{ol}\right) M_{\text{unit}}$ in which R_{ol} is the number of ester units of all the short chains per unit volume that are produced by chain scissions. R_{ol} is related to the number of chain scissions, R_s, through Equation [2.9]. The number of short chains per unit volume is given by R_{ol}/m where m is the average number of ester units of the short chains. The total number of long chains is given by $N_{\text{chain0}} + R_s - \left(R_{ol}/m\right)$. The average molecular weight discounting the short chains is then given by

$$M_n = \frac{\left(C_{e0} + \omega X_{c0} - R_{ol}\right) M_{\text{unit}}}{N_{\text{chain0}} + R_s - \left(R_{ol}/m\right)} = \frac{\left[C_{e0} + \omega X_{c0} - \alpha C_{e0}\left(R_s/C_{e0}\right)^{\beta}\right] M_{\text{unit}}}{N_{\text{chain0}} + R_s - \frac{\alpha}{m} C_{e0}\left(R_s/C_{e0}\right)^{\beta}} \quad [4.37]$$

Assuming the polymer contains no short chains before degradation, the initial molecular weight is given by Equation [4.35]. The molecular weight can be written into a normalised format as

$$\bar{M}_n = \frac{M_n}{M_{n0}} = \frac{1 + \bar{\omega} X_{c0} - \alpha \bar{R}_s^{\beta}}{\left(1 + \bar{\omega} X_{c0}\right)\left[1 + \left(C_{e0}/N_{\text{chain0}}\right)\left(\bar{R}_s - (\alpha/m)\bar{R}_s^{\beta}\right)\right]} \quad [4.38]$$

The definitions of all the symbols in Equation [4.38] are listed as following

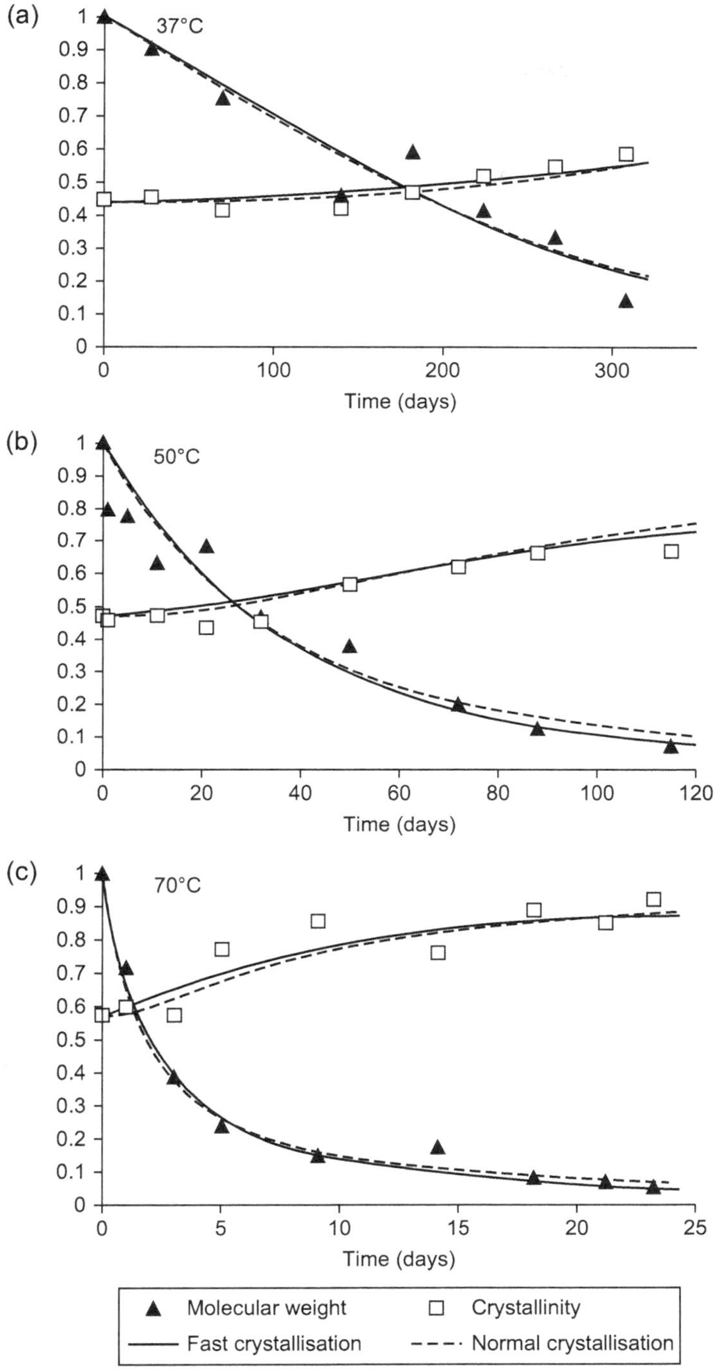

Figure 4.5 Best fits of the experimental data obtained by Weir *et al.* (2004) for PLLA using the model assuming fast crystallisation (solid lines) and the model without the assumption (dashed lines), respectively. The degradation data (discrete symbols) of molecular weight and degree of crystallinity as functions of time were obtained at three temperatures: (a) 37°C (b) 50°C and (c) 70°C. (*Source*: Taken from Gleadall *et al.*, 2012.)

- C_{e0} – initial number of ester units of long chains in the amorphous phase per unit volume of the semi-crystalline polymer.
- $\bar{R}_s = R_s / C_{eC}$ – number of chain scissions per unit volume normalised by C_{e0}
- X_{c0} – initial volume degree of crystallinity
- m – average degree of polymerisation of short chains
- α, β – empirical parameters for oligomer production
- $\bar{\omega} = \omega / C_{eC}$ – number of ester units per unit volume of crystalline phase normalised by C_{e0}
- N_{chain0} – initial number of all polymer chains per unit volume

4.7 Comparison between models assuming fast and normal crystallisation

The theory presented in this chapter has been shown to be able to fit a wide range of experimental data in the literature (Han and Pan, 2009; Gleadall *et al.*, 2012). Figures 4.5a to 4.5c present a comparison between fittings obtained by Gleadall *et al.* (2012) using the two models with a set of experimental data obtained by Weir *et al.* (2004) for PLLA. In these figures, the discrete symbols represent the experimental data for molecular weight and degree of crystallinity as functions of time. The solid lines represent the best fit obtained using the model assuming fast crystallisation. The dashed lines represent the best fit obtained using the model assuming normal crystallisation. It is clear from observing these figures that both models can fit the data for PLLA well. It is likely that this conclusion is generally valid, considering the extremely small size of the crystallites. The model assuming fast crystallisation is much easier to use, because the degree of crystallinity is explicitly related to the number of chain scissions.

The degradation experiments were carried out in phosphate buffer solution (PBS) with pH 7.4 at three temperatures: 37°C 50°C, and 70°C. Further details of the experimental study can be found in the original paper by Weir *et al.* (2004). In the fittings, it was assumed that only the –COOH end groups on the short chains act as the catalyst for the hydrolysis reaction. The temperature dependence of the kinetic parameters in the model was assumed to follow the Arrhenius relation. The full set of values for the model parameters that achieved the best fits can be found in the original paper by Gleadall *et al.* (2012), which are not repeated here.

4.8 Concluding remarks

The model presented in this chapter ignored the spherulite structure of the crystalline phase which exists in all semi-crystalline polymers unless being deliberately destroyed by manufacturing process (such as pulling of fibres). The amorphous phases inside a spherulite and between the spherulites are different in many ways. It is possible to account for this difference by modifying the model (Gleadall *et al.*, 2012). However this introduces more parameters into the model. The model assuming fast crystal growth and ignoring the spherulite structure is able to fit experimental data well. This indicates that the simpler model is perhaps good enough as a tool for device design.

References

Avrami M (1939) Kinetics of phase change. I. General theory. *Journal of Chemical Physics*, **7**(12):1103–1112.

Avrami M (1940) Kinetics of phase change. II. Transformation-time relations for random distribution of nuclei. *Journal of Chemical Physics*, **8**(2):212–224.

Avrami, M (1941) Kinetics of phase change. III. Granulation, phase change, and microstructure'. *Journal of Chemical Physics*, **9**(2):177–184.

Gleadall A, Pan J and Atkinson H (2012) A simplified theory of crystallisation induced by polymer chain scissions for biodegradable polyesters. *Polymer Degradation and Stability*, **97**:1616–1620.

Han X and Pan J (2009) A model for simultaneous degradation and crystallisation in biodegradable polymers. *Biomaterials*, **30**:423–430.

Tsuji H and Ikada Y (2000) Properties and morphology of poly(L-lactide) 4: effects of structural parameters on long-term hydrolysis of poly(L-lactide) in phosphate-buffered solution. *Polymer Degradation and Stability*, **67**:179–189.

Tsuji H and Muramatsu H (2001) Blends of aliphatic polyesters: V Non-enzymatic and enzymatic hydrolysis of blends from hydrophobic poly(L-lactide) and hydrophilic poly(vinyl alcohol). *Polymer Degradation and Stability*, **71**:403–413.

Weir NA, Buchanan FJ, Orr JF and Dickson GR (2004) Degradation of poly-L-lactide. Part1: *in vitro* and *in vivo* physiological temperature degradation. *Proceedings of the Institution of Mechanical Engineers, Part H: Journal of Engineering in Medicine*, **218**:307–319.

Zong XH, Wang ZG, Hsiao BS, Chu B, Zhou JJ, Jamiolkowski DD, Muse E and Dormier E (1999) Structure and morphology changes in absorbable poly(glycolide) and poly(glycolide-co-lactide) during *in vitro* degradation. *Macromolecules*, **32**:8107–8114.

Modelling biodegradation of composite materials made of biodegradable polyesters and tricalcium phosphates (TCPs)

5

J. Pan
University of Leicester, Leicester, UK

5.1 Introduction

It is well known that poly(lactides) (PLAs) or poly(glycolide) (PGA) generates an acidic environment during degradation which can induce inflammatory tissue response, resulting in osteolytic reactions and delaying bone healing or fusion. On the other hand tricalcium phosphate (TCP) is an ideal material for healing bone defects because of its biocompatibility and osteoconductivity. TCP in porous form is suitable for implants used in bone reconstruction or as bone substitutes. They have been used to replace or complement autologous bone in bone grafts. However, TCP is very brittle and poor in tensile strength. It is then natural to develop a composite material using PLAs and/or PGA as the matrix and TCP particles as the second phase. The hope is that devices made of the composite material can have good bone-bonding properties due to the osteoconductivity of the calcium phosphates, as well as good mechanical properties due to the polyester matrix (Heidemann *et al.*, 2001). The local acidity can be reduced or delayed by the buffering reactions between the dissolved phosphate ions and H^+ disassociated from the carboxylic end groups.

Furthermore, poor mechanical strength has been a major obstacle to using biodegradable polymeric devices for fixation of load bearing bones. A promising technology is to use TCP fibres as reinforcement in a PLA and/or PGA matrix in order to achieve the required high strength. Similar attempt is also being made using bioglass fibres. Composite materials, such as laminates made of carbon fibre reinforced epoxy, have been successfully used in many engineering areas such as the aerospace industry. Similar to carbon fibres, TCP or bioglass fibres can be made to have a tensile strength of about 1000 MPa by eliminating the microscopic defects. The design of biodegradable devices made of composite materials can benefit from the rich resource of research on the mechanics of composite materials over the last 40 years. Currently embedding the fibres in a controlled manner in tiny medical devices such as screws or stents remains a challenge. Fast loss of the interfacial strength between the fibres and matrix during degradation is another challenge. Unlike traditional composite materials, controlling the degradation rate of the biodegradable composites is a primary concern in device design. This chapter presents a model for the degradation of

Modelling Degradation of Bioresorbable Polymeric Medical Devices. http://dx.doi.org/10.1533/9781782420255.1.71

biodegradable composites between PLA/PGA and TCP. The model was originally developed by Pan *et al.* (2011). The general approach can also be applied for composite materials made of PLA/PGA and bioglass.

5.2 TCP dissolution and buffering reactions

TCP dissolves in aqueous solution to produce calcium and phosphate ions:

$$Ca_3(PO_4)_2 \Leftrightarrow 3Ca^{2+} + 2PO_4^{3-} \qquad [5.1]$$

At equilibrium the dissolution stops and the equilibrium concentrations of calcium and phosphate ions can be calculated from a solubility product, which is defined as

$$\left[Ca^{2+}\right]_{eq}^{3}\left[PO_4^{3-}\right]_{eq}^{2} = K_s \qquad [5.2]$$

Here the standard notation for concentration in chemistry is used, i.e. [X] represents the concentration of X in the polymer phase and is exchangeable for C_X. At 37°C, $K_s = 3.162 \times 10^{-26}\,(\text{mole/L})^5$ for α-TCP and $3.162 \times 10^{-30}\,(\text{mole/L})^5$ for β-TCP, respectively (Fernández *et al.*, 1999), which indicates that the solubility is rather poor. If H^+ are present in the aqueous solution, then the following reactions take place to produce phosphoric acid (H_3PO_4):

$$PO_4^{3-} + H^+ \Leftrightarrow HPO_4^{2-} \qquad [5.3]$$

$$PO_4^{2-} + H^+ \Leftrightarrow H_2PO_4^- \qquad [5.4]$$

$$H_2PO_4^- + H^+ \Leftrightarrow H_3PO_4 \qquad [5.5]$$

which are known as buffering reactions because they reduce H^+, and hence the acidity of the solution. The equilibrium expressions for these reactions are given by

$$K_1 = \frac{[H^+]\times[H_2PO_4{}^-]}{[H_3PO_4]} \qquad [5.6]$$

$$K_2 = \frac{[H^+]\times[HPO_4{}^{2-}]}{[H_2PO_4{}^-]} \qquad [5.7]$$

$$K_3 = \frac{[\mathrm{H}^+]\times[\mathrm{PO}_4{}^{3-}]}{[\mathrm{HPO}_4{}^{2-}]} \qquad [5.8]$$

in which, $\mathrm{p}K_1 = 2.33$, $\mathrm{p}K_2 = 6.82$ and $\mathrm{p}K_3 = 11.27$ at 37°C (Karickhoff *et al.*).

The buffering reactions consume PO_4^{3-} so that in the solution we have

$$[\mathrm{Ca}^{2+}]^3[\mathrm{PO}_4^{3-}]^2 < K_s \qquad [5.9]$$

i.e. the equilibrium is broken and Reaction [5.1] continuously shifts to the right, leading to further dissolution of TCP. It is useful to define strength of undersaturation, σ, for the calcium and phosphate ions in the solution such that

$$\sigma = 1 - \left(\frac{[\mathrm{Ca}^{2+}]^3[\mathrm{PO}_4{}^{3-}]^2}{K_s}\right)^{1/5} \qquad [5.10]$$

The further away from equilibrium, the larger the strength of undersaturation becomes. It is straightforward to understand that the rate of TCP dissolution depends on the value of σ. The dissolution rate is also linearly proportional to the total area of interface between the TCP phase and the polymer phase because the dissolution occurs at this interface. It is therefore convenient to define a dissolution rate, J, as the number of TCP molecules dissolved off a unit area of the interface per unit time. A mathematical relation between J and σ is needed, which can be generally expressed as

$$J = A_d f(\sigma) \qquad [5.11]$$

in which A_d is a constant and f represents a general mathematical function. The actual expression of f can be related to the underlying mechanism that controls the dissolution. Several controlling mechanisms have been suggested. For example, the dissolution rate could be controlled by the diffusion of calcium and phosphate ions. The ion concentrations in a small layer next to the interface are expected to be higher than those in the aqueous solution. The concentration gradient drives diffusion of the ions away from the interface. It is possible that this diffusion rate controls the overall rate of TCP dissolution. Another possibility is that the dissolution is controlled by the formation and growth of surface pits. It is beyond the scope of the current book to discuss these dissolution mechanisms. Table 5.1 provides some examples for f which are taken from Bohner *et al.* (1997). There is no generally agreed controlling mechanism in the literature. In practice, several mechanisms may act together. It is therefore practical to take an empirical expression following Tang *et al.* (2001).

Table 5.1 **TCP dissolution rate for different mechanisms**

Dissolution mechanism	$f(\sigma)$
Ion diffusion	σ
Surface spiral dissolution	σ^2
Nucleation of surface pits	$\sigma^{2/3}\left(-\ln\left(1-\sigma\right)\right)^{1/6} e^{k/\ln(1-\sigma)}$

$$J = A_d\sigma^\theta = A_d\left[1-\left(\frac{[Ca^{2+}]^3[PO_4^{3-}]^2}{K_s}\right)^{1/5}\right]^\theta \qquad [5.12]$$

in which A_d and θ are material constants. The power law expression covers several dissolution mechanisms and can approximate more sophisticated relations fairly well.

5.3 Rate equation for chain scission in presence of buffering reactions

For simplicity only amorphous polymers are considered in this chapter. As explained in Section 2.2, the hydrolysis reaction between the ester bonds and water molecules is responsible for the chain cleavage of the polyesters. The reaction is catalysed by H^+ and produces hydroxyl alcohol and carboxylic acid end groups. Following Section 2.2, the hydrolysis reaction can be schematically described as:

$$\text{ESTER BONDS} + H_2O \xrightarrow{H^+} R-COOH + R'-OH \qquad [2.1]$$

and the chain session rate can be written as

$$\frac{dR_s}{dt} = k_1C_e + k_2'C_eC_{H^+} \qquad [2.2]$$

where R_s, C_e and C_{H^+} represent the concentrations of chain scission, ester bonds of the long chains and H^+, respectively; and k_1 and k_2' represent the reaction constants for the non-catalytic and auto-catalytic hydrolysis reactions, respectively. The chain scissions produce short and water-soluble chains. As shown in Section 2.3, the number of ester units of the short chains produced by chain scission, referred to as R_{ol}, can be related to the number of scissions R_s by

$$\frac{R_{ol}}{C_{e0}} = \alpha\left(\frac{R_s}{C_{e0}}\right)^{\beta} \qquad [2.9]$$

in which C_{e0} is the initial value of C_e, and α,β are empirical constants. The ester bonds of the long chains are consumed by the production of short chains which can be expressed as

$$C_e = C_{e0} - R_{ol} = C_{e0}\left[1 - \alpha\left(\frac{R_s}{C_{e0}}\right)^{\beta}\right] \qquad [2.11]$$

Substituting Equation [2.11] into [2.2] gives

$$\frac{dR_s}{dt} = C_{e0}\left[1 - \alpha\left(\frac{R_s}{C_{e0}}\right)^{\beta}\right](k_1 + k_2' C_{\mathrm{H^+}}) \qquad [5.13]$$

The carboxylic end groups have a high degree of acid dissociation

$$\mathrm{R{-}COOH} \Leftrightarrow \mathrm{R{-}COO^-} + \mathrm{H^+} \qquad [2.3]$$

which accelerates the hydrolysis reaction. The equilibrium expression of Reaction [2.3] is given by

$$K_a = \frac{[\mathrm{H^+}]\times[\mathrm{R{-}COO^-}]}{[\mathrm{R{-}COOH}]} \qquad [2.4]$$

in which K_a is the equilibrium constant. For poly(D-Lactic acid) (PDLA) and PGA pK_a= 3.87 at 37°C. For polyesters without the buffering TCP phase, we have $[\mathrm{H^+}] = [\mathrm{R{-}COO^-}]$ and Equation [2.4] leads to $C_{\mathrm{H^+}} = (K_a C_{\mathrm{COOH}})^{0.5}$, i.e. Equation [2.5] in Section 2.2. For the two-phase composites, the hydrogen ions are consumed by the buffering reactions and consequently this expression for $C_{\mathrm{H^+}}$ is no longer valid. Instead, Equation [5.13] will be used directly.

5.4 Governing equations for degradation of polyester-TCP composites

Now consider a representative unit of a composite material made of a polyester and TCP, as illustrated in Figure 5.1. Two special but important cases are considered here.

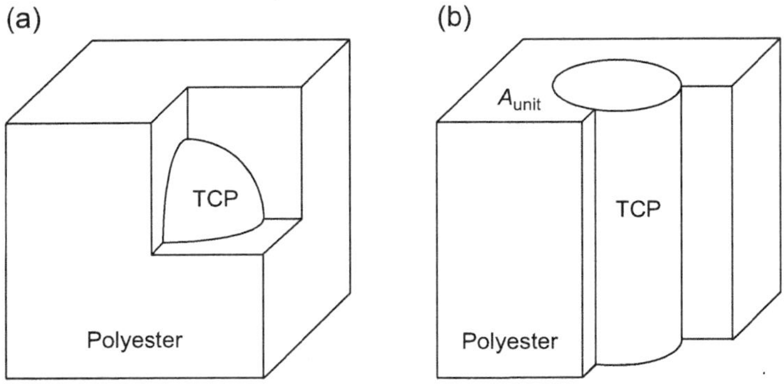

Figure 5.1 (a, b) Representative units of composite materials made of polyester and TCP.

Figure 5.1a shows a TCP phase made of uniform and spherical particles of radius r, while Figure 5.1b shows a TCP phase made of uniform fibres of radius r.

5.4.1 Geometric relations

The volume fraction of the TCP phase is denoted as f_{TCP}. For the particulate reinforced composite, its volume fraction can be calculated using

$$f_{TCP} = \frac{4\pi}{3}\frac{r^3}{V_{unit}} \quad [5.14]$$

in which V_{unit} represents the volume of the representative unit. For the fibre reinforced composite, the volume fraction can be calculated using

$$f_{TCP} = \frac{\pi r^2}{A_{unit}} \quad [5.15]$$

in which A_{unit} represents the cross-section area normal to the fibre direction of the representative unit. The total area of interface between the two phases per unit volume of the composite is denoted a_{TCP}. For particulate reinforced composite, we have

$$a_{TCP} = \frac{4\pi r^2}{V_{unit}} \quad [5.16]$$

For fibre reinforced composite, we have

$$a_{TCP} = \frac{2\pi r}{A_{unit}} \quad [5.17]$$

These geometric relations will be useful when developing the model.

5.4.2 TCP dissolution rate

TCP dissolution leads to an increase in the concentration of calcium ions in the polymer phase, which can be calculated as

$$\frac{d[\mathrm{Ca}^{2+}]}{dt}=\frac{3\times J\times a_{\mathrm{TCP}}\times V_{\mathrm{unit}}}{V_{\mathrm{polymer}}} \qquad [5.18]$$

in which the factor of 3 is due to the fact that each TCP molecule has three calcium ions, and V_{polymer} is the volume of the polymer phase in the representative unit. It should be pointed out that all the concentrations are defined in the polymer phase, hence the factor of $1/V_{\mathrm{polymer}}$ in Equation [5.18] is required. It is assumed that the volume of the polymer phase remains constant (no swelling) during degradation, so we have

$$\frac{a_{\mathrm{TCP}}\times V_{\mathrm{unit}}}{V_{\mathrm{polymer}}}=\frac{a_{\mathrm{TCP}}}{1-f_{\mathrm{TCP0}}} \qquad [5.19]$$

where f_{TCP0} is the initial volume fraction of TCP in the composite. Combining Equations [5.12], [5.18] and [5.19] leads to

$$\frac{d[\mathrm{Ca}^{2+}]}{dt}=3\frac{a_{\mathrm{TCP}}}{1-f_{\mathrm{TCP0}}}A_d\left[1-\left(\frac{[\mathrm{Ca}^{2+}]^3[\mathrm{PO}_4^{3-}]^2}{K_s}\right)^{1/5}\right]^{\theta} \qquad [5.20]$$

in which a_{TCP} is a function of time and can be calculated from the reduction in the volume of the TCP phase. The reduction in the TCP volume, V_{TCP}, is balanced by dissolution of the TCP phase, i.e. we have

$$\frac{dV_{\mathrm{TCP}}}{dt}=-\frac{\Omega_{\mathrm{TCP}}}{3}\frac{d[\mathrm{Ca}^{2+}]}{dt}\times V_{\mathrm{polymer}} \qquad [5.21]$$

where Ω_{TCP} represents the molecular volume of solid TCP. Equation [5.21] can be rewritten as

$$\frac{df_{\mathrm{TCP}}}{dt}=-\left(1-f_{\mathrm{TCP0}}\right)\frac{\Omega_{\mathrm{TCP}}}{3}\frac{d[\mathrm{Ca}^{2+}]}{dt} \qquad [5.22]$$

For particulate reinforced composite, differentiating Equations [5.14] and [5.16] with respect to time gives

$$\frac{df_{\mathrm{TCP}}}{dt}=\frac{4\pi r^2}{V_{\mathrm{unit}}}\frac{dr}{dt} \tag{5.23}$$

and

$$\frac{da_{\mathrm{TCP}}}{dt}=\frac{8\pi r}{V_{\mathrm{unit}}}\frac{dr}{dt} \tag{5.24}$$

Eliminating dr/dt from Equations [5.23] and [5.24], we obtain

$$\begin{aligned}\frac{da_{\mathrm{TCP}}}{dt}&=2\frac{1}{r}\frac{df_{\mathrm{TCP}}}{dt}=2\left(\frac{4\pi}{a_{\mathrm{TCP}}V_{\mathrm{unit}}}\right)^{1/2}\frac{df_{\mathrm{TCP}}}{dt}\\&=-\frac{4\pi^{1/2}}{3}\left(\frac{1}{a_{\mathrm{TCP}}V_{\mathrm{unit}}}\right)^{1/2}\Omega_{\mathrm{TCP}}\left(1-f_{\mathrm{TCP0}}\right)\frac{d[\mathrm{Ca}^{2+}]}{dt}\end{aligned} \tag{5.25}$$

in which we have used Equation [5.22] and $r=\left(a_{\mathrm{TCP}}V_{\mathrm{unit}}/4\pi\right)^{1/2}$ according to Equation [5.16]. Similarly for the fibre reinforced composite it can be shown that

$$\frac{da_{\mathrm{TCP}}}{dt}=\frac{1}{r}\frac{df_{\mathrm{TCP}}}{dt}=\frac{2\pi}{a_{\mathrm{TCP}}A_{\mathrm{unit}}}\frac{df_{\mathrm{TCP}}}{dt}=-\frac{2\pi}{3}\frac{\Omega_{\mathrm{TCP}}\left(1-f_{\mathrm{TCP0}}\right)}{a_{\mathrm{TCP}}A_{\mathrm{unit}}}\frac{d[\mathrm{Ca}^{2+}]}{dt} \tag{5.26}$$

5.4.3 Conservation of ions

In the polymer phase, each polymer chain terminates with a carboxylic end group, some of which lose H^+ due to acid disassociation, which can be expressed as

$$[\mathrm{R-COO^-}]+[\mathrm{R-COOH}]=C_{\mathrm{chain}}=C_{\mathrm{chain0}}+R_s \tag{5.27}$$

in which C_{chain} and C_{chain0} represent the concentrations of polymer chains at time t and the beginning of degradation respectively, and R_s represents number of chain scissions. The charge balance in the buffering reactions gives

$$\frac{\left([\mathrm{PO_4^{3-}}]+[\mathrm{HPO_4^{2-}}]+[\mathrm{H_2PO_4^-}]+[\mathrm{H_3PO_4}]\right)}{2}=\frac{[\mathrm{Ca}^{2+}]}{3} \tag{5.28}$$

and

$$[H^+]+[HPO_4^{2-}]+2[H_2PO_4^-]+3[H_3PO_4]=[R-COO^-]+[H^+]_0 \quad [5.29]$$

in which $[H^+]_0$ represents the initial concentration of H^+ in the polymer phase.

5.4.4 Collection of the governing equations

For clarity, the ten variables that change with time in the model are collected together and named as x_1, x_1, …, and x_{10}:

$$x_1 = R_{s,}\ x_2 = [H^+] = C_{H^+}, x_3 = [Ca^{2+}],\ x_4 = [PO_4^{3-}], x_5 = [R-COOH],$$
$$x_6 = [R-COO^-],\ x_7 = [HPO_4^{2-}],\ x_8 = [H_2PO_4^-],\ x_9 = [H_3PO_4] \text{ and } x_{10} = a_{TCP} \quad [5.30]$$

The governing equations for these variables can then be collected together as following:

$$\frac{dx_1}{dt} = C_{e0}\left[1-\alpha\left(\frac{x_1}{C_{e0}}\right)^{\beta}\right](k_1 + k_2' x_2) \quad [5.31]$$

$$\frac{dx_3}{dt} = 3\frac{1}{(1-f_{TCP0})}x_{10}A_d\left[1-\left(\frac{x_2^3x_4^2}{K_s}\right)^{1/5}\right]^{\theta} \quad [5.32]$$

for particulate composite, use

$$\frac{dx_{10}}{dt} = -\frac{4\pi^{1/2}}{3}\left(\frac{1}{V_{unit}}\right)^{1/2}\Omega_{TCP}(1-f_{TCP0})\left(\frac{1}{x_{10}}\right)^{1/2}\frac{dx_3}{dt} \quad [5.33]$$

for fibre reinforced composite, use

$$\frac{dx_{10}}{dt} = -\frac{2\pi}{3}\frac{\Omega_{TCP}(1-f_{TCP0})}{A_{unit}}\frac{1}{x_{10}}\frac{dx_3}{dt} \quad [5.34]$$

$$K_1 = \frac{x_2x_8}{x_9} \quad [5.35]$$

$$K_2 = \frac{x_2 x_7}{x_8} \quad [5.36]$$

$$K_3 = \frac{x_2 x_4}{x_7} \quad [5.37]$$

$$K_a = \frac{x_2 x_6}{x_5} \quad [5.38]$$

$$x_6 + x_5 - x_1 = C_{\text{chain}0} \quad [5.39]$$

$$x_4 + x_7 + x_8 + x_9 - \frac{2}{3}x_3 = 0 \quad [5.40]$$

$$x_2 + x_7 + 2x_8 + 3x_9 - x_6 = [\text{H}^+]_0 \quad [5.41]$$

These are a set of ten governing equations for the ten variables. The initial conditions for the governing equations are at $t = 0$

$$\begin{aligned} &x_1 = R_s = 0,\ x_2 = [\text{H}^+]_0 = [\text{R}-\text{COO}^-] = \left(K_a C_{\text{chain}0}\right)^{1/2},\ x_3 = [\text{Ca}^{2+}] = 0 \\ &x_4 = [\text{PO}_4{}^{3-}] = 0, x_5 = [\text{R}-\text{COOH}] = C_{\text{chain}0}, x_6 = x_2 = \left(K_a C_{\text{chain}0}\right)^{1/2} \\ &x_7 = [\text{HPO}_4{}^{2-}] = 0, x_8 = [\text{H}_2\text{PO}_4{}^-] = 0, x_9 = [\text{H}_3\text{PO}_4] = 0, x_{10} = a_{\text{TCP}0} \end{aligned} \quad [5.42]$$

The governing equations can be integrated using a numerical method. Care needs to be taken since some of the equations are non-linear. For the convenience of the readers, parameters in the equations are listed here:

1. Parameters that describe properties of the polymer phase
- C_{e0} – initial concentration of ester bonds of long chains. Using ρ_{pl} and M_{unit} to represent the density of the polymer phase and the mass of a repeating unit of the polymer phase, respectively, we have

$$C_{e0} = \frac{\rho_{pl}}{M_{\text{unit}}} \quad [5.43]$$

- $C_{\text{chain}0}$ – initial concentration of polymer chain ends, using M_{n0} to represent the initial molecular weight, we have

$$C_{\text{chian}0} = \frac{\rho_{pl}}{M_{n0}} \quad [5.44]$$

- $[H^+]_0$ – initial concentration of H^+ in the polymer phase which can be taken as $\left(K_a C_{\text{chain}0}\right)^{1/2}$.

2. Parameters that describe properties of the composite
- V_{unit} – volume of repeating unit of composite for spherical TCP phase
- A_{unit} – cross-sectional area of repeating unit of composite for fibre TCP phase
- $a_{\text{TCP}0}$ – initial interface area per unit volume of composite

If the TCP phase is made of uniform spherical particles of radius r_0 with a volume fraction of f_{TCP}, then we have

$$V_{\text{unit}} = \frac{4\pi}{3}\frac{r_0^3}{f_{\text{TCP}}} \quad [5.45]$$

$$a_{\text{TCP}0} = \frac{3 f_{\text{TCP}}}{r_0} \quad [5.46]$$

If the TCP phase is made of uniform fibres of radius r_0 with a volume fraction of f_{TCP}, then we have

$$A_{\text{unit}} = \frac{\pi r_0^2}{f_{\text{TCP}}} \quad [5.47]$$

$$a_{\text{TCP}0} = \frac{2 f_{\text{TCP}}}{r_0} \quad [5.48]$$

3. Parameters that describe properties of TCP
- Ω_{TCP} – volume of a single TCP molecule; use molar volume in practical calculations.

4. Equilibrium constants for chemical reactions
- K_s, K_a, K_1, K_2, K_3

5. Kinetic parameters
- k_1, k_2' – reaction rate constants for non-catalytic and auto-catalytic hydrolysis
- A_d, θ – rate constant and power for TCP dissolution

6. Empirical parameters
- α, β – empirical parameters for short chain production by chain scission.

5.4.5 Molecular weight of the polymer phase

Following Section 2.4 the number-averaged molecular weight of the polyester, excluding the short chains, can be calculated as

$$M_n = M_{n0}\frac{1-\alpha\left(R_s / C_{e0}\right)^{\beta}}{1+N_{dp0}\left[R_s / C_{e0} - (\alpha / m)\left(R_s / C_{e0}\right)^{\beta}\right]} \qquad [2.20]$$

in which M_{n0} is the initial molecular weight of the polymer, N_{dp0} is the initial average degree of polymerisation which can be calculated from M_{n0} and the mass of a repeating unit, M_{unit}, of the polymer using

$$N_{dp0} = \frac{M_{n0}}{M_{\text{unit}}} \qquad [2.16]$$

and m is the average degree of polymerisation of the short chains, which is usually taken as 4.

5.5 Normalised equations

It will prove useful to write the governing equations in a non-dimensional format. However non-dimensionalisation of the equations is not unique. Here we chose to use the autocatalytic hydrolysis as a reference for all the other time-dependant processes (non-catalytic hydrolysis and TCP dissolution). This is because autocatalytic hydrolysis is expected always to occur in the polyesters considered in this chapter. The scission rate equation,

$$\frac{dR_s}{dt} = C_{e0}\left[1-\alpha\left(\frac{R_s}{C_{e0}}\right)^{\beta}\right]\left(k_1 + k_2' C_{H^+}\right) \qquad [5.13]$$

can be rewritten as

$$\frac{d\left(R_s / C_{e0}\right)}{d\left(t \times k_2' \times (C_{H^+})_{pH=7.4}\right)} = \left[1-\alpha\left(\frac{R_s}{C_{e0}}\right)^{\beta}\right]\left(\frac{k_1}{k_2' \times (C_{H^+})_{pH=7.4}} + \frac{C_{H^+}}{(C_{H^+})_{pH=7.4}}\right) \qquad [5.49]$$

in which $(C_{H^+})_{pH=7.4}$ represents the concentration of H^+ at $pH = 7.4$ and is used to normalise the concentration of H^+, and C_{e0} represents the initial concentration of ester bonds of the long chains and is used to normalise the number of scissions R_s. These choices of normalisation for the concentrations are obviously not unique and can be replaced by different choices. Similarly the TCP dissolution rate equation,

$$\frac{d[\mathrm{Ca}^{2+}]}{dt} = 3\frac{a_{\mathrm{TCP}}}{1-f_{\mathrm{TCP0}}}A_d\sigma^\theta \qquad [5.20]$$

can be rewritten as

$$\frac{d\left([\mathrm{Ca}^{2+}]/[\mathrm{Ca}^{2+}]_{\mathrm{eq}}\right)}{d\left(t\times k_2'\times(C_{\mathrm{H}^+})_{\mathrm{pH}=7.4}\right)} = \frac{3\left(a_{TCP0}/1-f_{\mathrm{TCP0}}\right)A_d}{k_2'\times(C_{\mathrm{H}^+})_{\mathrm{pH}=7.4}\times[\mathrm{Ca}^{2+}]_{\mathrm{eq}}}\frac{a_{\mathrm{TCP}}}{a_{\mathrm{TCP0}}}\sigma^\theta, \qquad [5.50]$$

in which $[Ca^{2+}]_{\mathrm{eq}}$ is used to normalise $[Ca^{2+}]$ and a_{TCP0} is used to normalise a_{TCP}. Defining the following non-dimensional variables:

$$\bar{R}_s = \frac{R_s}{C_{e0}} \qquad [5.51]$$

$$\bar{C}_{\mathrm{H}^+} = \frac{C_{\mathrm{H}^+}}{(C_{\mathrm{H}^+})_{\mathrm{pH}=7.4}} \qquad [5.52]$$

$$[\bar{C}a^{2+}] = \frac{[Ca^{2+}]}{[Ca^{2+}]_{\mathrm{eq}}} \qquad [5.53]$$

$$\bar{a}_{\mathrm{TCP}} = \frac{a_{\mathrm{TCP}}}{a_{\mathrm{TCP0}}} \qquad [5.54]$$

$$\bar{t} = t\times k_2'\times(C_{\mathrm{H}^+})_{\mathrm{pH}=7.4} \qquad [5.55]$$

and two non-dimensional groups of material parameters

$$\bar{k}_1 = \frac{k_1}{k_2'\times(C_{\mathrm{H}^+})_{\mathrm{pH}=7.4}} \qquad [5.56]$$

$$S_{\text{TCP}} = \frac{3\left(a_{\text{TCP0}}/1 - f_{\text{TCP0}}\right)A_d}{k_2' \times (C_{\text{H}^+})_{\text{pH}=7.4} \times \left[\text{Ca}^{2+}\right]_{\text{eq}}} \quad [5.57]$$

the two rate equations can be non-dimensionalised as

$$\frac{d\bar{R}_s}{d\bar{t}} = \left(1 - \alpha \bar{R}_s^{\beta}\right)\left(\bar{k}_1 + \bar{C}_{\text{H}^+}\right) \quad [5.58]$$

and

$$\frac{d\left[\bar{\text{C}}\text{a}^{2+}\right]}{d\bar{t}} = S_{\text{TCP}}\bar{a}_{\text{TCP}}\sigma^{\theta} \quad [5.59]$$

Equations [5.33] to [5.41] can all be non-dimensionalised similarly.

The two non-dimensional groups of material parameters, $\bar{k}_1$ and S_{TCP}, control the degradation behaviour of the composite. In the expression for $\bar{k}_1$ (Equation [5.56]), $k_2' \times (C_{\text{H}^+})_{\text{pH}=7.4}$ represents the rate of auto-catalytic hydrolysis at pH = 7.4. $\bar{k}_1$ reflects the relative rate of non-catalytic hydrolysis to the auto-catalytic hydrolysis. A very large value of $\bar{k}_1$ means that the hydrolysis is non-catalytic. Similarly S_{TCP} reflects the relative rate of TCP dissolution with respect to the auto-catalytic hydrolysis. In the expression for S_{TCP} (Equation [5.57]), the term $a_{\text{TCP0}}/(1-f_{\text{TCP0}})$ represents the interface area per unit volume of the polymer phase, that is, S_{TCP} also contains information about the interface area in the composite. The dissolution constant A_d and the interface area acts together to give the total rate of TCP dissolution. $[\text{Ca}^{2+}]_{\text{eq}}$ appears in the expression to normalise the concentration of Ca^{2+}. A very large value of S_{TCP} indicates fast TCP dissolution relative to polymer chain scission. S_{TCP} is referred to as the strength of TCP dissolution.

5.6 TCP effectiveness map

Ehrenfried *et al.* (2008) and Yang *et al.* (2009) observed a saturation phenomenon when introducing a TCP phase in polylactide-co-glycolides (PLGAs). Their data indicate that there may be an upper limit to the total area of TCP/PLGA interface beyond which further increasing the area cannot further reduce the degradation rate of the polymer phase. To characterise the effectiveness of introducing TCP to reduce the degradation rate, a half degradation time, $t_{0.5}$, can be defined which is the time taken by the polymer phase to halve its average molecular weight. Introducing TCP reduces the acidity and hence increases the half degradation time. The larger the value of $t_{0.5}$, the more effective the TCP buffering is. By numerically solving the governing equations in Section 5.4, Pan *et al.* (2011) showed that the mathematical model also

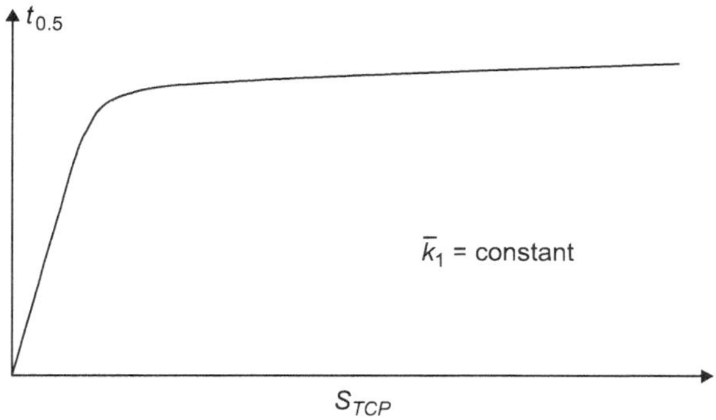

Figure 5.2 Half degradation time of the composite as a function of S_{TCP} for a fixed value of $\bar{k}_1$ showing the saturation effect.

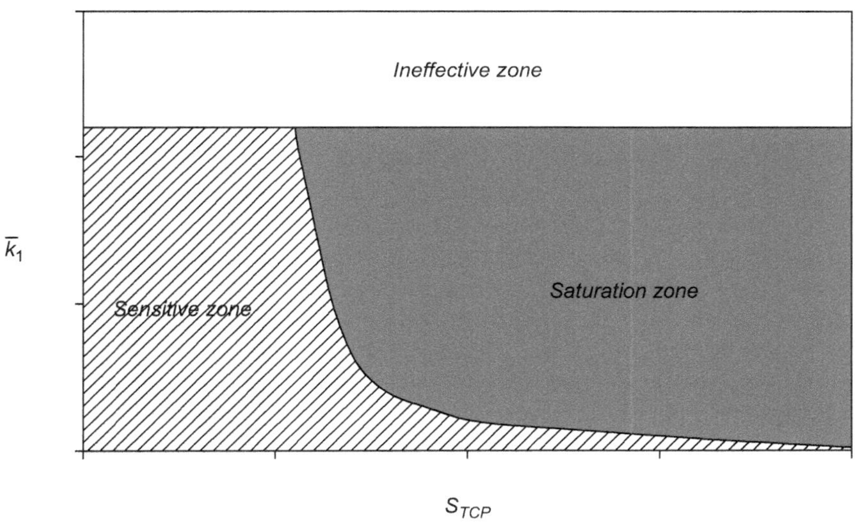

Figure 5.3 Effectiveness map of incorporating TCP to reduce degradation rate of the polymer phase. Taken from Pan *et al.* (2011).

predicts the saturation phenomenon. As illustrated in Figure 5.2. for any fixed value of $\bar{k}_1$, the calculated $t_{0.5}$ increases sharply with S_{TCP} initially, indicating a strong effect of the TCP on slowing down the polymer degradation. However, as S_{TCP} increases further $t_{0.5}$ reaches a limiting value showing that adding more TCP phase would have little further effect, i.e. a saturation has been reached.

The ability of reducing the degradation rate by the TCP phase is also strongly affected by $\bar{k}_1$. As an extreme example, if the hydrolysis is non-catalytic ($\bar{k}_1 = \infty$)

then the TCP phase has no effect on the degradation rate of the polymer phase. The effectiveness of the TCP phase on reducing degradation rate of the polymer phase is therefore controlled by both S_{TCP} and $\bar{k}_1$. By solving the governing equations covering a wide range of values of S_{TCP} and $\bar{k}_1$, Pan *et al.* (2011) obtained an 'effectiveness map' which is illustrated schematically in Figure 5.3. The horizontal axis is S_{TCP} and the vertical axis is $\bar{k}_1$. Roughly speaking, more and more TCP dissolves as one moves from left to the right on the map, and the hydrolysis reaction becomes more and more non-catalytic as one moves from the bottom to the top. The very top region represents polymers which degrade by non-catalytic hydrolysis. Incorporating TCP in these polymers is ineffective because their degradation is insensitive to the local pH. The left bottom region is where the degradation rate can be significantly altered by changing S_{TCP}, through changing the volume fraction and/or reducing the particle size of the TCP. The saturation region is where changing S_{TCP} has little effect on further changing the degradation rate. The map is illustrative and the boundaries between the various regions are only indicative rather than absolute because the numerical results always show a gradual transition across these boundaries between the different behaviours.

5.7 Concluding remarks

Diffusion processes are ignored in the model presented in this chapter which could be important. For example, if diffusion of the calcium and phosphate ions in the polymer phase is slow comparing with the polymer scission rate, then the model would over-predict the effect of the TCP phase and hence under-predict the degradation rate. On the other hand, if the short chains can diffuse out of the device quickly such as in a very thin sample, then the TCP phase will be less useful and the model will over-predict the degradation rate of the polymer. It is possible to build these diffusion processes into the model to analyse all the different possible scenarios.

References

Bohner M, Lemaitre J and Ring TA (1997), Kinetics of dissolution of β-tricalcium phosphate. *J Colloid Interface Sci*, **190**:37–48.

Ehrenfried LM, Munnawwar HP and Cameron RE (2008), The effect of tri-calcium phosphate (TCP) addition on the degradation of polylactide-co-glycolide (PLGA). *J Mater Sci Mater Med*, **19**:459–466.

Fernández E, Gil FJ, Ginebra MP, Driessens FC, Planell JA and Best SM (1999), Calcium phosphate bone cements for clinical applications. Part I: solution chemistry. *J Mater Sci Mater Med*, **10**:169–176.

Heidemann W, Jeschkeit S, Ruffieux K, Fischer JH, Wagner M, Kruger G, Wintermantel E and Gerlach KL (2001), Degradation of poly(D,L)lactide implants with or without addition of calcium phosphates *in vivo*. *Biomaterials*, **22**:2371–2381.

Karickhoff SW, Carreira LA and Hilal SH (2003), The SPARC on-line calculator, http://sparc.chem.uga.edu/sparc/.

Pan J, Han X, Niu W and Cameron RE (2011), A model for biodegradation of composite materials made of polyesters and tricalcium phosphates. *Biomaterials*, **32**:2248–2255.

Tang R, Wu W, Haas M and Nancollas GH (2001), Kinetics of dissolution of β-tricalcium phosphate. *Langmuir*, **17**:3480–3488.

Yang Z, Best SM and Cameron RE (2009), The influence of α-tricalcium phosphate nanoparticles and microparticles on the degradation of poly(D,L-lactide-co-glycolide). *Adv Mater*, **21**:3900–3904.

Modelling heterogeneous degradation of polymeric devices due to short chain diffusion

6

J. Pan, X. Chen
University of Leicester, Leicester, UK

6.1 Introduction

In the previous chapters, rate equations for chain scission have been presented in which the long and short chains are carefully separated. This chapter completes these equations by coupling them with a diffusion equation for the short chains. Grizzi *et al.* (1995) were probably the first to propose a schematic reaction–diffusion model to explain heterogeneous degradation. The driving force for short chain diffusion is the difference in concentration of the short chains at different locations. Water-soluble monomers and oligomers migrate from where their concentration is high to where it is low. This difference is initiated at the surface of a device by dissolution of the short chains into the aqueous media.

The fundamental element of a diffusion model is the diffusion law that relates the diffusion flux to the driving force. A linear relationship, i.e. Fick's law, is often used in the literature which is expected to be valid for the short chain diffusion. The proportional 'constant' in Fick's law is known as the diffusion coefficient. There are two complications regarding the diffusion coefficient when modelling short chain diffusion. The first is that the diffusion coefficient is sensitive to the size of the short chains. In reality short chains of different numbers of ester units diffuse with different diffusion coefficients. It is impractical to measure all the diffusion coefficients for all the different sizes of short chains. A major simplification in this chapter is that the short chains are treated as a single diffusing species with a single diffusion coefficient. The calculated diffusion rate reflects an average over the size range of the short chains. The second complication is that the loss of short chains generates porosity in the polymer which leads to a significant increase in the diffusion coefficient. This is an important but lengthy topic, which is dealt with in Chapter 8. In the current chapter, only the result from Chapter 8 is used.

Modelling Degradation of Bioresorbable Polymeric Medical Devices. http://dx.doi.org/10.1533/9781782420255.1.89

6.2 Scission rate of long chains affected by short chain diffusion

The rate equation for polymer chain scission was presented in Chapter 3 for amorphous polymers and Chapter 4 for semi-crystalline polymers. These equations are summarised in this section. The terms in these equations that are affected by the diffusion of short chains are highlighted.

6.2.1 Amorphous polymers

In Section 3.2, the hydrolysis rate equation,

$$\frac{dR_s}{dt} = k_1 C_e + k_2' C_e C_{\mathrm{H}^+} \qquad [2.2]$$

was rewritten as

$$\frac{dR_s}{dt} = k_1 C_e + k_2 C_e \left(\chi_1 C_{\mathrm{COOH}}^{\mathrm{long}} + \chi_2 C_{\mathrm{COOH}}^{\mathrm{short}}\right)^n \qquad [6.1]$$

in which the concentration of carboxylic acid end groups was divided into two types: those of the longer polymer chains denoted by $C_{\mathrm{COOH}}^{\mathrm{long}}$ and those of the shorter chains denoted by $C_{\mathrm{COOH}}^{\mathrm{short}}$. The difference between the short and long chains is that the short chains are water soluble and can diffuse out of a device, while the long chains cannot. Each chain scission produces one more carboxylic end groups, but by chance some of the chain scissions produce a short chain. Using R_{ol} to represent the number of ester units of short chains that have been produced, we have

$$C_{\mathrm{COOH}}^{\mathrm{long}} = C_{\mathrm{chain0}} + R_s - \frac{R_{ol}}{m} \qquad [3.2]$$

in which m is the average number of ester units of the short chains. R_{ol} is a historical record and cannot be altered by short chain diffusion. It can be related to the total number of chain scission R_s through an empirical relation

$$R_{ol} = \alpha C_{e0} \left(\frac{R_s}{C_{e0}}\right)^{\beta} \qquad [2.9]$$

On the other hand, using C_{ol} to represent the number of ester units of short chains that currently remain in the polymer per unit volume, we have

$$C_{\mathrm{COOH}}^{\mathrm{short}} = \frac{C_{ol}}{m} \qquad [3.4]$$

C_{ol} represents the current concentration and can be altered by short chain diffusion. Figure 3.1 illustrates the difference between R_{ol} and C_{ol}. The short chains are generated at the expense of the long chains which can be expressed as

$$C_e = C_{e0} - R_{ol} = C_{e0}\left[1-\alpha\left(\frac{R_s}{C_{e0}}\right)^{\beta}\right] \quad [2.11]$$

Combining all the above equations leads to the rate equation for chain scission:

$$\frac{dR_s}{dt} = C_{e0}\psi(R_s)\left\{k_1 + k_2 C_{e0}^n\left[\chi_1\phi(R_s)+\frac{\chi_2}{m}\left(\frac{C_{ol}}{C_{e0}}\right)\right]^n\right\} \quad [6.2]$$

in which

$$\psi(R_s) = 1-\alpha\left(\frac{R_s}{C_{e0}}\right)^{\beta} \quad [6.3]$$

and

$$\varphi(R_s) = \frac{C_{\text{chain0}}}{C_{e0}} + \frac{R_s}{C_{e0}} - \frac{\alpha}{m}\left(\frac{R_s}{C_{e0}}\right)^{\beta} \quad [6.4]$$

All the symbols in the above equations are defined in Section 3.2.

6.2.2 Semi-crystalline polymers

For semi-crystalline polymers, following Section 4.2 the rate Equation [4.6] for chain scission can be rewritten as

$$\frac{dR_s}{dt} = C_{e0}\psi(R_s)\left\{k_1 + k_2 C_{e0}^n\left[\left(\chi_1\varphi(R_s)+\frac{\chi_2}{m}\left(\frac{C_{ol}}{C_{e0}}\right)\right)\frac{1}{1-X_c}\right]^n\right\} \quad [6.5]$$

in which $\varphi(R_s)$ is given by Equation [6.4], X_c is given by Equations [4.17] or [4.18], and

$$\psi(R_s) = 1-\alpha\left(\frac{R_s}{C_{e0}}\right)^{\beta} - \frac{\omega}{C_{e0}}(X_c - X_{c0}) \quad [6.6]$$

All the symbols are defined in Section 4.5.1.

In the previous chapters, it has been assumed that the diffusion of short chains is prohibited, and consequently

$$C_{ol} = C_{ol0} + R_{ol} \tag{3.6}$$

where C_{ol0} represents the concentration of residual short chains at the beginning of degradation. Equation [3.6] is no longer valid if the short chains can diffuse and C_{ol} in Equations [6.2] and [6.5] is subject to change by diffusion.

6.3 Diffusion equation for short chains

Wang *et al.* (2008) and Han and Pan (2009) introduced a diffusion equation into the degradation model. Figure 6.1 illustrates the diffusion process of the short chains using an infinitely large plate that is placed in an aqueous media, as an example. In Figure 6.1a a rectangular unit of the plate is isolated. The left and right surfaces are exposed to the aqueous media and all the other surfaces can be considered as symmetry planes. Because of symmetry, diffusion occurs only in the thickness direction, marked x in the figure. Figure 6.1b shows the section highlighted in Figure 6.1a and the change in distribution of the short chains over time in the section. At the beginning, the short chains are generated everywhere in the plate and dissolve into the media off the left and right surfaces. As chain scission proceeds, more and more short chains are generated while some of them diffuse into the aqueous media. The concentration of short chains at the core of the plate reaches a peak value at some inter-medium time of the degradation. Towards the end of the degradation, a large amount of long chains have been turned into short ones and diffused out.

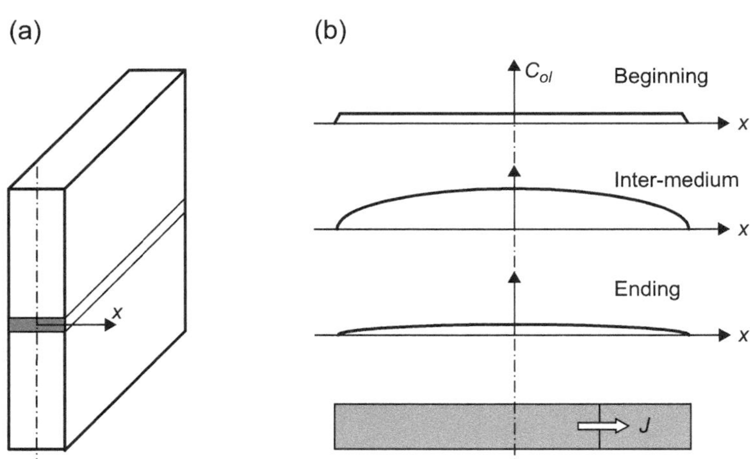

Figure 6.1 Short chain diffusion in a plate showing distributions of short chain concentration over thickness of the plate at different stages of degradation. (a) A representative unit of the plate and (b) change of short chain concentration over time.

The diffusion flux, J, is defined as number of ester units of short chains passing through a unit area per unit time, as illustrated in Figure 6.1b. The driving force for the chain diffusion is the gradient of concentration: dC_{ol} / dx. Fick's diffusion law assumes that

$$J = -D\frac{dC_{ol}}{dx} \quad [6.7]$$

in which D is the diffusion coefficient. The minus sign is because chains diffuse from where their concentration is high to where it is low. Fick's law has been widely used because of its simplicity and its ability to capture general trend observed in experiments. More sophisticated diffusion laws are sometime necessary, which does not pose any problem to solving the equations because the finite element method can deal with any diffusion law conveniently.

At any location x, the change in the concentration of short chains comes from two parts: (i) production of short chains due to chain scissions at that location and (ii) deposit or removal of chains from this location by diffusion. (i) can be calculated by differentiating Equation [2.9] as

$$\frac{dR_{ol}}{dt} = \alpha\beta\left(\frac{R_s}{C_{e0}}\right)^{\beta-1}\frac{dR_s}{dt} \quad [6.8]$$

To calculate (ii), let us consider a small section, Δx, along the diffusion route as illustrated in Figure 6.2. In the figure, $J(x)$ and $J(x+\Delta x)$ represent diffusion fluxes entering and leaving the section, respectively. If $J(x) > J(x+\Delta x)$, then some short chains are deposited on the small section, and if $J(x) < J(x+\Delta x)$ then some short chains are removed from the section, both of which lead to a change in the concentration of short chains in the section. The changing rate of the concentration can be calculated from the following statement of matter conservation:

$$J(x) - J(x+\Delta x) = \Delta x \times \left(\frac{dC_{ol}}{dt}\right)_{\text{diffusion}}. \quad [6.9]$$

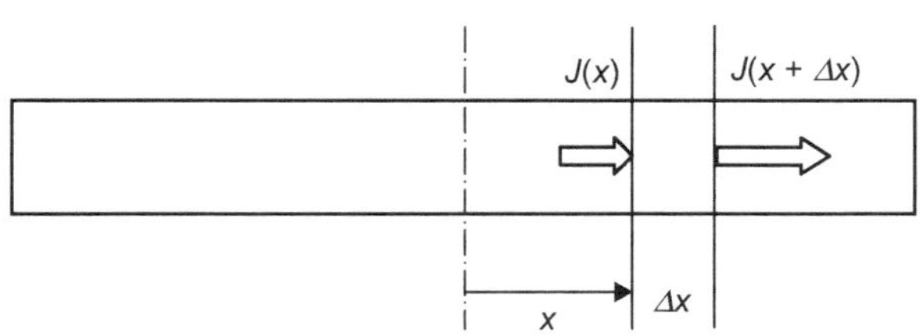

Figure 6.2 Removing or depositing short chains due to difference in the diffusion flux J on either sides of a small section Δx.

For a very small Δx, Equation [6.9] can be written as

$$\left(\frac{dC_{ol}}{dt}\right)_{\text{diffusion}} = -\frac{dJ}{dx} \quad [6.10]$$

The total change in the concentration is given by summation of the short chain production due to chain scissions and the change due to diffusion, i.e. we have

$$\frac{dC_{ol}}{dt} = \frac{dR_{ol}}{dt} - \frac{dJ}{dx} \quad [6.11]$$

Substituting Equations [6.7] and [6.8] into Equation [6.11] gives

$$\frac{dC_{ol}}{dt} = \alpha\beta\left(\frac{R_s}{C_{e0}}\right)^{\beta-1}\frac{dR_s}{dt} + \frac{d}{dx}\left(D\frac{dC_{ol}}{dx}\right) \quad [6.12]$$

For a three-dimensional device, such as a screw or scaffold, using x_1, x_2, x_3 to represent the three coordinates in the space, Equation [6.7] can be expanded as

$$J_1 = -D\frac{\partial C_{ol}}{\partial x_1} \quad [6.13]$$

$$J_2 = -D\frac{\partial C_{ol}}{\partial x_2} \quad [6.14]$$

$$J_3 = -D\frac{\partial C_{ol}}{\partial x_3} \quad [6.15]$$

in which J_1, J_2 and J_3 represent diffusion fluxes in the three directions, respectively. Equation [6.11] can be expanded as

$$\frac{dC_{ol}}{dt} = \frac{dR_{ol}}{dt} - \left(\frac{\partial J_1}{\partial x_1} + \frac{\partial J_2}{\partial x_2} + \frac{\partial J_3}{\partial x_3}\right) \quad [6.16]$$

Substituting Equations [6.8] and [6.13]–[6.15] into Equation [6.16] gives

$$\frac{dC_{ol}}{dt} = \alpha\beta\left(\frac{R_s}{C_{e0}}\right)^{\beta-1}\frac{dR_s}{dt} + \frac{\partial}{\partial x_1}\left(D\frac{\partial C_{ol}}{\partial x_1}\right) + \frac{\partial}{\partial x_2}\left(D\frac{\partial C_{ol}}{\partial x_2}\right) + \frac{\partial}{\partial x_3}\left(D\frac{\partial C_{ol}}{\partial x_3}\right)$$

[6.17]

This type of equation is referred to as a reaction–diffusion equation in the literature.

6.4 Collection of the governing equations

For the convenience of readers and sake of absolute clarity, the governing equations are collected together with a list of definitions of all their variables and parameters.

6.4.1 Amorphous polymers

For amorphous polymers, the governing equations for the scission of long chains and the diffusion of short chains are

$$\frac{dR_s}{dt} = C_{e0}\psi(R_s)\left\{k_1 + k_2 C_{e0}^n\left[\chi_1\phi(R_s) + \frac{\chi_2}{m}\left(\frac{C_{ol}}{C_{e0}}\right)\right]^n\right\} \qquad [6.2]$$

and

$$\frac{dC_{ol}}{dt} = \alpha\beta\left(\frac{R_s}{C_{e0}}\right)^{\beta-1}\frac{dR_s}{dt} + \sum_{i=1}^{3}\frac{\partial}{\partial x_i}\left(D\frac{\partial C_{ol}}{\partial x_i}\right) \qquad [6.17]$$

in which

$$\psi(R_s) = 1 - \alpha\left(\frac{R_s}{C_{e0}}\right)^{\beta} \qquad [6.3]$$

and

$$\varphi(R_s) = \frac{C_{\text{chain}0}}{C_{e0}} + \frac{R_s}{C_{e0}} - \frac{\alpha}{m}\left(\frac{R_s}{C_{e0}}\right)^{\beta} \qquad [6.4]$$

Equations [6.2] and [6.17] are subject to the following initial conditions:

$$R_s = 0 \text{ and } C_{ol} = C_{ol0} \text{ at } t = 0 \qquad [6.18]$$

and boundary condition:

$$C_{ol} = 0, \text{ at device surface.} \qquad [6.19]$$

A degrading polymer can be considered as a two-phase material made of a polymer phase and a porous phase. Using Equation [8.41] in Section 8.5 for a two-phase material made of a polymer phase and a porous phase, the diffusion coefficient D can be related to porosity V_{pore} through

$$D = D_{\text{polymer}} + \left(1.3V_{\text{pore}}^2 - 0.3V_{\text{pore}}^3\right)\left(D_{\text{pore}} - D_{\text{polymer}}\right) \qquad [6.20]$$

in which D_{polymer} (replacing D_{matrix} in Equation [8.41]) is the diffusion coefficient of short chains in a fresh amorphous polymer, and D_{pore} is the diffusion coefficient of short chains in liquid-filled pores. The porosity is due to the loss of short chains and can be calculated using

$$V_{\text{pore}} = \frac{R_{ol} - (C_{ol} - C_{ol0})}{C_{e0}} = \alpha\left(\frac{R_s}{C_{e0}}\right)^{\beta} - \frac{C_{ol} - C_{ol0}}{C_{e0}} \qquad [6.21]$$

The average molecular weight is calculated using

$$\overline{M}_n = \frac{M_n}{M_{n0}} = \frac{1 - \alpha\overline{R}_s^{\beta}}{1 + N_{dp0}\left(\overline{R}_s - (\alpha / m)\overline{R}_s^{\beta}\right)} \qquad [2.20]$$

in which $\overline{R}_s = R_s / C_{e0}$.

6.4.2 Semi-crystalline polymers

For semi-crystalline polymers, the governing equation for chain scission rate and short chain diffusion are

$$\frac{dR_s}{dt} = C_{e0}\psi(R_s)\left\{k_1 + k_2 C_{e0}^n\left[\left(\chi_1\varphi(R_s) + \frac{\chi_2}{m}\left(\frac{C_{ol}}{C_{e0}}\right)\right)\frac{1}{1 - X_c}\right]^n\right\} \qquad [6.5]$$

and

$$\frac{dC_{ol}}{dt} = \alpha\beta\left(\frac{R_s}{C_{e0}}\right)^{\beta-1}\frac{dR_s}{dt} + \sum_{i=1}^{3}\frac{\partial}{\partial x_i}\left(D\frac{\partial C_{ol}}{\partial x_i}\right) \qquad [6.17]$$

in which

$$\varphi(R_s) = \frac{C_{\text{chain}0}}{C_{e0}} + \frac{R_s}{C_{e0}} - \frac{\alpha}{m}\left(\frac{R_s}{C_{e0}}\right)^{\beta} \qquad [6.4]$$

$$\psi(R_s) = 1 - \alpha\left(\frac{R_s}{C_{e0}}\right)^{\beta} - \frac{\omega}{C_{e0}}(X_c - X_{c0}) \qquad [6.6]$$

and

$$X_c = \begin{cases} X_{c\max} - (X_{c\max} - X_{c0})e^{-k_c\left(\frac{R_s}{C_{e0}}\right)} & \lambda = 1 \\ X_{c\max} - \left[(\lambda - 1)k_c\left(\frac{R_s}{C_{e0}}\right) + (X_{c\max} - X_{c0})^{1-\lambda}\right]^{\frac{1}{1-\lambda}} & \lambda \neq 1 \end{cases} \qquad [4.17, 4.18]$$

Equations [6.5] and [6.17] are subject to the following initial conditions:

$$R_s = 0,\ C_{ol} = C_{ol0} \text{ at } t = 0 \qquad [6.18]$$

and boundary condition

$$C_{ol} = 0, \text{ at device surface.} \qquad [6.19]$$

A degrading semi-crystalline polymer can be considered as a two-phase material made of a polymer phase and a porosity phase. Using Equation [8.41] in Section 8.5, the diffusion coefficient D can be related to porosity V_{pore} through

$$D = D_{\text{matrix}} + \left(1.3V_{\text{pore}}^2 - 0.3V_{\text{pore}}^3\right)\left(D_{\text{pore}} - D_{\text{matrix}}\right) \qquad [6.22]$$

in which

$$V_{\text{pore}} = (1 - X_{c0})\left[\alpha\left(\frac{R_s}{C_{e0}}\right)^{\beta} - \frac{C_{ol} - C_{ol0}}{C_{e0}}\right] + (X_c - X_{c0})(1 - \omega/C_{e0}) \qquad [6.23]$$

and D_{matrix} is diffusion coefficient of the semi-crystalline matrix. The first term in Equation [6.23] reflects porosity generated by the diffusion of short chains while the second term reflects porosity generated by the difference in density between the amorphous and crystalline phases. The semi-crystalline matrix can also be considered as a two-phase material made of an amorphous phase and a crystalline phase. The diffusion coefficient of the crystalline phase is very small, and taken as zero. Using Equation [8.41] in Section 8.5, D_{matrix} can be calculated as

$$D_{\text{matrix}} = \left(1.3V_{\text{am}}^2 - 0.3V_{\text{am}}^3\right)D_{\text{polymer}} \qquad [6.24]$$

where

$$V_{\text{am}} = \frac{1 - V_{\text{pore}} - X_c}{1 - V_{\text{pore}}} \quad [6.25]$$

The average molecular weight at any location can be calculated using Equation [4.38]

$$\bar{M}_n = \frac{M_n}{M_{n0}} = \frac{1 + \bar{\omega} X_{c0} - \alpha \bar{R}_s^{\beta}}{\left(1 + \bar{\omega} X_{c0}\right)\left[1 + \frac{C_{e0}}{N_{\text{chain0}}}\left(\bar{R}_s - (\alpha / m)\bar{R}_s^{\beta}\right)\right]} \quad [4.38]$$

in which $\bar{R}_s = R_s / C_{e0}$ and $\bar{\omega} = \omega / C_{e0}$.

For thin samples used in most degradation experiments, the diffusion of short chains only occurs in the thickness direction of the sample and the problem is one-dimensional. In such cases, the governing equations can be solved either analytically using a weighted residual method (Wang *et al.*, 2008) or numerically using a finite difference method (Han and Pan, 2011). For general three-dimensional devices however, the equations have to be solved using the finite element method which is the topic of Chapter 7.

6.4.3 Definition of variables and parameters in the governing equations

The definitions of all the symbols used in the governing equations are listed here for clarity and convenience of the readers.

(I) Variables that depend on time t and location (x_1, x_2, x_3) and need to be found by solving the governing equations

- R_s – number of chain scissions per unit volume
- C_{ol} – number of ester units of short chains per unit volume
- X_c – volume percentage of crystalline phase
- M_n – number-averaged molecular weight

Only R_s and C_{ol} are independent variables.

(II) Parameters that describe polymer properties:

- C_{e0} – initial number of ester units of long chains in amorphous phase per unit volume
- C_{chain0} – initial number of amorphous chains per unit volume
- N_{chain0} – initial number of polymer chains including the crystalline phase per unit volume
- N_{dp0} – initial average degree of polymerisation of amorphous polymers
- C_{ol0} – initial number of ester units of residual short chains per unit volume
- M_{n0} – initial number-averaged molecular weight
- X_{c0} – initial volume degree of crystallinity
- $X_{c\max}$ – maximum volume degree of crystallinity
- ω – number of ester units of crystalline phase per unit volume

(III) Empirical parameters

- α, β – empirical parameters for short chain production
- χ_1, χ_2 – partitioning parameters for – COOH groups on long and short chains
- m – average degree of polymerisation of short chains, usually set as 4–6

(IV) Kinetic parameters

For amorphous polymers:

- n – exponent for acid dissociation of –COOH end groups, usually taken as 0.5
- k_1 – rate constant of non-catalytic reaction
- k_2 – rate constant of autocatalytic reaction
- D_{polymer} – diffusion coefficient of short chains in non-degraded amorphous polymer.
- D_{pore} – diffusion coefficient of short chains in liquid-filled pores

For semi-crystalline polymers, add

- λ – impingement exponent for crystal growth
- $k_c = pv_cC_{e0}$ in which p is the probability for a cleaved chain to form a crystallite and v_c is the average size of the crystallites.

6.5 A numerical study of size effect

Grizzi *et al.* (1995) demonstrated strong size dependence in the degradation of poly(DL-lactic acid) samples. They showed that plate samples of 2 mm in thickness degrade faster than thin film samples of 0.3 mm. There is some uncertainty in the reported experimental data. In particular, the amount of residual monomers was not reported for the samples. Their data shows that the thin samples lost 5% of their weights within the first week. This number of monomers could not have been produced by chain scissions. It is therefore logical to assume that these samples contained 5% residual monomers which are lost by fast dissolution and diffusion. The thick samples had very little weight loss until week 9, by which time the samples had already broken up. It is therefore logical to assume these samples had very few residual monomers. Using these assumed initial conditions, Han and Pan (2013) solved Equations [6.2] and [6.12] for the two types of samples. Figure 6.3 shows the average molecular weight as a function of time for the thin and thick samples obtained by Grizzi *et al.* (1995) (discrete symbols) and by the mathematical model (lines). A very large diffusion coefficient was used to mimic the dissolution of the residual monomers. In the numerical results, all the monomers left the thin sample on the first day, which is reflected by a sharp turn on the curve of molecular weight as function of time. Figure 6.4 shows comparison between the model calculation and the experimental data for weight loss. It can be observed from both figures that the model can capture the experimental data fairly well. The numerical solution also provides distribution of the average molecular weight across the thickness of the samples at any chosen time. The average molecular weight shown in Figure 6.3 is the value of the average molecular weight that is averaged over the entire thickness of the samples. The mathematical model assumes that the samples remain as a continuum solid during degradation. It cannot deal with sample disintegration and the corresponding

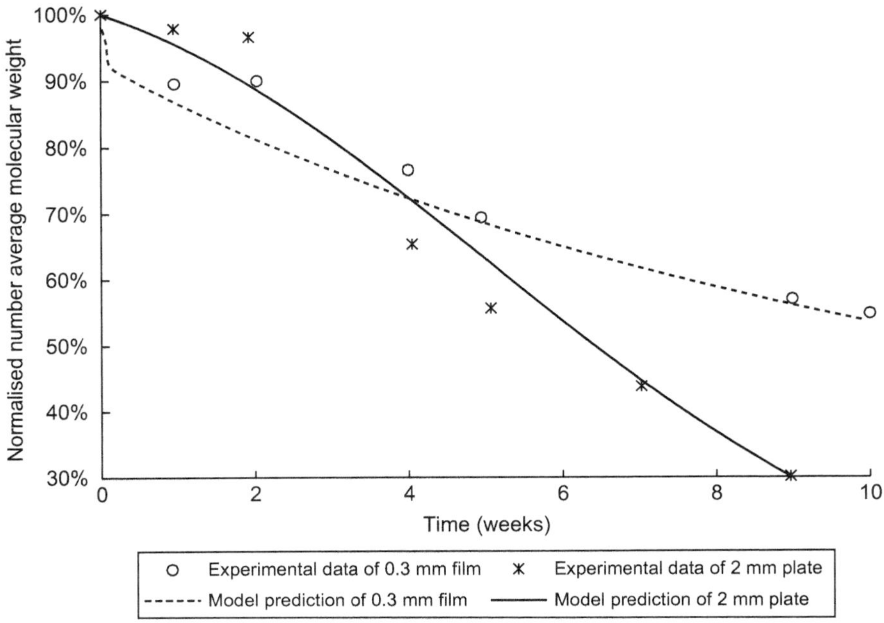

Figure 6.3 Normalised average molecular weights of plate and film samples as functions of time. Discrete symbols are the experimental data by Grizzi *et al.* (1995) and the lines are the best fitting using Equations [6.2] and [6.12]. (*Source*: Taken from Han and Pan, 2014.)

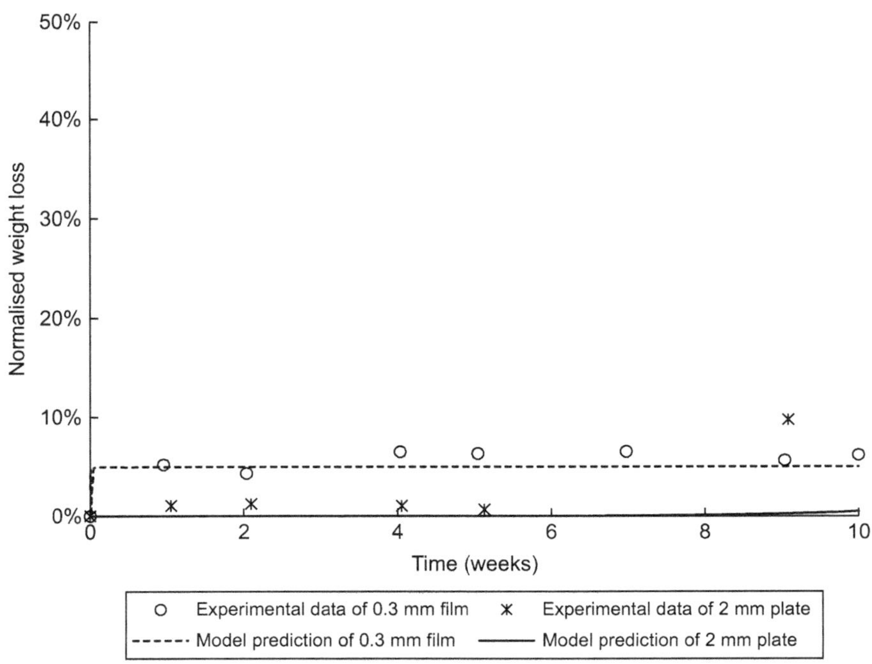

Figure 6.4 Mass loss of plate and film samples as functions of time. Discrete symbols are the experimental data by Grizzi *et al.* (1995) and the lines are the best fit using Equations [6.2] and [6.12]. (*Source*: Taken from Han and Pan, 2014.)

Table 6.1 Model parameters used in the numerical analysis for Figures 6.3 and 6.4

$C_{e0} = 17\,300$ mol/m^3	$k_1 = 1.4 \times 10^{-4}$/week
$M_0 = 72$ g/mol	$k_2 = 0.0019 \left(\sqrt{(m^3/\text{mol})}/\text{week}\right)$
$M_{n0} = 20000$ g/mol for plate sample	$D_{\text{polymer}} = 8 \times 10^{-7}$ m^2/week
$M_{n0} = 34000$ g/mol for film sample	$D_{\text{pore}} = 1000 \times D_{\text{polymer}}$
$m = 4$	$C_{ol0} = 5\% \, C_{e0}$ for film sample
$\alpha = 28, \beta = 2$	$C_{ol0} = 0$ for plate sample

Source: Taken from Han and Pan (2014).

weight loss. The calculation is therefore terminated at week 10. Parameters used in the model to achieve the best fit are provided in Table 6.1. In the table, the values for C_{e0} and M_0 are typical values for PLA. The values for M_{n0} are directly taken from the paper by Grizzi *et al.* (1995). It is widely recognised that short poly(lactide) (PLA)/ poly(glycolide) (PGA) chains of less than eight repeating units are water soluble. Hence, the average degree of polymerisation for the small molecules is set as $m = 4$. The values for α and β were chosen such that these values correspond to the assumption that the molecular weight reduction is dominated by random scission. The values of k_1, k_2 and D_{polymer} are obtained by fitting the numerical predictions with the experimental data. In the calculation it is further assumed that only the short chains act as catalysts in the hydrolysis reaction.

6.6 Non-dimensionalisation and degradation map

For a simple device such as a plate or a pin, it is possible to graphically illustrate the conditions that lead to different behaviours of degradation using a 'degradation map' (Wang *et al.*, 2008). These conditions also indicate when the diffusion of the short chains can be ignored in the mathematical model. If the short chain diffusion can be ignored, then the analytical or numerical solutions provided in Chapters 2–5 can be used. The governing equations in Section 6.4 contain quite a few parameters. By performing a non-dimensionalisation exercise, it is possible to identify two non-dimensional groups of these parameters that control the degradation behaviour. The thickness of the plate or the diameter of the pin is one of the key parameters in the analysis. For devices of sophisticated shape, finite element analysis as discussed in Chapter 7 has to be carried out to determine the different degradation behaviours. However it is often possible to identify a characteristic diffusion distance (the outer diameter of a screw for example) to replace the plate thickness or pin diameter in the following analysis. This then allows the degradation map to be used for general devices as a rough guide on whether short chain diffusion can be ignored.

6.6.1 Non-dimensionalisation of governing equations

Considering the very large plate, as illustrated in Figure 6.1, that has a thickness l and is made of an amorphous polymer; the governing Equations [6.2] and [6.12] can be rearranged as follows without changing them:

$$\frac{d(R_s / C_{e0})}{d(tk_2C_{e0}^n)} = \psi(R_s)\left\{\frac{k_1}{k_2C_{e0}^n} + \left[\chi_1\phi(R_s) + \frac{\chi_2}{m}\left(\frac{C_{ol}}{C_{e0}}\right)\right]^n\right\} \quad [6.2]$$

and

$$\frac{d(C_{ol} / C_{e0})}{d(tk_2C_{e0}^n)} = \alpha\beta\left(\frac{R_s}{C_{e0}}\right)^{\beta-1}\frac{d(R_s / C_{e0})}{d(tk_2C_{e0}^n)} + \frac{\partial}{\partial(x/l)}\left(\frac{D}{l^2k_2C_{e0}^n}\frac{\partial(C_{ol} / C_{e0})}{\partial(x/l)}\right) \quad [6.17]$$

Such rearrangement is not unique and one can chose different parameters to normalise the equations. Here all the concentrations are normalised by C_{e0} and all the lengths are normalised by the thickness of the plate. These are rather obvious choices of normalisation. Furthermore both sides of the equations are divided by $k_2C_{e0}^n$. This is because we chose to use the rate of autocatalytic hydrolysis as a reference for the rates of diffusion and noncatalytic hydrolysis. This is a sensible choice because autocatalytic hydrolysis always occurs in the polyesters that are considered in this book while diffusion and noncatalytic hydrolysis may or may not be important depending on the device and polymers.

Defining the following non-dimensional variables (Wang *et al.*, 2008)

$$\overline{R}_s = \frac{R_s}{C_{e0}} \quad [6.26]$$

$$\overline{C}_{ol} = \frac{C_{ol}}{C_{e0}} \quad [6.27]$$

$$\overline{t} = k_2C_{e0}^n t \quad [6.28]$$

$$\overline{x} = \frac{x}{l} \quad [6.29]$$

and kinetic parameters

$$\overline{k}_1 = \frac{k_1}{k_2C_{e0}^n} \quad [6.30]$$

$$\bar{D} = \bar{D}_{\text{polymer}} + \left(1.3V_{\text{pore}}^2 - 0.3V_{\text{pore}}^3\right)\left(\bar{D}_{\text{pore}} - \bar{D}_{\text{polymer}}\right) \quad [6.31]$$

in which

$$\bar{D}_{\text{polymer}} = \frac{D_{\text{polymer}}}{k_2 C_{e0}^n l^2}, \quad \bar{D}_{\text{pore}} = \frac{D_{\text{pore}}}{k_2 C_{e0}^n l^2} \quad [6.32, 6.33]$$

the governing equations can be non-dimensionalised as

$$\frac{d\bar{R}_s}{d\bar{t}} = \psi\left(\bar{R}_s\right)\left\{\bar{k}_1 + \left[\chi_1\varphi\left(\bar{R}_s\right) + \frac{\chi_2}{m}\bar{C}_{ol}\right]^n\right\} \quad [6.34]$$

and

$$\frac{d\bar{C}_{ol}}{d\bar{t}} = \alpha\beta\bar{R}_s^{\beta-1}\frac{d\bar{R}_s}{d\bar{t}} + \frac{\partial}{\partial\bar{x}}\left(\bar{D}\frac{\partial\bar{C}_{ol}}{\partial\bar{x}}\right). \quad [6.35]$$

The expressions for functions ψ and ϕ in Equations [6.3] and [6.4], and number-averaged molecular weight given by Equation [2.20], are already in non-dimensional format.

There are three kinetic parameters in the non-dimensionalised equations: $\bar{k}_1$, $\bar{D}_{\text{polymer}}$ and $\bar{D}_{\text{pore}}$. $\bar{D}_{\text{pore}}$ reflects the diffusion rate of short chains in liquid and can be set as a value much larger than $\bar{D}_{\text{polymer}}$. The remaining two parameters, $\bar{D}_{\text{polymer}}$ and $\bar{k}_1$, control the degradation behaviour of a plate. $\bar{k}_1$ reflects the non-catalytic hydrolysis rate relative to the autocatalytic hydrolysis rate. The larger $\bar{k}_1$ is, the faster is the non-catalytic hydrolysis is in comparison with the auto-catalytic hydrolysis. $\bar{D}_{\text{polymer}}$ reflects the diffusion rate of short chains in non-degraded polymer relative to the autocatalytic hydrolysis rate. It also includes the effect of thickness of the plate. The effect of a faster diffusion, thinner plate or slower autocatalytic hydrolysis is equivalent as long as $\bar{D}_{\text{polymer}}$ remains the same.

The values of n, α and β also affect the degradation behaviour although these parameters are not expected to change as much as the kinetic parameters from polymer to polymer.

6.6.2 Degradation map

Considering the very large plate shown in Figure 6.1, the effect of changing $\bar{D}_{\text{polymer}}$ on its degradation behaviour is computed by solving Equations [6.34] and [6.35] numerically. Figure 6.5 shows the effect of changing $\bar{D}_{\text{polymer}}$ on molecular weight $\bar{M}_n$ at $\bar{t} = 27$ for a fixed value of $\bar{k}_1 = 0.001$. The choice of $\bar{t} = 27$ is arbitrary and will be explained later. The average molecular weight in the plate is a function of x as indicated in Figure 6.1. The value of $\bar{M}_n$ shown in Figure 6.5 is calculated by

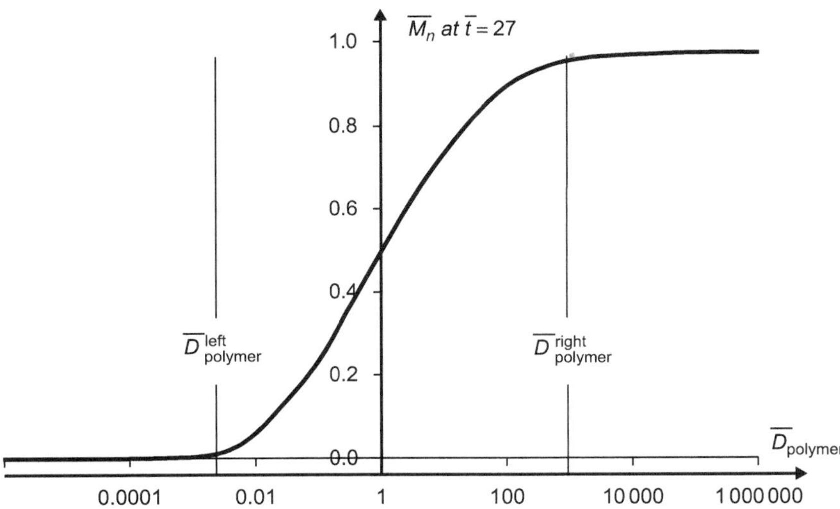

Figure 6.5 Molecular weight (vertical axis) averaged across the plate at $\overline{t} = 27$ as a function of $\overline{D}_{\text{polymer}}$ (horizontal axis). $\overline{k}_1 = 0.001$. (By Xinpu Chen, third year undergraduate project, University of Leicester.)

averaging the molecular weight across the thickness of the plate. Observing the left section of the curve in Figure 6.5, it can be seen that if $\overline{D}_{\text{polymer}}$ is very small, then $\overline{M}_n$ has already reached zero at $\overline{t} = 27$. This means if either the diffusion is very slow or the plate is very thick, degradation is fast because the short chains accumulate inside the plate and generate an acidic environment. Moving from left to right, as $\overline{D}_{\text{polymer}}$ gradually increases $\overline{M}_n$ at $\overline{t} = 27$ also increases. This indicates that degradation is slowed down by the diffusion process. At the right-most section, where either diffusion is very fast or the plate is very thin, the plate degrades very slowly because the short chains can leave the plate quickly. It is interesting to observe that $\overline{M}_n$ does not change with $\overline{D}_{\text{polymer}}$ on either the left-most section or the right-most section. Two thresholds, referred to as $\overline{D}^{\text{left}}_{\text{polymer}}$ and $\overline{D}^{\text{right}}_{\text{polymer}}$ in the figure, can be identified such that $\overline{M}_n$ only changes with $\overline{D}_{\text{polymer}}$ if $\overline{D}^{\text{left}}_{\text{polymer}} < \overline{D}_{\text{polymer}} < \overline{D}^{\text{right}}_{\text{polymer}}$.

Choosing a different value for $\overline{t}$ does not affect the values of $\overline{D}^{\text{left}}_{\text{polymer}}$ and $\overline{D}^{\text{right}}_{\text{polymer}}$. However if $\overline{t}$ is set at a too large value, $\overline{M}_n$ will be almost zero at this time for all values of $\overline{D}_{\text{polymer}}$. If $\overline{t}$ is set at a too small value, $\overline{M}_n$ will have not changed very much at this time for all values $\overline{D}_{\text{polymer}}$. Consequently, these choices of $\overline{t}$ would make the identification of $\overline{D}^{\text{left}}_{\text{polymer}}$ and $\overline{D}^{\text{right}}_{\text{polymer}}$ difficult.

It is expected that the values of $\overline{D}^{\text{left}}_{\text{polymer}}$ and $\overline{D}^{\text{right}}_{\text{polymer}}$ depend on $\overline{k}_1$. To account for the effect of $\overline{k}_1$, the above calculation was repeated for a wide range of values of $\overline{k}_1$, and the numerical results are graphically presented using a degradation map as shown in Figure 6.6. The vertical axis of the map represents $\overline{D}_{\text{polymer}}$ and the horizontal axis represents $\overline{k}_1$. The bottom part of the map corresponds to the left side of the curve in Figure 6.5 and the top part of the map corresponds to the right side of the curve. For any fixed value of $\overline{k}_1$, regions *C, A* and *B* on the map corresponds to the left flat

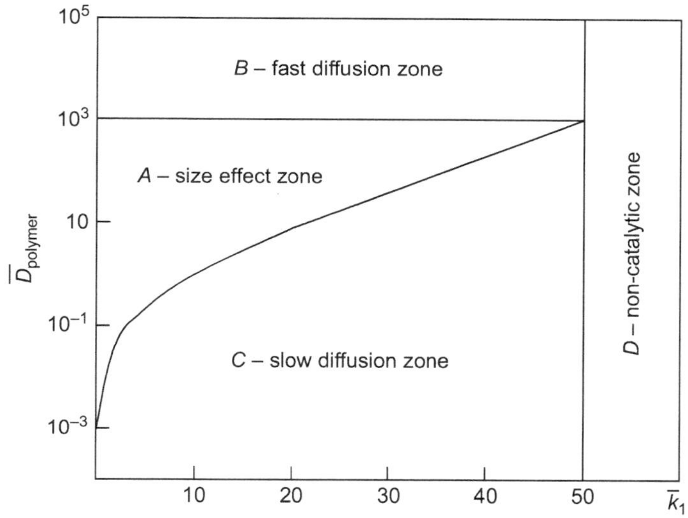

Figure 6.6 Degradation map showing different behaviours of degradation of a infinitively large plate controlled by $\overline{D}_{\text{polymer}}$ and $\overline{k}_1$. Other parameters used in the calculation are $\alpha = 1$, $\beta = 1$, $\chi_1 = 0$, $\chi_2 = 1$, $m = 4$, $n = 0.5$, $\overline{D}_{\text{pore}} = 1000\overline{D}_{\text{polymer}}$, $N_{dp0} = 2307$ and $C_{\text{ol0}} = 0$. (Original version obtained by Wang *et al.* (2008). Recalculated by Xinpu Chen, undergraduate third year project, the University of Leicester.)

section, the middle ascending section and the right flat section of the curve, respectively. The boundary between regions *C* and *A* corresponds to $\overline{D}^{\text{left}}_{\text{polymer}}$, and the boundary between regions *A* and *B* corresponds to $\overline{D}^{\text{right}}_{\text{polymer}}$.

The top zone *B* represents where $\overline{D}_{\text{polymer}}$ is large, which means either diffusion is fast or the plate is very thin. Under these conditions, the short chains cannot remain inside the plate long enough to act as catalyst for the hydrolysis reaction. The polymer degrades at the non-catalytic rate and the degradation of the plate is uniform. Above the boundary between zones *A* and *B*, further increasing $\overline{D}_{\text{polymer}}$ (by reducing the thickness, for example) cannot change the degradation rate. An interesting numerical result is that this boundary, i.e. $\overline{D}^{\text{right}}_{\text{polymer}}$, is very weakly affected by $\overline{k}_1$ and located at approximately $\overline{D}^{\text{right}}_{\text{polymer}} = 1000$. The absolute location of the boundary is however fuzzy because the curve in Figure 6.5 shows a gradual transition between the two zones. Rearranging Equation [6.32] gives

$$l_{th} = \sqrt{\frac{D_{\text{polymer}}}{D^{\text{right}}_{\text{polymer}} k_2 C^n_{e0}}} \approx \sqrt{\frac{D_{\text{polymer}}}{1000 k_2 C^n_{e0}}} \qquad [6.36]$$

where l_{th} is a threshold for the thickness of the plate under which the degradation rate is no longer affected by the thickness. Equation [6.36] indicates that the faster the short chain diffusion or the slower the autocatalytic hydrolysis, the larger l_{th} becomes.

In zone *C*, $\bar{D}_{\text{polymer}}$ is small, although the definition of 'small' depends on $\bar{k}_1$. In this zone, despite the short chains near the surface of the plate diffusing into the aqueous media, the effect remains very local to the surface layer throughout the life time of the plate and does not affect its overall degradation rate. Degradation of the plate is heterogeneous and a hard skin can be expected to form, while the inside degrades faster due to the acidic environment. It is interesting to note that $\bar{k}_1$ has a significant effect on the upper boundary of this region. The larger is $\bar{k}_1$, the easier it is for a plate to enter this zone from zone *A*.

The right zone *D* is where $\bar{k}_1$ is very large and the hydrolysis is dominantly non-catalytic. In this zone diffusion of the short chains plays no role in the degradation rate, the plate degrades uniformly, and the concept of a threshold thickness does not exist. The numerical results show that the boundary between zone *D* and other zones is located at $\bar{k}_1 = 50$. Again, this absolute location is fuzzy because the numerical results show a gradual transition. Rearranging Equation [6.30] gives $k_1 \geq 50 k_2 C_{e0}^n$ in zone *D*. $k_2 C_{e0}^n$ represents the rate of autocatalytic hydrolysis with a catalyst concentration of C_{e0}. Noting that C_{e0} is the initial number of ester units of all the long chains, we have $C_{e0} >> C_{ol}$, i.e. for practical polymers the number of short chains available as catalyst should be much less than C_{e0}. This means that $k_2 C_{e0}^n$ represents an unrealistically fast rate of autocatalytic hydrolysis. It is therefore unlikely that a typical biodegradable polymer, such as PLA or PGA, will fall into zone *D*.

In zones *B*, *C* and *D*, there is no need to involve the diffusion equation in order to calculate the degradation rate. In the governing equations one should set $C_{ol} = 0$ for zone *B*, $C_{ol} = R_{ol}$ for zone *C* and $k_2 = 0$ in zone *D*. The analytical and numerical solutions provided by Chapters 2–5 can be used for these zones.

Zone *A* is where the diffusion of short chains and the hydrolysis reaction strongly interact with each other and the size effect on degradation rate is expected. Although the degradation map was calculated for a plate, the same principle applies for all sophisticated devices such as screws or stents. Unfortunately, this is probably the zone into which most devices fall, and the device design has to be carefully analysed because changing the size has a major effect on its degradation rate.

The degradation map presented in Figure 6.6 was first obtained by Wang *et al.* (2008). It was recalculated, as explained in the current section, by Xinpu Chen as his third year (undergraduate) research project at the University of Leicester. The calculation by Chen confirmed that the map was not affected by using the updated version of the mathematical model.

6.7 Effect of other factors on the degradation map

The degradation map shown in Figure 6.6 was calculated using a specific set of parameters of $\alpha = 1$, $\beta = 1$, $\chi_1 = 0$, $\chi_2 = 1$, $m = 4$, $n = 0.5$, $N_{dp0} = 2307$, $C_{ol0} = 0$ and $\bar{D}_{\text{pore}} = 1000 \bar{D}_{\text{polymer}}$. It was also assumed that the polymer is amorphous. The choice

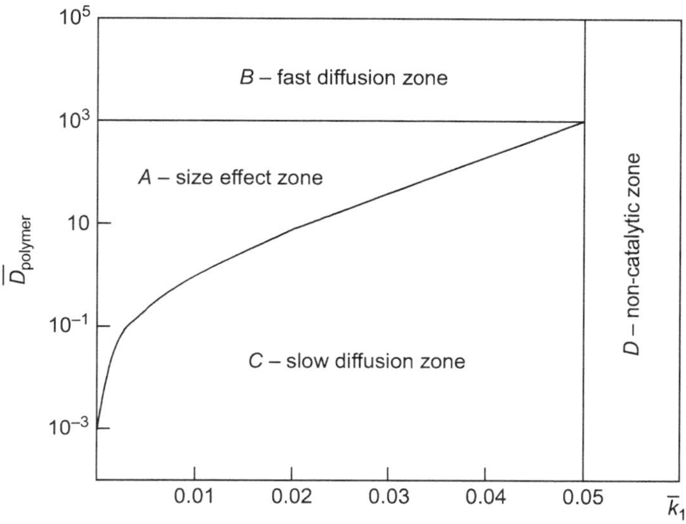

Figure 6.7 Degradation map obtained using $\alpha = 28$ and $\beta = 2$ with all other parameters identical to that for Figure 6.6. (By Xinpu Chen, undergraduate third year project, the University of Leicester.)

of some of these parameters does have a significant effect on the degradation map, although the concept of the four zones is generally valid.

6.7.1 Effect of α and β

As discussed in Section 2.3, the values of α and β determine the number of short chains produced by chain scissions through Equation [2.9]. For end scission, $\alpha = 1$ and $\beta = 1$. At this extreme, each scission produces a monomer and the chain scission is very efficient in producing short chains. For random scission, $\alpha = 28$ and $\beta = 2$, which reflects that the chain scission is rather ineffective in producing short chains. The real situation is somewhere between the two extremes. The degradation map is recalculated using $\alpha = 28$ and $\beta = 2$ and presented in Figure 6.7. All the other parameters remain unchanged. It can be observed that the degradation map for $\alpha = 28$ and $\beta = 2$ is identical in its shape to that for $\alpha = 1$ and $\beta = 1$, except that the vertical boundary between zone D and other regions shifts to the left by three orders of magnitude. This reflects the fact that if much fewer short chains are produced it is far more likely for a plate to degrade through non-catalytic hydrolysis.

6.7.2 Effect of crystallisation induced by chain scission

Han and Pan (2009) compared degradation maps for amorphous (dashed lines) and semi-crystalline polymers (solid lines), which is reproduced in Figure 6.8. Full details of the calculation can be found in the paper by Han and Pan (2009). It can be observed

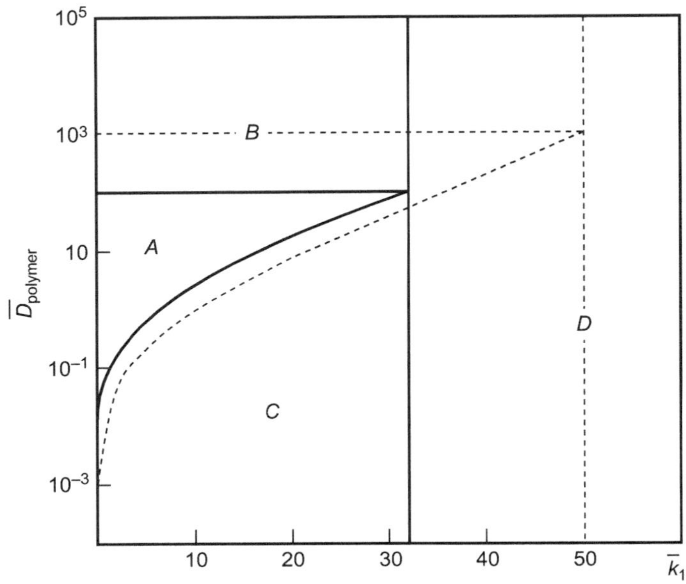

Figure 6.8 Effect of crystallisation on degradation map. The solid lines show the four zones for semi-crystalline polymer while the dashed lines are for amorphous polymers. (*Source*: Taken from Han and Pan, 2009.)

that zone *A* shrinks in all directions for semi-crystalline polymers. This indicates that for semi-crystalline polymers it is more likely to degrade uniformly than amorphous polymers, i.e. semi-crystalline polymers are expected to show less size effect than amorphous ones. The underlying reason for this phenomenon is simple – the crystalline phase resists degradation, which reduces the difference in degradation rate at different locations of a device.

6.7.3 Effect of device geometry

The degradation map can be calculated for devices of any sophisticated shape if the dimensions of the device scale by a single parameter. This parameter can be called the characteristic size of the device. In the case of the very large plate, its thickness is the characteristic size. For a sphere or a very long solid cylinder, the radius is the characteristic size. Replacing l in the definition of $\bar{D}_{polymer}$ in Equation [6.23] with the characteristic size, a similar map can be calculated. Figure 6.9 shows a degradation map for solid pins. All the parameters are the same as those for the map in Figure 6.6. It can be observed from Figure 6.9 that the vertical boundary of zone *D* shifts to the left by half comparing with the map for the plate. This is because for a solid pin, more material per unit volume is located at the surface, making it easier for the short chains to leave. Consequently, a pin behaves in a more non-catalytic manner in comparison to the plate.

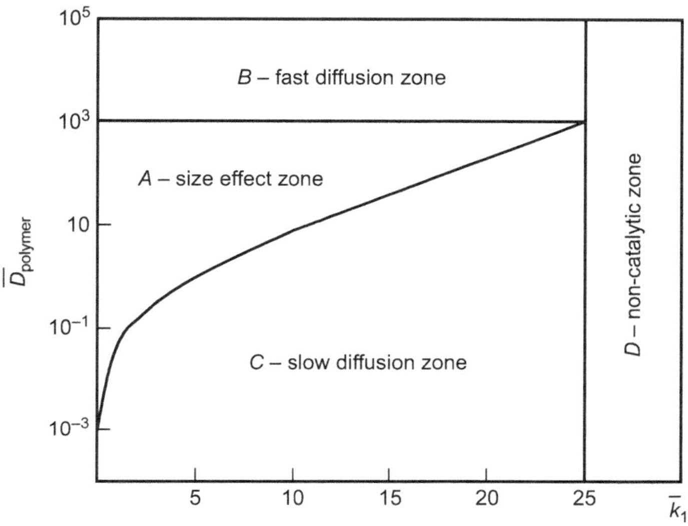

Figure 6.9 Degradation map for solid cylinder using the same parameters as those used for the large plate in Figure 6.6. (By Xinpu Chen, undergraduate third year project, the University of Leicester.

6.8 Concluding remarks

Although it is generally recognised that the hydrolysis of PLAs and PGA is autocatalytic, there is surprisingly little data on the size effect of device degradation in the literature. The lack of control on residual monomers in some of the early experiments contributes to further uncertainty in our understanding. The effect of short chain diffusion on device degradation is therefore still an open issue. The mathematical models and degradation maps presented in this chapter could serve as a useful guide for the future research.

References

Grizzi I, Garreau H, Li S and Vert M (1995) Hydrolytic degradation of devices based on poly [DL-lactic acid] size dependence. *Biomaterials* **16**:305–311.

Han X and Pan J (2009) A model for simultaneous degradation and crystallisation in biodegradable polymers. *Biomaterials* **30**:423–430.

Han X and Pan J (2011) Polymer chain scission, oligomer production and diffusion – a two scale model for degradation of bioresorbable polyesters. *Acta Biomaterialia* **7**: 538–547.

Han X and Pan J (2013) Finite element analysis of degradation of biodegradable medical devices. *OA Biotechnology* **2**(3):22.

Wang Y, Pan J, Han X, Sinka IC and Ding L (2008) A phenomenological model for the degradation of biodegradable polymers. *Biomaterials* **29**:3393–3401.

Part Two

Advanced methods of modelling degradation of bioresorbable polymeric medical devices

Finite element analysis (FEA) of biodegradation of polymeric medical devices

7

X. Han
Loughborough University, Loughborough, UK

7.1 Introduction

Biodegradable polymers have found great attractions in a board range of medical applications: they were firstly used to made sutures successfully in 1970s,[1] afterward they drew great interests in fields of orthopaedic fixation devices, controlled drug release and scaffolds in tissue engineering. Biodegradable polymers gradually replace conventional biomaterials in many medical applications owing to their nature of degradation. Degradation of biodegradable devices is, however, a complicated chemical–physical process. It depends on the chemical structure of polymer, the shape and size of the device and the degradation environment. Heterogeneous degradation and size effect (thicker plates degrade faster than thin films) were demonstrated by researchers[2–4] which were believed to be results of auto-catalytic hydrolysis reactions. Following the mathematical framework developed in Part One, this chapter is to show that how the mathematical model can be implemented in commercial finite element analysis (FEM) package COMSOL Multiphysics® and used for the design of medical implant of any sophisticated shapes. Four cases are demonstrated in this chapter. These include (a) a simple cube to demonstrate the three-dimensional effect of device degradation, (b) a typical scaffold for tissue engineering, (c) a fixation screw for orthopaedic surgery and (d) a coronary stent.

7.1.1 Finite element method

Partial differential equations (PDE) that arise in the mathematical modelling of many physical, chemical and biological phenomena are frequently too complicated to find their solutions analytically. In order to develop approximations of PDEs, the finite element method (FEM) is introduced in this section. FEM is a numerical technique to find the approximate solutions of PDEs, especially for problems to be solved in complicated and irregular geometries. PDEs are not solved directly using FEM. Instead, they are transformed to a set of equivalent variationals or weak forms based on the variational principle. Global variables in the variationals or weak forms are discretised and expressed by local variables using definite shape functions. Discrete variationals or weak forms can be, then, solved using different algorithms. Detailed introduction regarding FEM is beyond the scope of this chapter. One who is interested in FEM can

Modelling Degradation of Bioresorbable Polymeric Medical Devices. http://dx.doi.org/10.1533/9781782420255.2.113

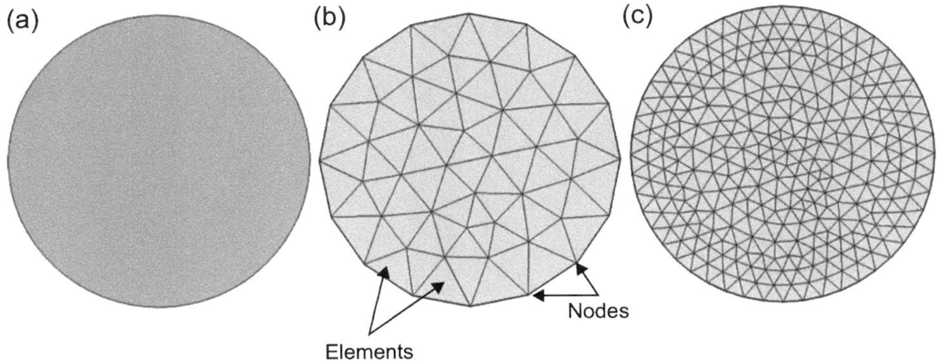

Figure 7.1 Geometry discretisation: (a) original domain; (b) coarse mesh; (c) refined mesh.

refer to the book.[5] As an alternative, generic steps of applying FEM to solve PDEs numerically for biodegradation of bioresorbable polymers are described as follows:

a. Transforming PDEs into a variational format using $\delta\Pi = 0$, where Π is obtained using the variational principle (see Reference 6).

b. Geometry discretisation: A domain (Figure 7.1a) is divided into smaller regions as shown in Figure 7.1b and Figure 7.1c. Each small triangular region is called an element. Different types of elements can be used in the meshing procedure, for example segments of lines for 1D problems, triangles and squares for 2D problems, and tetrahedra for 3D problems. In each element, there are some vertices, which are called nodes in FEM (see Figure 7.1b). Triangular elements, as illustrated in Figure 7.1b, are the most used elements in 2D problems. The total number of nodes determines the final matrix size to be solved. Figures 7.1b and 7.1c show two different sizes of meshing, representing a coarse meshing and a refined meshing, respectively.

c. Discretisation of equations: Variables in PDEs at any given position inside an FEM element can be described as functions of that at each node, and an example is shown in Equation [7.1].

$$R_s = [\mathrm{N}]\{\mathrm{R}_s^e\} \qquad [7.1]$$

in which R_s is the total number of chain scissions per unit volume defined in Section 3.2.1, $[\mathrm{N}]$ is the matrix of shape functions and $\{\mathrm{R}_s^e\}$ is the nodal vector of R_s for element e. A shape function can usually be selected as a polynomial; for example, a first order polynomial (known as linear element) or a second order polynomial (quadratic element) is mostly used in a FEM.

d. Equation assembling and boundary conditions: Substituting variables for element e, such as R_s in Equation [7.1], into functional Π, Π for the eth element can be expressed as Π^e. Elemental stiffness matrix $[\mathrm{K}]_e$ and elemental forces vector $\{\mathrm{f}^e\}$ can, thus, be derived (see Reference 2). Global stiffness matrix $[\mathrm{K}]$ and force vector $\{\mathrm{f}\}$ are gained by assembling elemental stiffness matrix $[\mathrm{K}]_e$ and forces vector $\{\mathrm{f}^e\}$ over all elements. A tricky issue when assembling is that neighbouring elements have shared nodes so that they need to be added into one term. Generally speaking, if a system contains M nodes, the final global stiffness matrix $\left[K\right]$ has a size of M × M while the size of vector {f} is M. There are two types of boundary conditions used in FEM: (1) Dirichlet boundary condition (the first type boundary condition); and (2) Neumann boundary condition (the second type boundary condition). The former specifies the value of the solution on boundaries while the latter specifies the derivative of the solution on boundaries, which can be automatically satisfied through the variational principle.

e. Solve the system of equations: A number of methods can be used in solving the global variational both for steady state and transient problems.[5] In this chapter, degradation process is considered as a time dependent problem, so that Euler's method or the Runge-Kutta method can be utilised.

7.1.2 COMSOL Multiphysics®

A large number of either open source software or commercial packages are available which implement FEM for solving PDEs and provide pre- and post-processing of finite element models. COMSOL Multiphysics® is one of commercial finite element analysis simulation packages for physics and engineering applications. It is very reliable in solving coupled phenomena (or multiphysics). COMSOL Multiphysics® allows users to input PDEs for coupled physics directly or use corresponding weak forms.[7] It also provides interfaces to MATLAB for further simulation and post-processing and to CAD packages so that users can import complex CAD geometries for finite element analysis. In this chapter, four degradation analysis cases will be carried out using FEM, and **PDE interfaces** in COMSOL Multiphysics® software (v4.3) are utilised to perform the modelling.[8] In the first two cases, step-by-step user guides are provided, while readers are encouraged to practise their own modelling skills by following the brief introductions for Case 3 and Case 4.

7.1.3 The PDEs for polymer degradation

The PDEs for polymer degradation that are introduced in this chapter are taken from Chapter 6:

$$\frac{dR_s}{dt} = C_{e0}\left[1-\alpha\left(\frac{R_s}{C_{e0}}\right)^{\beta}\right]\left\{k_1 + k_2 C_{e0}^{n}\left[\frac{1}{m}\left(\frac{C_{ol}}{C_{e0}}\right)\right]^{n}\right\} \quad [7.2]$$

in which R_s is the mole concentration of polymer chain scissions, C_{ol} is the mole concentration of dissolvable small molecules, and C_{e0} is the initial mole concentration of ester bonds of the polymer chains. The reaction–diffusion equation for C_{ol} is

$$\frac{dC_{ol}}{dt} = \alpha\beta\left(\frac{R_s}{C_{e0}}\right)^{\beta-1}\frac{dR_s}{dt} + \sum_{i=1}^{3}\frac{\partial}{\partial x_i}\left(D\frac{\partial C_{ol}}{\partial x_i}\right) \quad [7.3]$$

In Equations [7.2] and [7.3], k_1 and k_2 are rates for the non-catalytic hydrolysis and auto-catalytic hydrolysis reactions, respectively, α and β are related to the production rate of the small molecules by chain scission, m is the average degree of polymerisation of the small molecules, and n is the exponent for acid dissociation, which is usually taken as 0.5. D is the diffusion coefficient of the small molecules in a degrading polymer, which is calculated by

$$D = D_{\text{polymer}} + \left(1.3V_{\text{pore}}^2 - 0.3V_{\text{pore}}^3\right)\left(D_{\text{pore}} - D_{\text{polymer}}\right) \quad [7.4]$$

in which V_{pore} is the porosity of the polymer caused by the loss of the small molecules given by

$$V_{\text{pore}} = \frac{R_{ol} - (C_{ol} - C_{ol0})}{C_{e0}} = \alpha\left(\frac{R_s}{C_{e0}}\right)^{\beta} - \frac{C_{ol} - C_{ol0}}{C_{e0}} \quad [7.5]$$

D_{polymer} and D_{pore} are diffusion coefficients of the small molecules in non-degraded polymer and liquid-filled pores, respectively. Here C_{ol0} is the concentration of residual monomers that may exist in the polymer. The average molecular weight is calculated using

$$\frac{M_n}{M_{n0}} = \frac{1 - \alpha\left(R_s/C_{e0}\right)^{\beta}}{1 + N_{\text{dp0}}\left(\left(R_s/C_{e0}\right) - \left(\alpha/m\right)\left(R_s/C_{e0}\right)^{\beta}\right)} \quad [7.6]$$

in which M_{n0} is initial number-averaged molecular weight, N_{dp0} is the initial average degree of polymerisation of the polymer, and $N_{\text{dp0}} = M_{n0} / M_0$ in which M_0 is the molecular weight of a single repeating unit of the polymer.

7.2 Case study A: a three-dimensional cube

A simple three-dimensional cube is created using COMSOL®'s own geometry tools in this case. Equations [7.2] and [7.3] are applied into PDE interfaces. Boundary conditions will also be determined. Post-processing is carried out, which can help us analyse the results.

7.2.1 Problem description

Geometry and boundary conditions

A 1 × 1 × 1 mm three-dimensional cube is demonstrated here. All boundaries of this cube are considered to be exposed to the aqueous medium, so that C_{ol} equals zero during degradation process at all boundaries.

Independent variables

Independent variables in an FEM include space and time variables: **x, y, z** and **t.**

Dependent variables

Master Equation [7.2] and diffusion Equation [7.3] yield two dependent variables: R_s and C_{ol}. Rest of the variables that can be expressed directly from these two dependent variables and material properties are known as secondary variables.

7.2.2 FEM implementation steps

A-I Starting a new model

1. Double click COMSOL Multiphysics®
2. In the **Model Wizard** page, select **3D** on the **Select Space Dimension** page (see Figure 7.2), and click **Next** button (⇨).

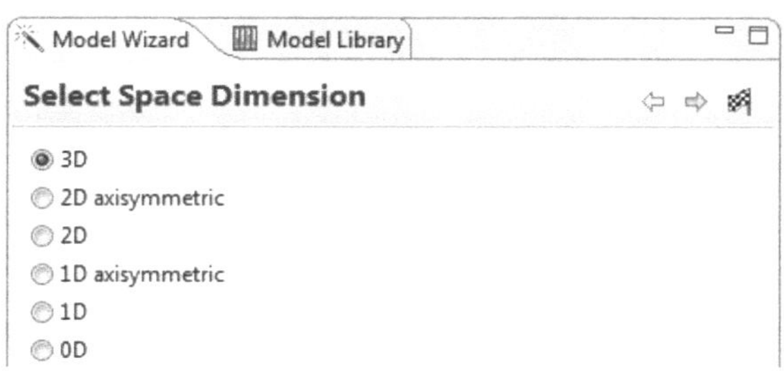

Figure 7.2

3. In **Add Physics**, expand the **Mathematics > PDE Interfaces** node in the list of physics interfaces and select **General From PDE** ***(g)***.
4. Click the **Add Selected** button (+) underneath the list to add the selected PDE interface to the model. The interface is now added to **Selected physics**.
5. Underneath **Selected physics**, you may define dependent variables in **Dependent variables.** We keep the **Field name** unchanged but alter **Number of dependent variables** to 2. Readers may name these two **Dependent variables** as **Rs** and **Col** as shown in Figure 7.3. Then click **Next** button (⇨) in the upper right corner of the **Model Wizard** window.
6. In **Studies**, click **Time Dependent** under the **Preset Studies** page and then click the Finish button (🏁) in the upper right corner of the **Model Wizard** window.

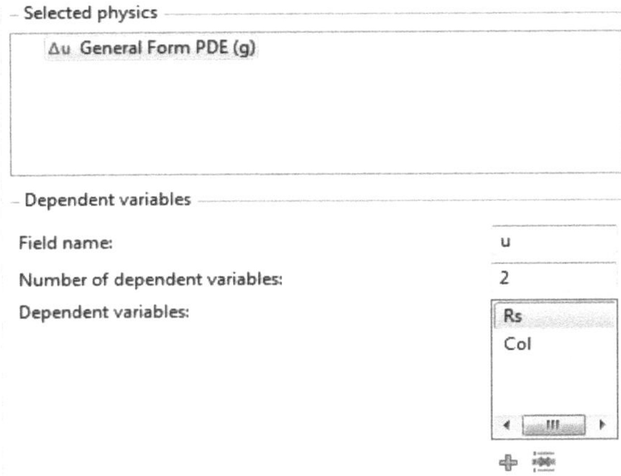

Figure 7.3

A-II Define global parameters

After step A-I, a new physics has been added into the model. Instead of defining a new material, we define all parameters (including material properties) in **Global Definitions**: right click **Global Definitions** and select **Parameters.** In **Parameters**, click **Load File**

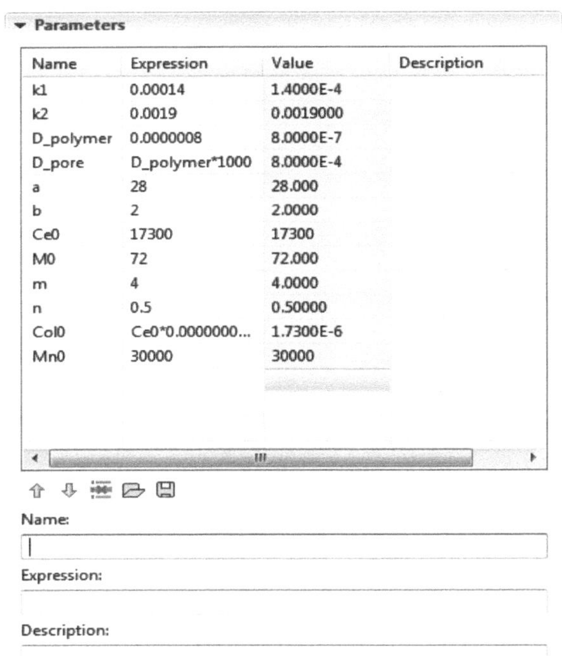

Parameters

Name	Expression	Value	Description
k1	0.00014	1.4000E-4	
k2	0.0019	0.0019000	
D_polymer	0.0000008	8.0000E-7	
D_pore	D_polymer*1000	8.0000E-4	
a	28	28.000	
b	2	2.0000	
Ce0	17300	17300	
M0	72	72.000	
m	4	4.0000	
n	0.5	0.50000	
Col0	Ce0*0.0000000...	1.7300E-6	
Mn0	30000	30000	

Figure 7.4

button (📂) to load a text file 'parameters.txt', which contains values of all parameters, see Figure 7.4. Alternatively, if the text is not available, readers may manually input every parameter one by one in the boxes underneath, as shown in Figure 7.4. Values of all the parameters shown in Figure 7.4 are fixed throughout the chapter.

A-III Define model variables

Right click **Definitions** under **Model1 (*mol1*)** and select **Variables.** We will enter two new variables in **Variables** manually, which are **Vpore** from Equation [7.5] and **D** from Equation [7.4], as shown in Figure 7.5.

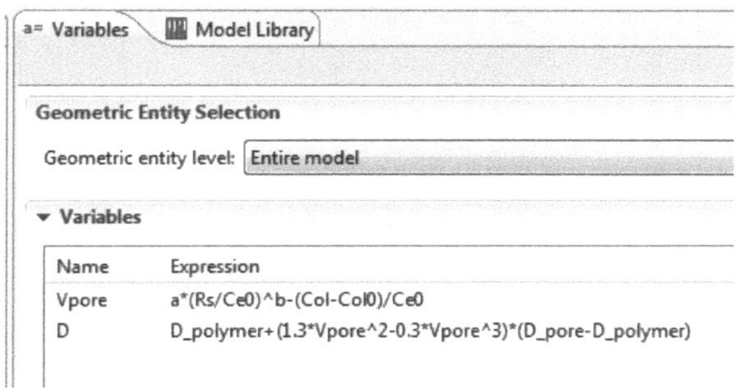

Figure 7.5

Click **Save to File** button (💾), save the defined variables as text file 'variables.txt' for future use.

A-IV Create Geometry

1. Click **Geometry1** in **Model1*(mod1)***, in **Units** page change **Length Unit** to 'mm'. Right click **Geometry1**, and select **Block** to insert a three-dimensional cube (see Figure 7.6).

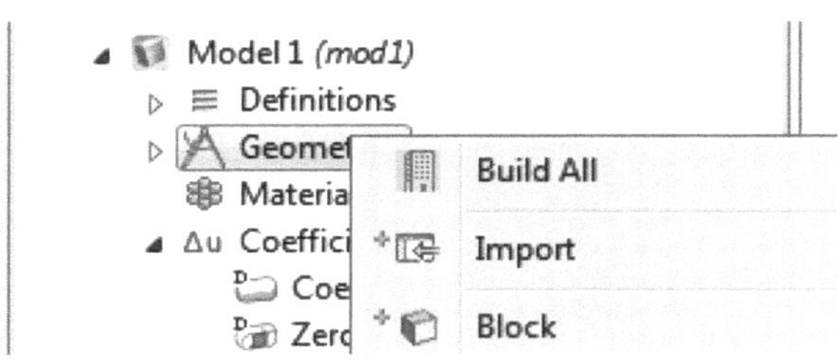

Figure 7.6

2. In **Block** page, enter **Width=Depth=Height=**1 mm. Then click **Build All** button (Build All) in the upper left corner of **Block** page. A 1×1×1 mm three-dimensional cube appears in the **Graphics** window as shown in Figure 7.7.

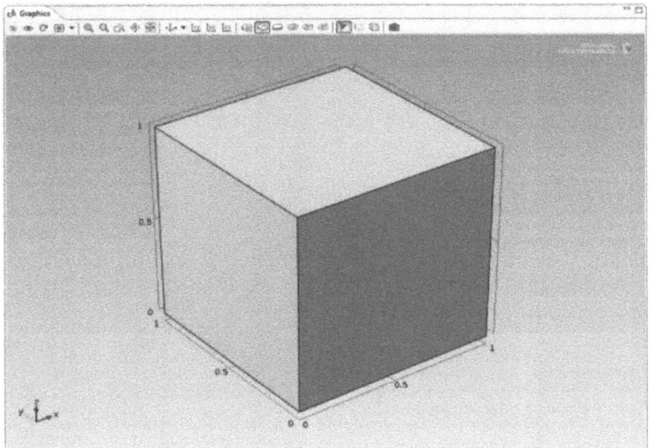

Figure 7.7

A-V Input PDEs in COMSOL®

In a **General Form PDE** module of COMSOL®, a transient general type of a PDE is[7]:

$$\begin{cases} e_a \dfrac{\partial^2 u}{\partial t^2} + d_a \dfrac{\partial u}{\partial t} + \nabla \cdot \Gamma = f & \text{in } \Omega \\ -\mathbf{n} \cdot \Gamma = G + \left(\dfrac{\partial R}{\partial u} \right)^T \mu & \text{on } \partial\Omega \\ 0 = R & \text{on } \partial\Omega \end{cases} \quad [7.7]$$

where Ω is the computational domain, $\partial\Omega$ is the domain boundaries, **n** is the outward unit normal vector on $\partial\Omega$. Term e_a is the mass coefficient, d_a is a damping coefficient or a mass coefficient, Γ is the conservative flux vector and f is the source term. In Equation set [7.7], the first equation is a PDE while the second and the third equations are the Neumann and Dirichlet boundary conditions, respectively. u is a PDE variable and in this case $u = [R_s, C_{ol}]^T$, and $\nabla = [\partial/\partial x, \partial/\partial y, \partial/\partial z]$. Rearranging Equations [7.2] and [7.3] we have:

$$1 \times \frac{dR_s}{dt} = C_{e0}\left[1 - \alpha\left(\frac{R_s}{C_{e0}}\right)^{\beta}\right]\left\{k_1 + k_2 C_{e0}^n \left[\frac{1}{m}\left(\frac{C_{ol}}{C_{e0}}\right)\right]^n\right\} \quad [7.8]$$

$$1 \times \frac{dC_{ol}}{dt} + (-\alpha\beta)\left(\frac{R_s}{C_{e0}}\right)^{\beta-1} \times \frac{dR_s}{dt} + \nabla \cdot \left(-D_x \frac{\partial C_{ol}}{\partial x} - D_y \frac{\partial C_{ol}}{\partial y} - D_z \frac{\partial C_{ol}}{\partial z}\right) = 0 \quad [7.9]$$

The matrix versions of Equations [7.8] and [7.9] are written as:

$$\begin{bmatrix} 1 & 0 \\ (-\alpha\beta)\left(\frac{R_s}{C_{e0}}\right)^{\beta-1} & 1 \end{bmatrix} \begin{bmatrix} \frac{\partial R_s}{\partial t} \\ \frac{\partial C_{ol}}{\partial t} \end{bmatrix} + \nabla\cdot\begin{bmatrix}\Gamma_{R_s} & \Gamma_{C_{ol}}\end{bmatrix} = \begin{bmatrix} C_{e0}\left[1-\alpha\left(\frac{R_s}{C_{e0}}\right)^{\beta}\right]\left\{k_1 + k_2 C_{e0}^{n}\left[\frac{1}{m}\left(\frac{C_{ol}}{C_{e0}}\right)\right]^{n}\right\} \\ 0 \end{bmatrix} \qquad [7.10]$$

By comparing Equation [7.10] with the first equation in Equations set [7.7], expressions for each coefficient in Equation [7.7] can be derived:

$$e_a = \begin{bmatrix} 0 & 0 \\ 0 & 0 \end{bmatrix},\quad d_a = \begin{bmatrix} 1 & 0 \\ (-\alpha\beta)\left(\frac{R_s}{C_{e0}}\right)^{\beta-1} & 1 \end{bmatrix},\quad \Gamma_{R_s} = \begin{bmatrix} 0 \\ 0 \\ 0 \end{bmatrix},\quad \Gamma_{C_{ol}} = \begin{bmatrix} -D_x \frac{\partial C_{ol}}{\partial x} \\ -D_y \frac{\partial C_{ol}}{\partial y} \\ -D_z \frac{\partial C_{ol}}{\partial z} \end{bmatrix}$$

$$f = \begin{bmatrix} C_{e0}\left[1-\alpha\left(\frac{R_s}{C_{e0}}\right)^{\beta}\right]\left\{k_1 + k_2 C_{e0}^{n}\left[\frac{1}{m}\left(\frac{C_{ol}}{C_{e0}}\right)\right]^{n}\right\} \\ 0 \end{bmatrix} \qquad [7.11]$$

To enter coefficients into COMSOL®, expand **General Form PDE (g)** and click **General Form PDE1.** In the **General Form PDE** page, expand **Conservative Flux** and enter each component in $\Gamma = \begin{bmatrix}\Gamma_{R_s} & \Gamma_{C_{ol}}\end{bmatrix}$ from Equation [7.11] into the box as shown in Figure 7.8. In Figure 7.8. Colx, Coly and Colz represent the gradient of C_{ol}. Expand the **Source Term**, enter each component of vector f as shown in Figure 7.9. In the **Damping or Mass Coefficient**, enter each component of matrix d_a as shown in Figure 7.10 using the expressions from Equation [7.11].

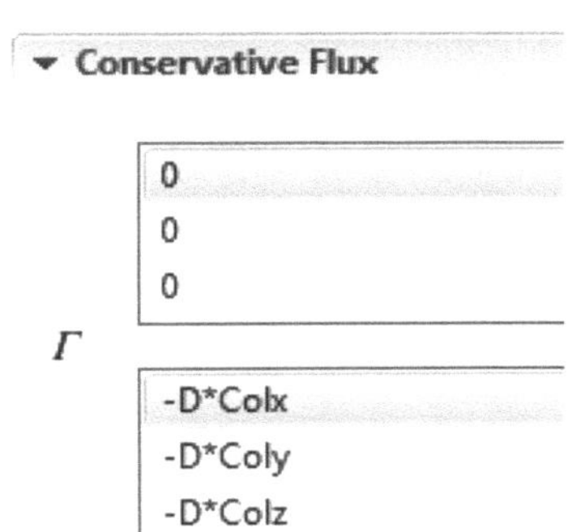

Figure 7.8

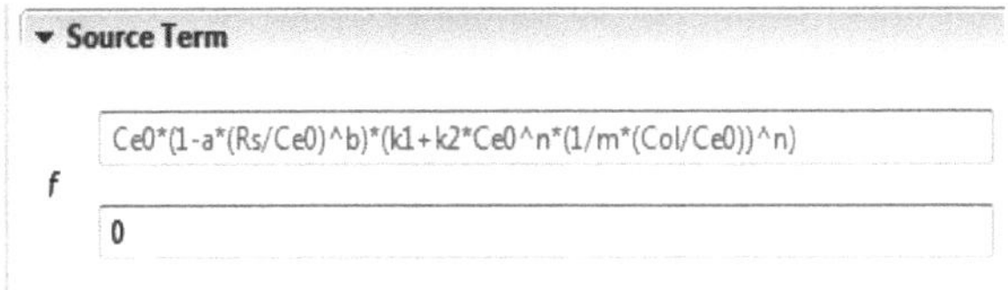

Figure 7.9

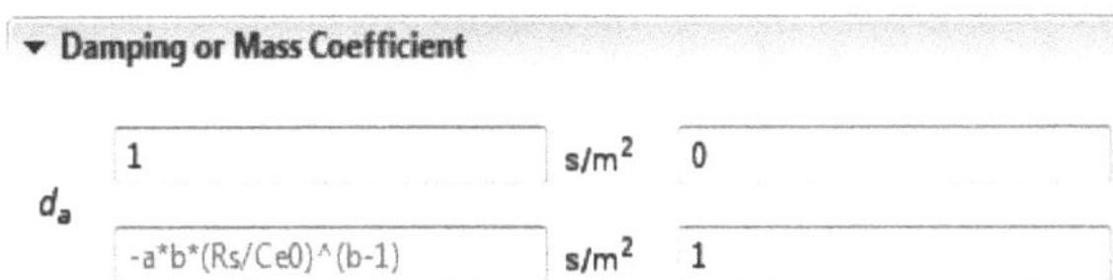

Figure 7.10

A-VI Set initial values

Click **Initial Values1** to add initial values for the dependent variables that serve as initial conditions for a transient simulation or as initial guesses for a non-linear solver. In **Domain Selection**, from the **Selection** list, choose **All domains** to define an initial value. Enter initial value for $C_{ol}(t=0) = C_{ol0}$only and keep other values as default zeros as shown in Figure 7.11.

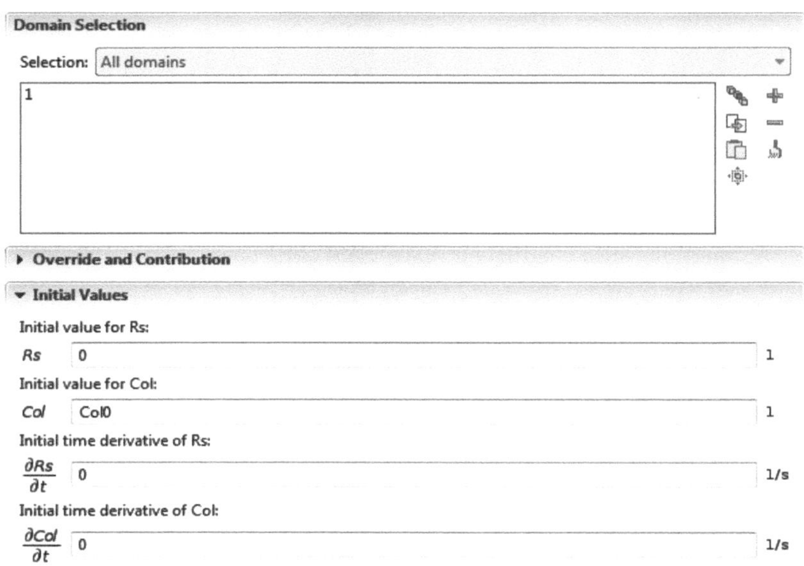

Figure 7.11

A-VII Boundary conditions for the PDE interfaces

Right click **General Form PDE** ***(g)***, select **Dirichlet Boundary Condition** (detailed information of each boundary condition can be found in COMSOL® Users Guide). Select **Dirichlet Boundary Condition1**, in **Boundary Selection**, and from **Selection** list choose **All boundaries** to define a Dirichlet boundary condition on each side. In **Dirichlet Boundary Condition**, tick check box of **Prescribed value of Col** to activate **Dirichlet Boundary Condition** for dependent variable C_{ol}, see Figure 7.12 for reference.

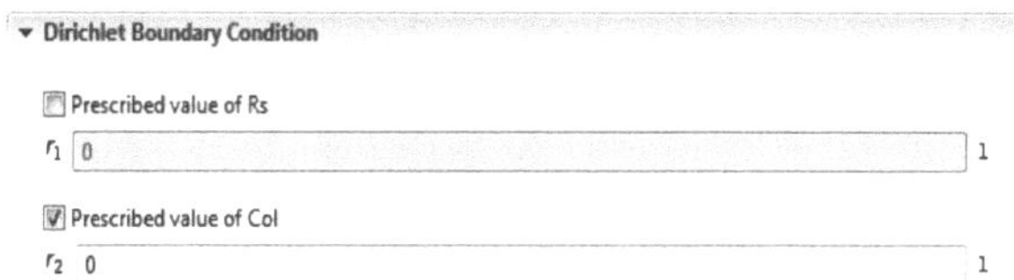

Figure 7.12

A-VIII Mesh

The **Mesh** features enable the discretisation of the geometry model into small units of simple shapes, referred to as elements. In the **Mesh** page, from **Sequence type** list, there are two mesh techniques, which are **Physics-controlled mesh** and **User-controlled mesh**, respectively. In this FEM case, we choose **Physics-controlled mesh** for simplicity. From **Element size** list, **Coarser** size is selected. Click **Build All** () button in the left upper corner of **Mesh** page. Now we have a discretised (meshed) model shown in Figure 7.13. In the **Messages** window, readers can find all kinds of information regarding the current command. It displays the number of elements in the current mesh, which is 2463 in this case, see Figure 7.14.

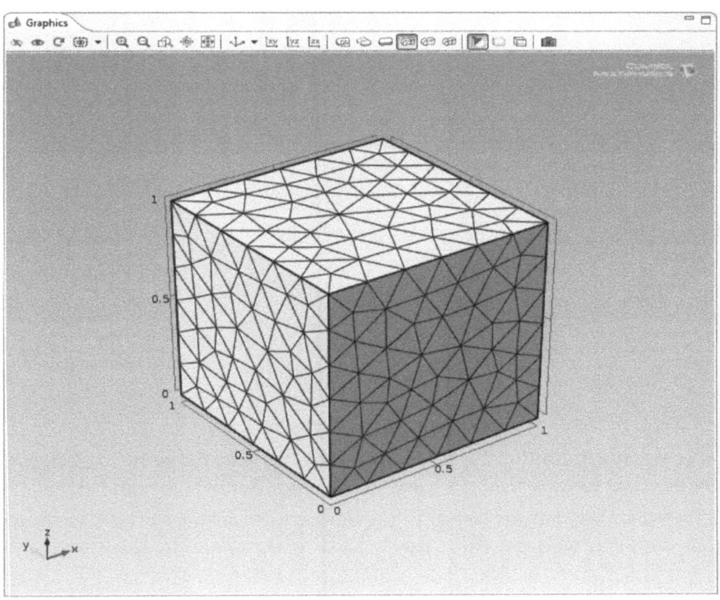

Figure 7.13

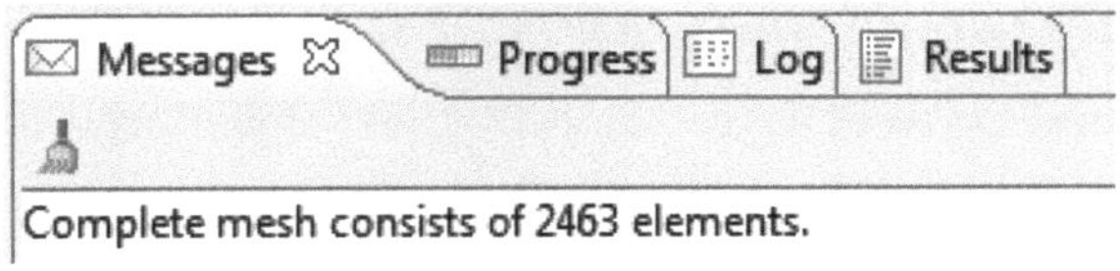

Figure 7.14

A-IX Solve PDEs

Under the **Study 1** node, click **Step 1: Time Dependent**. In **Study Settings**, change **Times** to range (0,0.01,10), in which 10 (weeks) is the total degradation time of this modelling. The time step is set to be 0.01 (week), as shown in Figure 7.15. The selection of the time step is dependent on the time integration schemes that are implemented in COMSOL®. However, a generic scheme that can be used to select the time step will be described in the **A-XI Convergence analysis** section. Go back to **Study1**, click **Compute** button ( ) in the left upper corner of **Study** page to solve PDEs using default solvers. During the solving process, readers can check the convergence status of each step by clicking the **Convergence Plot1** tap for **Nonlinear solver** or **Convergence Plot2** tap for **Time-dependent solver (BDF)**. After a few seconds of computation time, the default plot is displayed in the **Graphics** window. Other information of computations can be found by clicking the **Messages** or **Log** tabs, as shown in Figure 7.16.

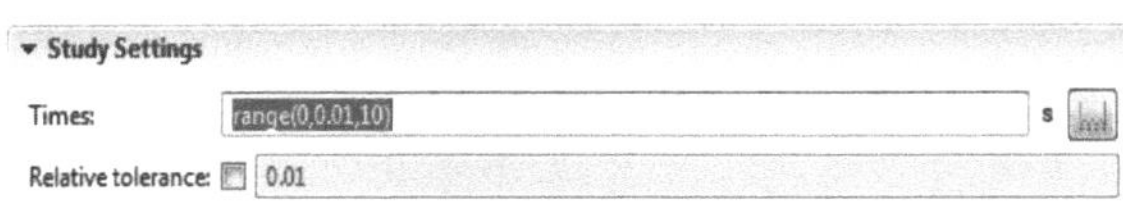

Figure 7.15

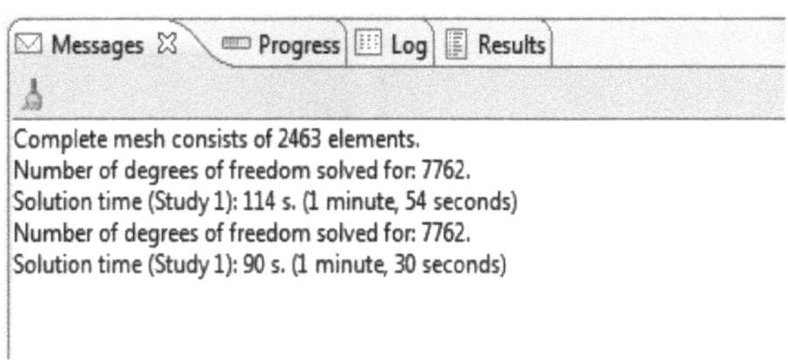

Figure 7.16

A-X Post-processing

The default distribution on slices at time 10 are displayed in the **Graphics** window. In the **Model Builder**, right click **Results>Data Sets**, add a section plane by clicking add **Cut Plane** (Cut Plane). In the **Cut Plane** page, enter the plane data as shown in Figure 7.17. Click **Plot** button (Plot) in the upper left corner of the **Cut Plane** page; a section view which is highlight lighted in grey is displayed in the **Graphics** window, see Figure 7.18. Right click **Results** node and add a **2D Plot Group**. In the **2D Plot**

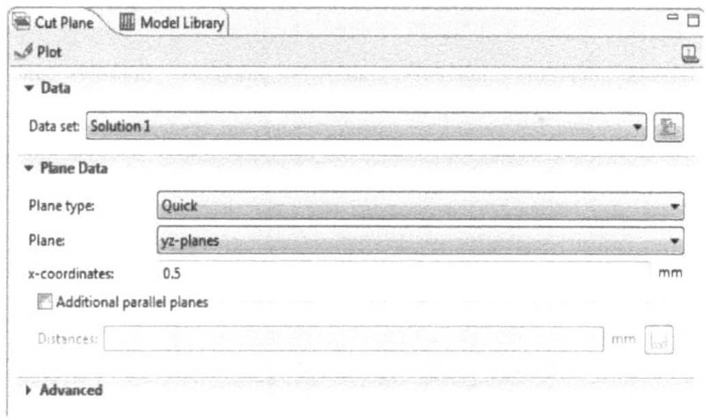

Figure 7.17

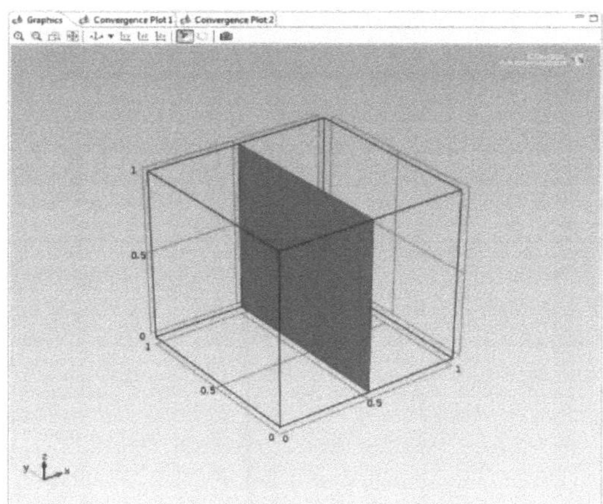

Figure 7.18

Group page, from **Data set** list select **Cut Plane 1**, and from the **Time** list, select **10**. Right click **2D Plot Group 2** (2D Plot Group 2) and add a **Surface** (Surface 1) node to it. Keep the default settings, and then click Plot button (Plot).R_s distribution on Cut Plane 1 is now displayed in the **Graphics** window as shown in Figure 7.19 (Plate II in the colour section between pages 130 and 131). In order to plot an average M_n over the entire volume as a function of time, we need to define M_n under **Results>Derived Values,** and then click **Integration>Volume Integration.** In the **Volume Integration** page, select the three-dimensional cube in the **Graphics** window and then click **Add to Selection** button (+) to add the cube into the **selection list**. In the **Expression** tab, enter the expression of M_n from Equation [7.6] as shown in Figure 7.20. Note that the expression in Equation [7.6] needs to be divided by the whole volume of the domain in order to get an averaged value. Click the **Evaluate** button (Evaluate) to display all integration values in the **Results** window under the **Graphics** window. Readers can either copy these values to **Clipboard** for further analysis, or plot them directly in COMSOL®. Click the **Graph Plot** button ( ) to plot these values as a function of time and a plot is now displayed in the **Graphics** window shown in Figure 7.21.

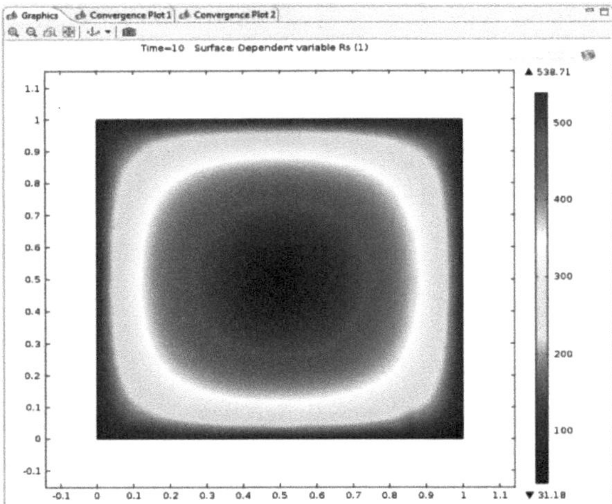

Figure 7.19

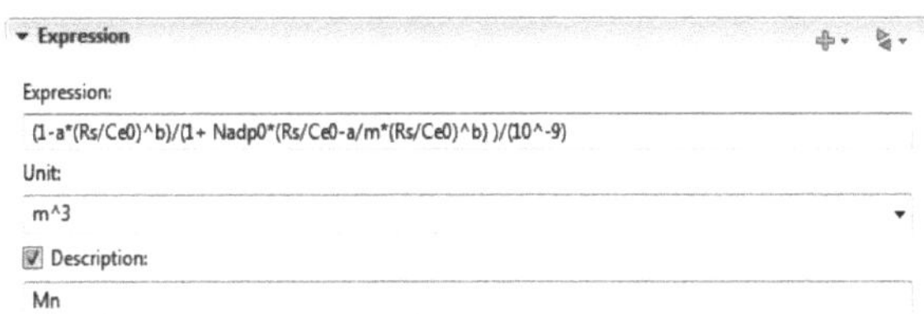

Figure 7.20

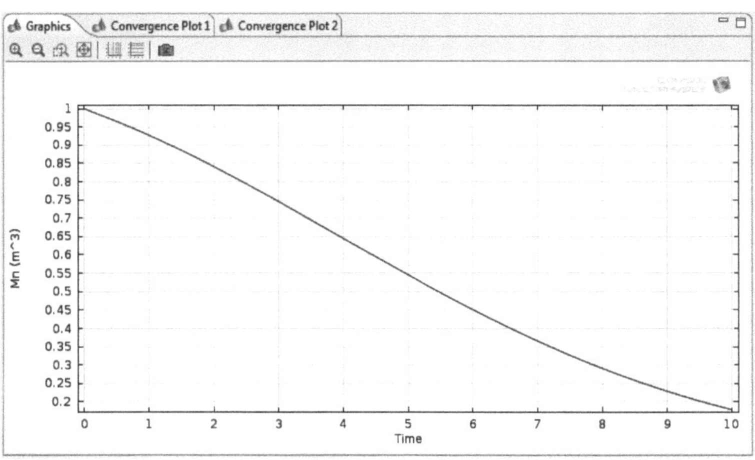

Figure 7.21

A-XI Convergence analysis

Both the spatial meshe and the temporal step need to be analysed so that a convergence solution can be guaranteed. Selections of a spatial mesh and a temporal step are dependent on the numerical solver implemented. Given the fact that different solvers may be used for different physical problems, it is not practical to provide a convergence analysis scheme for each problem. A generic scheme is, however, given here for readers to check the convergence of their own problem:

1. Select a mesh density d.
2. Select a time step Δt.
3. Solve the problem based on d and Δt, and obtain the solution, S.
4. Reduce Δt to $\Delta t'$ and obtain another solution S'.
5. Calculate $\Delta S = |S - S'|$ and select a very small number ε.
6. If $\Delta S < \varepsilon$, $\Delta t = \Delta t$, $S = S$ and go to Step 7; else $\Delta t = \Delta t'$, $S = S'$ and go to Step 4; (temporal convergence is achieved until this step).
7. Refine mesh by increasing d to d', and obtain another solution S''.
8. Calculate $\Delta S = |S - S''|$ and select a very small number ε'.
9. If $\Delta S < \varepsilon'$, $d = d$, $S = S$ and go to step 10; else $d = d'$, $S = S''$ and go to step 7; (spatial convergence is achieved).
10. End

Using this scheme to analyse the mesh elements generated in this case using **Coarser** size and the time step Δt, we found that they are both spatially and temporally converged.

7.2.3 Degradation analysis

Figure 7.22 (Plate III) illustrates three distributions of number-averaged molecular weights over the cross-section at Week 3, Week 5, and Week 7, respectively. The molecular weights have been normalised by its initial value. From Figure 7.22, it can be observed that obvious heterogeneous degradation starts at Week 3. At Week 5, M_n in the centre of the cube is reduced to 45% of the initial value while on the surface M_n is about 60–70% of the initial value. A shell-like structure emerges at Week 5 when the molecular weight averaged over the entire volume of the cube is about 50% of the initial value, see Figure 7.21. This centre–surface differentiation has been widely observed for devices made of PLA and PGA.[2–3, 9–10]

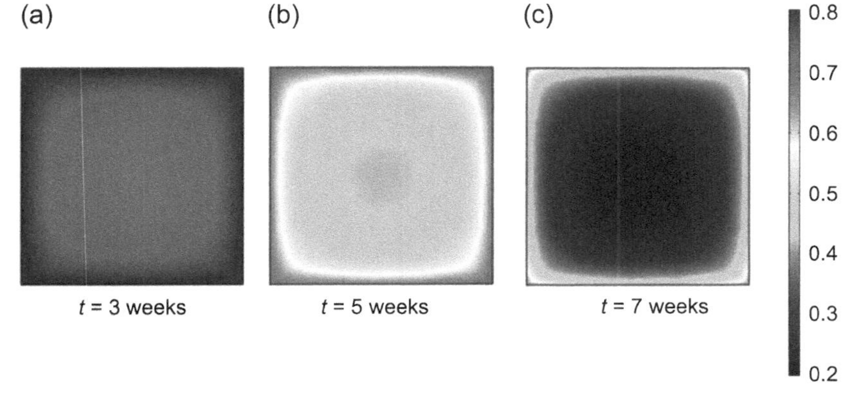

Figure 7.22 Distribution of normalised average molecular weight over the cross-section of the cube indicated by Figure 7.18 at (a) $t = 3$ weeks, (b) $t = 5$ weeks and (c) $t = 7$ weeks.

7.3 Case study B: scaffolds in tissue engineering

In this section, various representative units of scaffolds in bone tissue engineering are generated using COMSOL® with different pore sizes, and porosities. Similar to the Section 7.4, complete tutorials of generating scaffold geometry and implementing the finite element analysis are provided in this section. Finite element analysis is then carried out for each case and the correlations between various geometric parameters and corresponding degradation rates are discovered.

7.3.1 Problem description

In bone tissue engineering, PLA, PGA, and their copolymers are widely used to make scaffolds for tissue generation because of their manufacturability to highly porous foams. The microstructure of a scaffold plays an important role in nutrient transport and waste diffusion. The pore size and its distribution can be designed for different scaffold applications. The purpose in this section is to demonstrate how to use finite element analysis to evaluate the degradation rate in the design of a scaffold. Cases B-I, B-II, and B-III use the same physical equations and parameters in COMSOL® from Case A, but different geometries and boundary conditions are applied. This section will guide readers through the process of establishing new geometries and setting up new boundary conditions. Figure 7.23 illustrates three cases of a cube containing a spherical pore of different sizes. Each case can be regarded as a representative unit of either a uniform scaffold or a different part of the same scaffold that has non-uniform porosity. Case B-I has a pore of 650 μm in diameter and 64.85% porosity, Case B-II has a pore of 100 μm in diameter and 64.85% porosity, and Case B-III has a pore of 650 μm in diameter and 89.59% porosity. L is the unit length for each case whose values are shown in Figure 7.23. Although the representative units of Cases B-I and B-II look the same in geometry, their absolute sizes are different. The inner surface of the pore is where the scaffold is exposed to the aqueous medium. The boundary condition

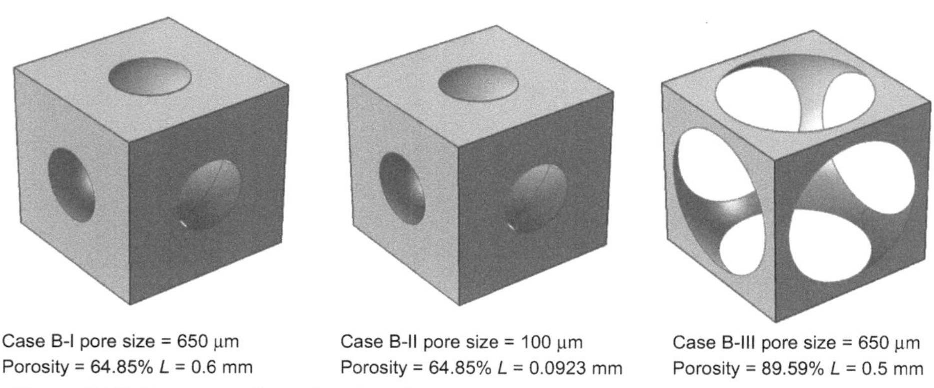

Figure 7.23 Representative units of scaffolds of three different porosities.

at the pore surface is set as $C_{ol} = 0$. Other 'surfaces' of the representative unit are actually local symmetry planes. It is assumed that the small molecules do not diffuse across these planes.

7.3.2 FEM Implementation

Implementation steps in this case are the same with those in Case A, except for the geometries and the boundary conditions. Please refer to Section 7.2.2 for detailed steps, including importing the values of parameters and defining the variables. Geometry creations and boundary conditions employment can be found step by step as follows.

B-I Create geometry of scaffold representative units

Go to **Geometry1**, click the **Block1** node and change the values of Width, Depth and Height to **0.6 mm** in the **Block** page for a block. Click **Build All** button (Build All) to activate the changes. Right click **Geometry1** and select the **Add sphere** button to add a sphere in the centre of the block. Click **Geometry1>Sphere1**, and change sphere coordinates and diameter in the **Sphere** page as shown in Figure 7.24. Click **Build All** button to activate this change. Now we have a geometry consisting of a block and a sphere inside, as shown in the **Graphics** window, see Figure 7.25. Right click **Geometry 1** and select **Boolean Operations>Differences**. In the **Difference** page, select **Block 1** and click **Add to Selection** button (⊕) to add the block into **Objects to add**. Select **Sphere1** and click **Add to Selection** button (⊕) to add the sphere into **Object to subtract**. Click **Build All** button to activate the difference operation. We have now obtained the geometry shown in Figure 7.26 of Case B-I. Repeat **step B-I** for Cases B-II and B-III by changing coordinates and dimensions for both block and sphere.

B-II Boundary conditions

Inner surfaces of the hollow pore inside are exposed to the aqueous medium while outer surfaces of the block are assumed as zero flux boundaries. To input these boundary conditions into our model, go to **Model1>General Form PDE** (g), click **Dirichlet Boundary Conditions1**, in the **Dirichlet Boundary Condition** page, select all inner boundaries **manually** and then click **Add to Selection** button (⊕) to add them into **Boundary Selection** for Dirichlet boundary conditions. Boundary conditions for all outside surfaces are set as the default zero flux boundaries.

B-III Mesh

In the **Mesh** page, select **Physics-controlled mesh**. From the **Element size** list, **Coarser** size is selected. Readers can use the convergence analysis skills mastered from Section 7.2.2, Step A-XI to check the convergence of the mesh. Click **Build All** ( ) button on the left upper corner of the **Mesh** page to activate the mesh.

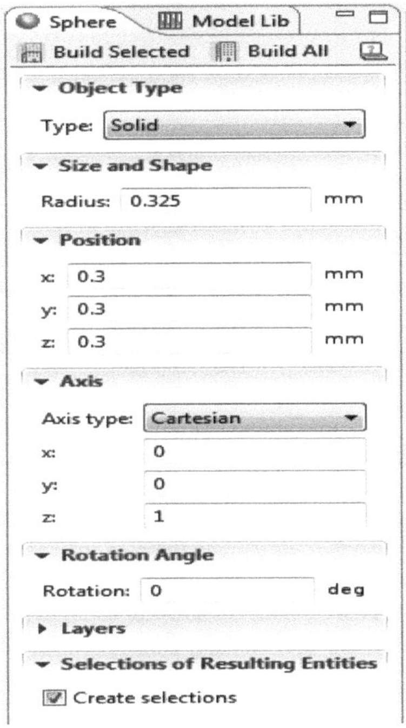

Figure 7.24

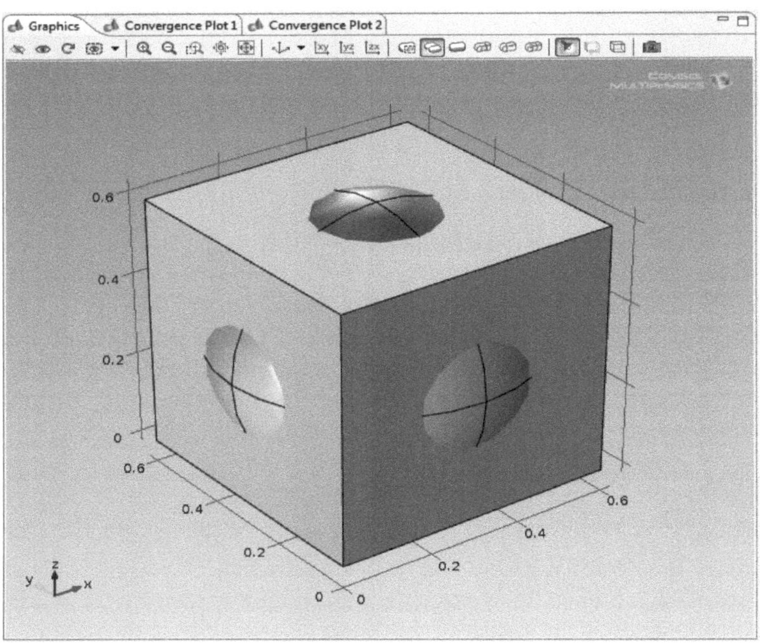

Figure 7.25

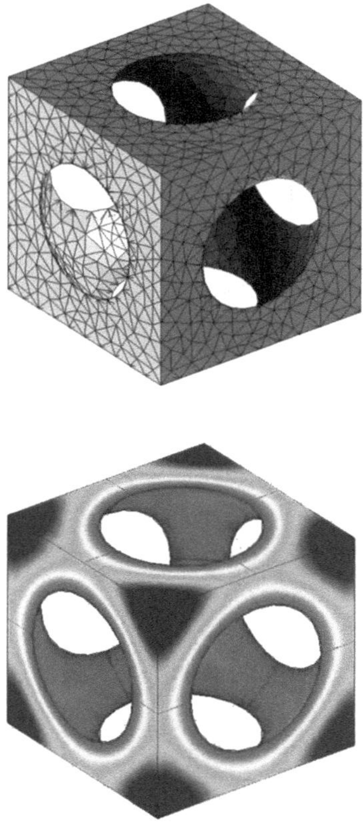

Plate I (Chapter 1) A finite element model for a representative unit of a scaffold.

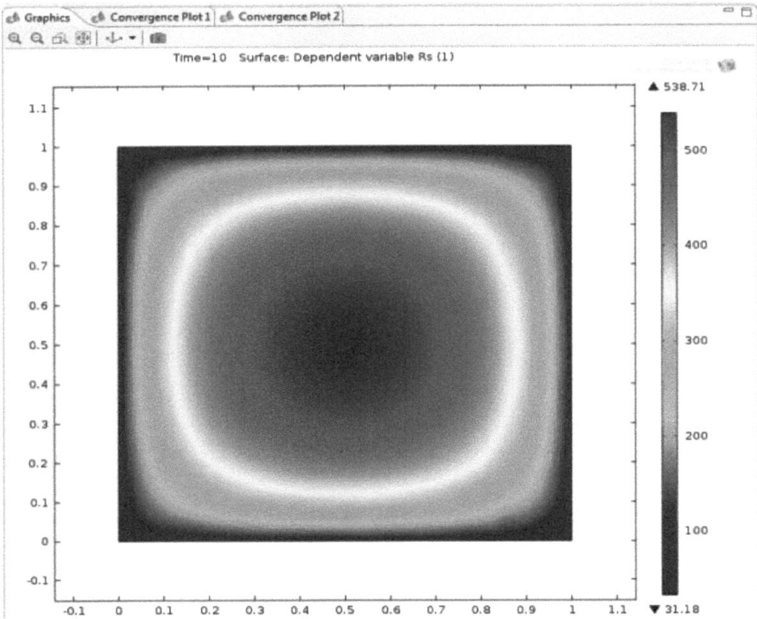

Plate II (Chapter 7) Screenshot from COMSOL®: RS distribution on Cut-plane 1 displayed in the Graphics window.

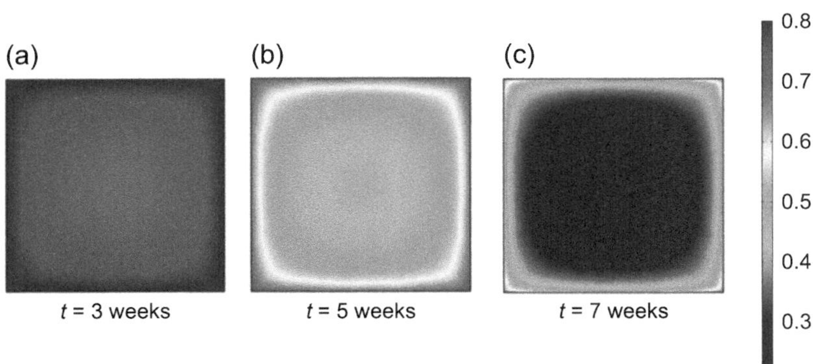

Plate III (Chapter 7) Distribution of normalised average molecular weight over the cross-section of the cube indicated by Fig. 7.5b at (a) $t = 3$ weeks, (b) $t = 5$ weeks and (c) $t = 7$ weeks.

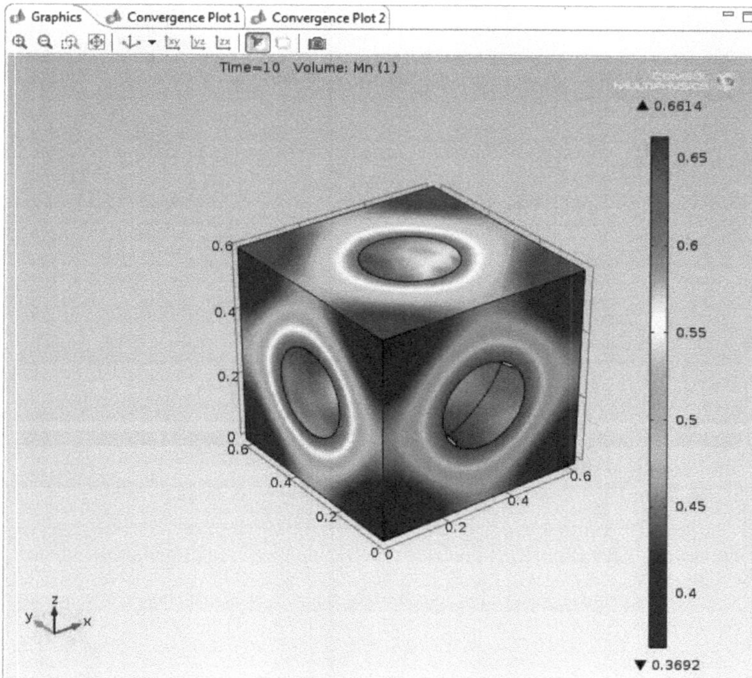

Plate IV (Chapter 7) Screenshot from COMSOL®: Spatial distribution of M is shown at week 10.

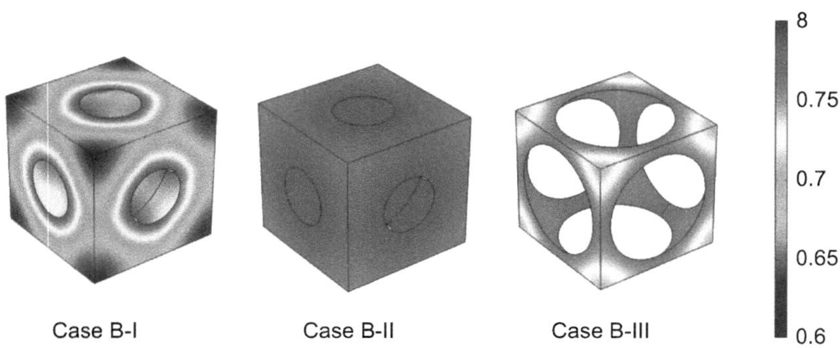

Plate V (Chapter 7) Distribution of normalised average molecular weight at week 5 calculated using finite element models for the three cases.

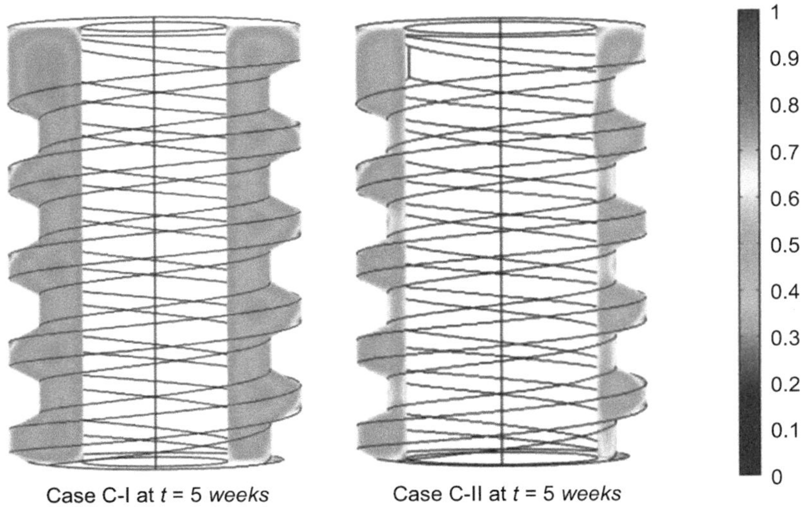

Plate VI (Chapter 7) Number average molecular weight distributions for two cases at week 5.

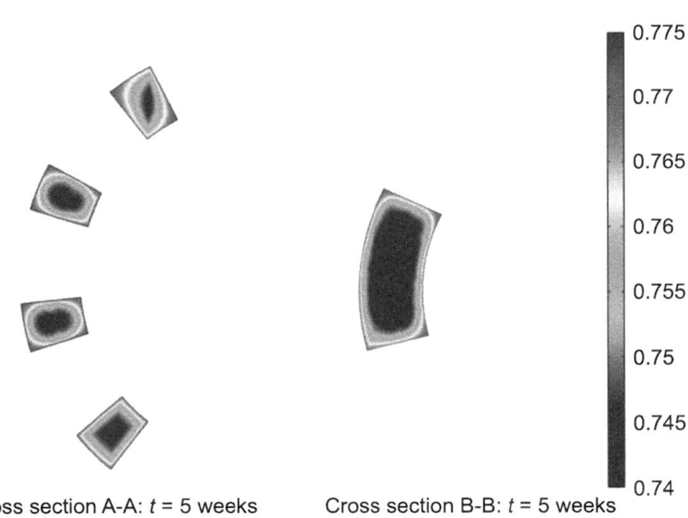

Plate VII (Chapter 7) Number average molecular weight distributions for two sections at 5 weeks.

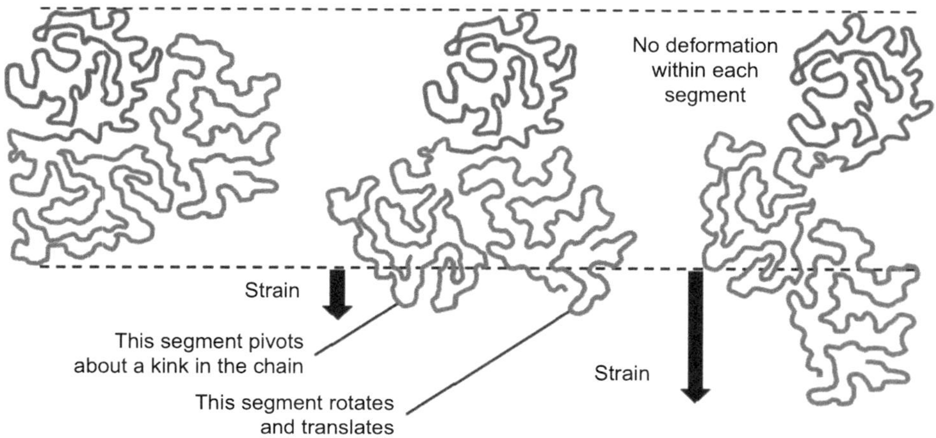

Plate VIII (Chapter 9) Segmental motion during plastic deformation of a glassy amorphous polymer.

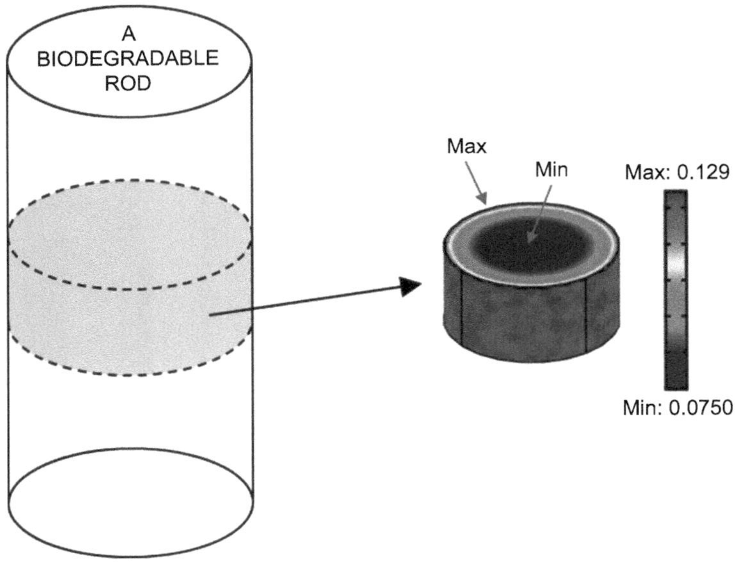

Plate IX (Chapter 9) Figure adapted from the original publication with permission from the publisher Elsevier and the author Wang[2] via the Copyright Clearance Centre. A mathematical model for degradation of molecular weight was implemented in a FEA simulation for a section of a biodegradable rod. The colour indicates normalised molecular weight part-way through degradation. The molecular weight degraded more rapidly in the centre of the rod than at the surface.

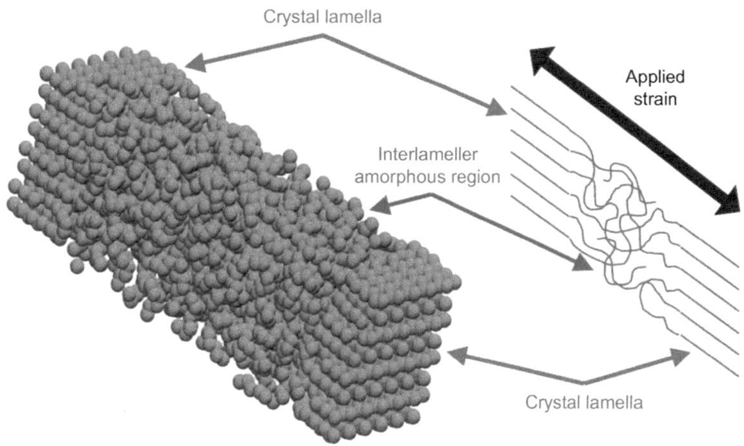

Plate X (Chapter 9) The polymer structure used in MD simulations by Ding *et al.*[34] consisted of an amorphous phase in between two crystalline phases which represent crystal lamellae. To calculate Young's modulus, the crystal lamellae were separated.

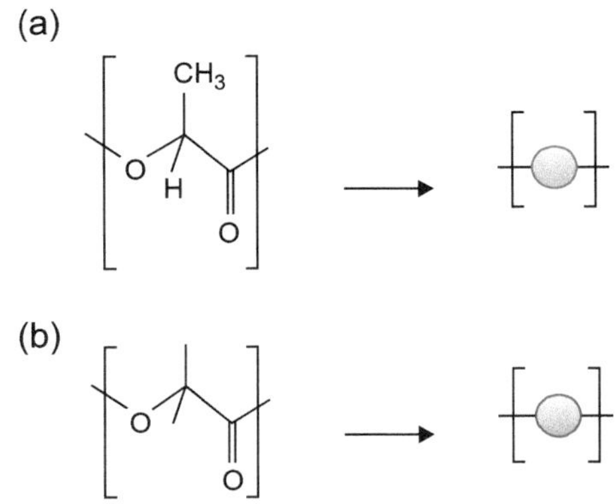

Plate XI (Chapter 10) Repeat units representations (lumped units) in molecular models for (a) PLA and (b) PGA.

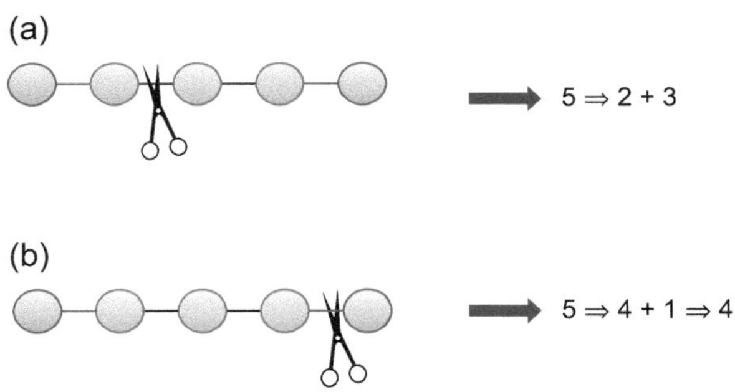

Plate XII (Chapter 10) Schematic diagrams for (a) random chain scission and (b) end chain scission implement methods.

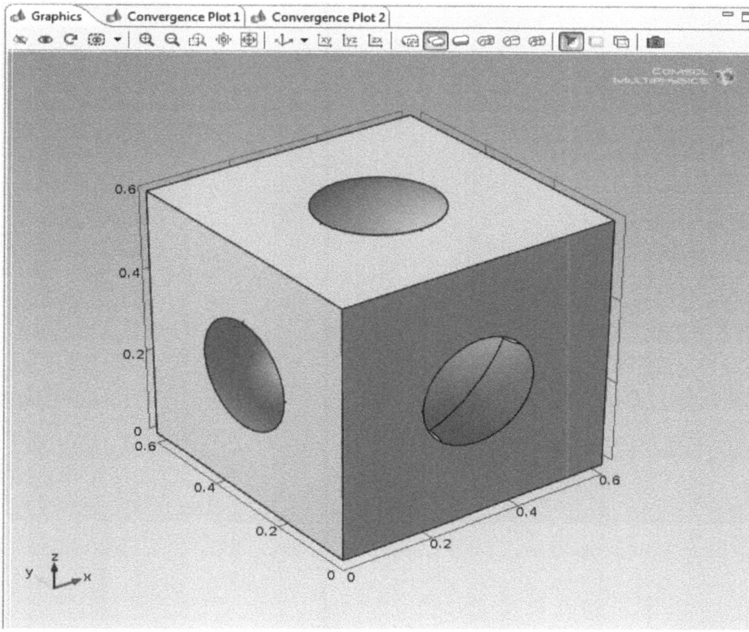

Figure 7.26

B-IV Calculation

Right click **Study1>Compute** to calculate the updated scaffold model. Default display shown in the **Graphics** page is a sliced plot. Right click **3D Plot Group 1>Volume** to add a volume display. Change the **Expression** in the **Volume** page to the number-average molecular weight M_n as shown in Figure 7.27. Spatial distribution of M_n is shown in Figure 7.28 (Plate IV) at week 10. The coloured legend range can be altered by expanding **Range** node in **Volume** page.

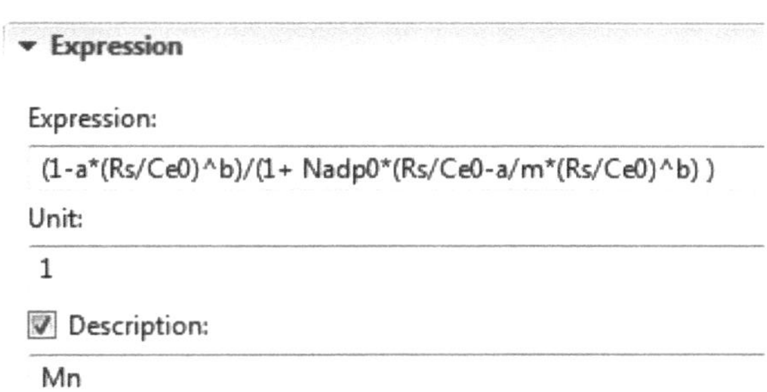

Figure 7.27

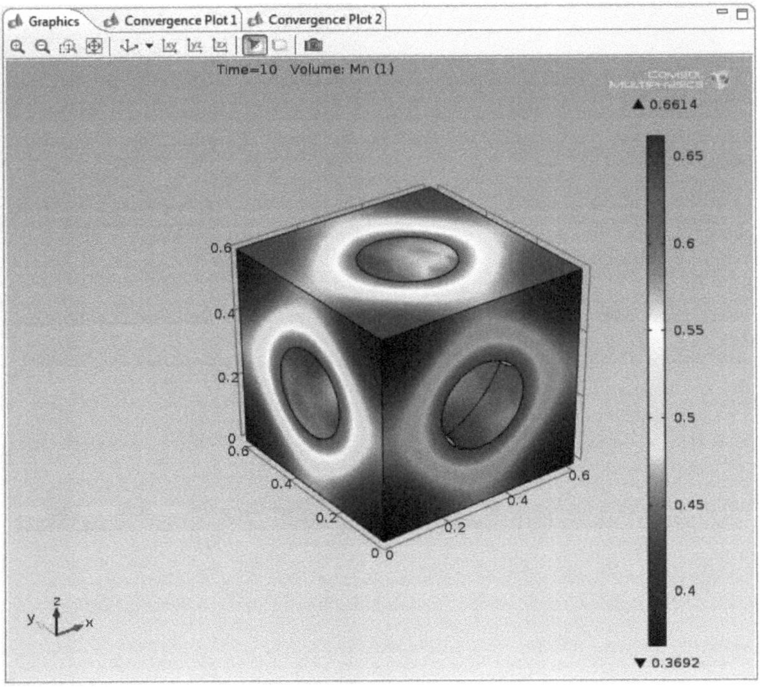

Figure 7.28

7.3.3 Degradation analysis

Repeat Step B-II to Step B-IV, for Case B-II and Case B-III, Figures 7.29 (Plate V) and 7.30 are generated. In Figure. 7.29, it can be found that the number-averaged molecular weight distributions of three cases are widely diverse at Week 5. It is easy to understand that significant difference is found in Case B-I and Case B-III because they have different porosities and geometries. Degradations of Cases B-I and B-III behave totally differently from each other although they seem to have the same geometry and the same porosity. It is their absolute wall thicknesses that affect the molecular weight distributions. In Case B-I, the minimal wall thickness is 0.175 mm, while that of Case B-II reduces to 0.02691 mm. In Figure 7.29, it can also be seen that heterogeneous degradation is not obvious in Case B-II, due to its small value of wall thickness. The characteristic diffusion path for small molecules produced from hydrolysis reactions during degradation is small enough in Case B-II so that these small molecules migrate out of the device instantly, resulting in a rather uniform M_n distribution. Figure 7.30 gives the plots from three cases of the average M_n over the entire domain as functions of time. The degradation rates for Cases B-I, B-II, and B-III are diverse, indicating that the degradation rate of a scaffold is mainly dependent on its average wall thickness. A conclusion can therefore be made that pore size and porosity of a scaffold combined together affect both degradation rate and M_n distribution. In scaffold designs, porosity is predesigned according to clinical demands, and pore size and its distribution thus become the most important controlled parameters.

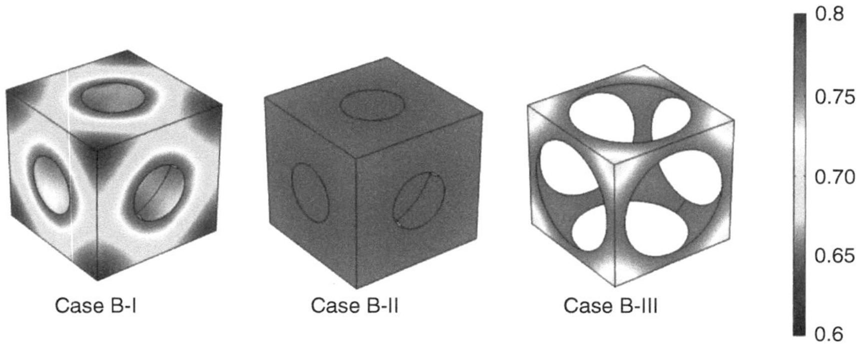

Figure 7.29 Distribution of normalised average molecular weight at week 5 calculated using finite element models for the three cases.

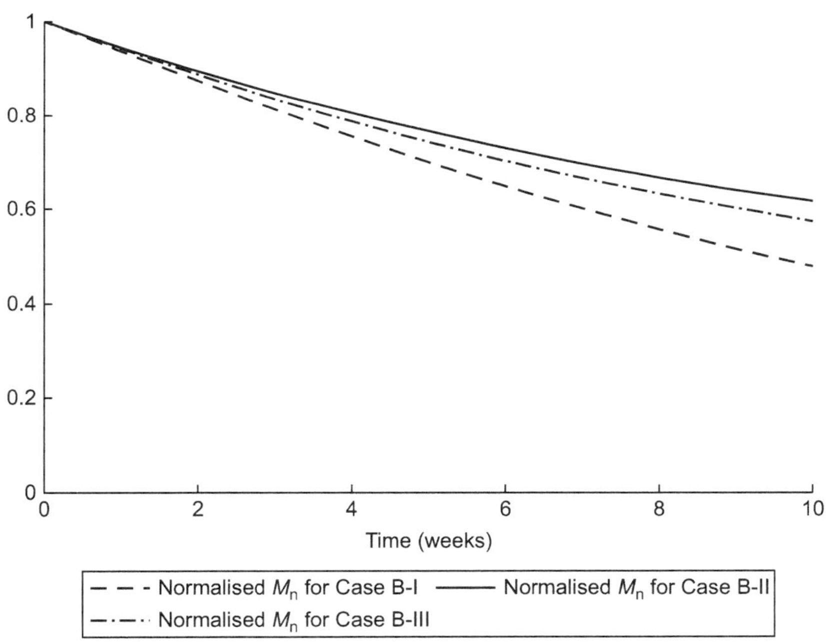

Figure 7.30 Molecular weight averaged over the polymer volume as functions of time for the three cases.

7.4 Case study C: internal bone-fixation screws

Biodegradable internal fixation devices such as screws, pins, and plates are already used in clinical applications such as orthopaedic surgery. The advantage of using biodegradable fixation devices instead of metallic counterparts in bone orthopaedic surgery is obvious – the device simply disappears after the bone heals. Loads

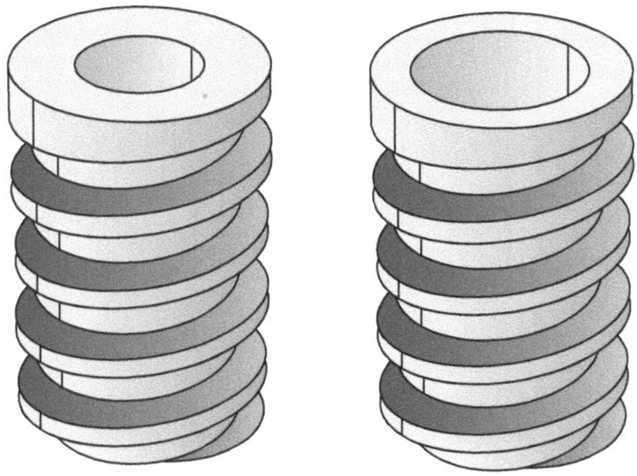

Figure 7.31 Screw geometries.

can slowly shift from the degrading polymer device to the healing bone in a bone remodelling process which ensures a complete healing of the bone. A study carried out by Wang *et al.*[11] suggest a close relationship between the number-average molecular weight and the Young's modulus of a degradable polymer. In order to design a biodegradable screw with the required mechanical demand, finite element analysis of degradation performance is carried out in this section. More specifically, we focus on the screw design with a hollow cavity inside serving as a material delivery channel. The dimensions of screws used in a specific orthopaedic surgery are determined based on the bone-fixation requirements. Those parameters of a screw include the major diameter, the minor diameter, the length, and the pitch angle. Apart from those, the only parameter that is allowed to change is the hollow cavity diameter. Two screw examples with the same dimension but different diameters of cavities are illustrated in Figure 7.31. The dimensions of these screws are: major diameter, 6 mm; minor diameter, 4.75 mm; length, 10 mm; pitch, 2 mm; angle, 60°; and the diameter of the hollow cavity for Case C-I is 3 mm, while that of Case C-II is 4 mm.

7.4.1 Finite element implementation

Readers can either draw geometries of screws in commercial CAD packages, such as Unigraphics NX® and then import them into COMSOL®, or draw them using the Geometry feature of COMSOL® directly. In Case C, all boundaries are outside surfaces that follow the boundary condition $C_{ol} = 0$. By repeating the steps in Case A, Figures 7.32 (Plate VI) and 7.33 can be produced using COMSOL® calculation.

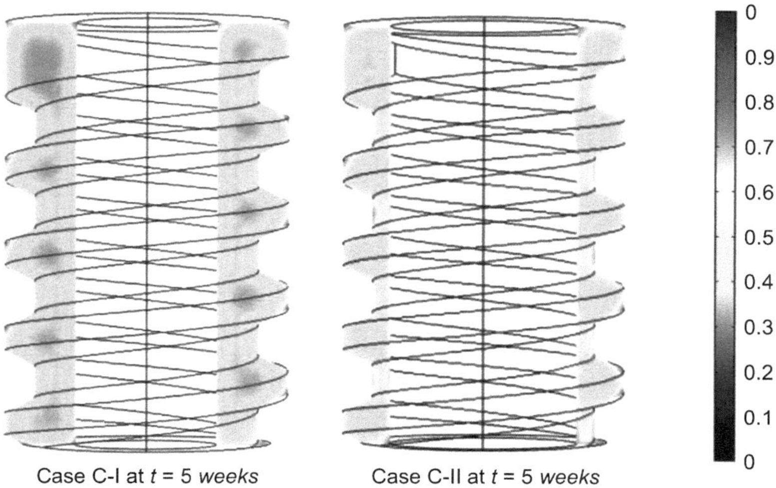

Figure 7.32 Number average molecular weight distributions for two cases at week 5.

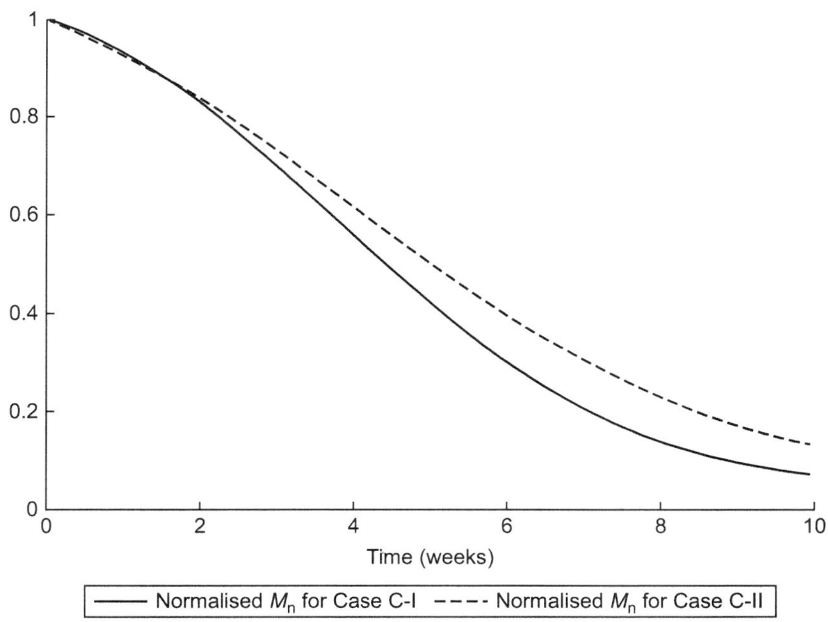

Figure 7.33 Average M_n over the entire volume as functions of time.

7.4.2 Finite element analysis

Figure 7.32 illustrates the calculated distributions of the average molecular weights over the central vertical cross-section of two screws at Week 5, while Figure 7.33 shows the average molecular weights averaged over the entire screw as functions of time. Obvious heterogeneous degradations and a clear size effect can be observed from Figures 7.32 and 7.33, respectively. The screw in Case C-I degrades faster and less uniformly than that in C-II because it has a larger wall thickness. Focusing on Case C-I shown in Figure 7.32 (Plate VI), it is interesting to note the dark blue spots at the core of the shred. This is the area of low average molecular weight caused by acid accumulation. The identical pattern of degradation was observed by Schwach and Vert[12] in their *in vivo* experiment.

7.5 Case study D: coronary stents

A stent is a meshed tube inserted into coronary arteries to prevent localised blood flow constrictions. It can be classified as metallic stents and polymer stents in terms of material, and polymer stents are sub-classified as non-degradable stents and degradable stents. The biodegradable polymer stent has been found advantageous compared to conventional metallic stents and non-degradable polymer stents, due to the nature of its biodegradation, high biocompatibility, and that it can be used as a drug loaded platform. Additionally, its tuneable degradation rate achieved by controlling copolymer ratio or initial molecular weight is very attractive. PLLA is found to be more applicable in human coronary artery disease.

7.5.1 Finite element implementation

In this case, the degradation rate of a representative unit of a 2 mm diameter degradable stent will be tested computationally using FEM by COMSOL®. A representative unit of a stent is shown in Figure 7.34. Again, its geometry can be obtained either from CAD packages or the COMSOL® geometry feature. Although a stent may look complicated in its three-dimensional shape, a large part of it is made of straight columns which degrade in a two-dimensional pattern. For these columns, their cross-sectional size is the characteristic diffusion distance for the small polymer chains and hence decides the degradation rate. The junctions of the columns, however, degrade in a full three-dimensional pattern. Because of their relatively large size, they also degrade faster than the columns. In Figure 7.34, boundaries rather than surfaces 1–5 are exposed to aqueous medium so that $C_{ol} = 0$ is applied as the boundary condition. Surfaces 1–5 are assumed to be zero flux boundaries. In order to identify the size effect at junctions, we cut this stent unit by two planes, and two sections are generated, Sections A-A and B-B, which are shown in Figure 7.35. Cross-section A–A is of a junction, while cross-section B–B is of a column.

7.5.2 Finite element analysis

At Week 5, the number-average molecular weight distributions on two sections are shown in Figure 7.36 (Plate VII). Figure 7.37 compares the molecular weights as functions of time for two points located at the centre of the column and the centre of

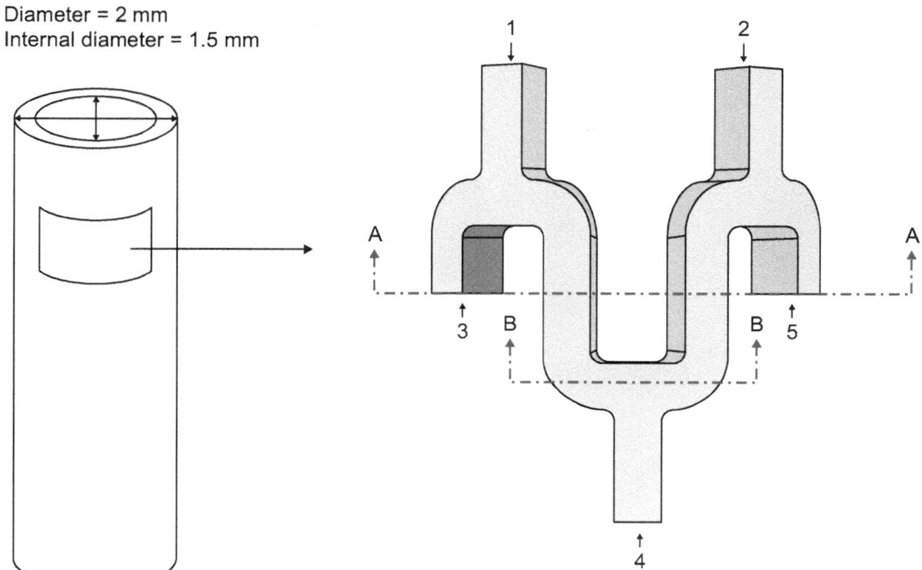

Figure 7.34 Geometry of a representative unit of a 2 mm diameter stent.

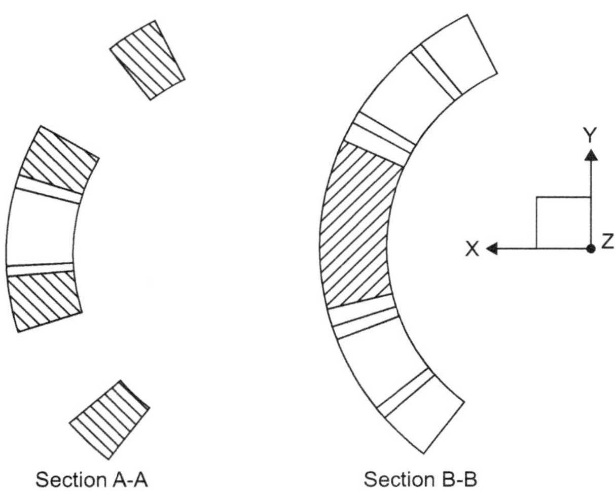

Figure 7.35 Section views A-A and B-B.

the junction, respectively. It is clear that the core of the junction degrades faster than the average rate of the device. If the junction fails, the stent will collapse and lose its ability to function as a complete stent. It is therefore important to design the junctions carefully, so that premature failure can be avoided.

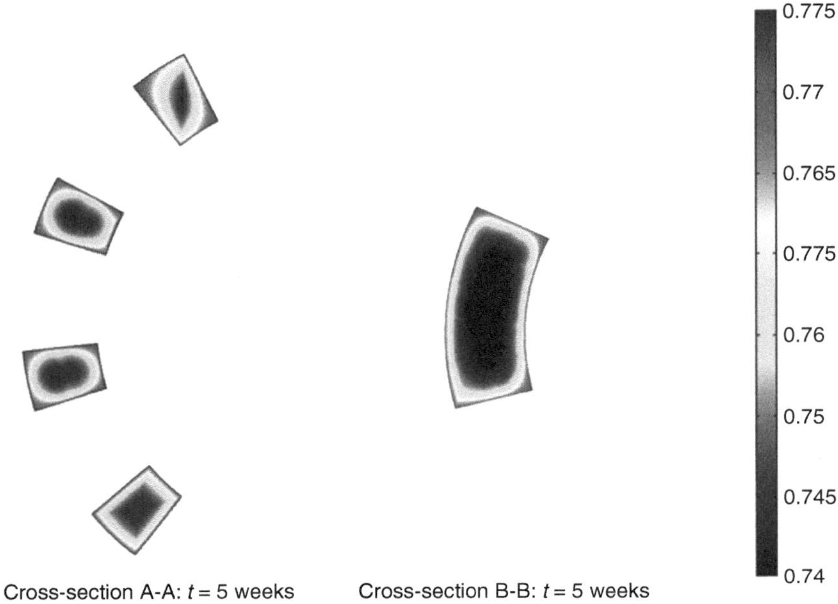

Figure 7.36 Number average molecular weight distributions for two sections at 5 weeks.

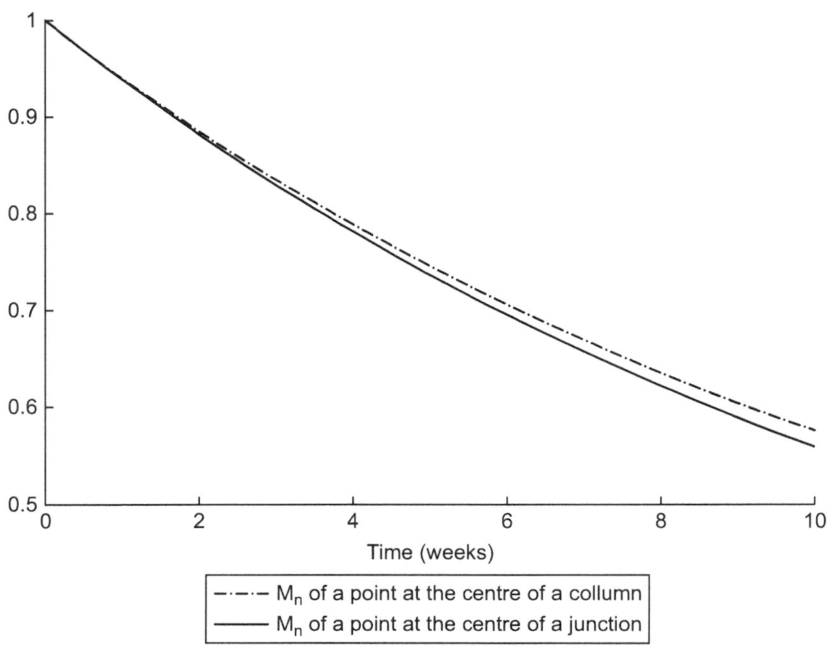

Figure 7.37 Normalised surface integrated M_ns as function of time for two cut planes.

7.6 Conclusions

The biodegradation behaviour of four biodegradable devices – Case A: a simple 3D cube; Case B: scaffolds for bone tissue engineering; Case C: fixation screws; and Case D: the stent – are simulated computationally using a set of PDEs derived from Chapter 6. These PDEs are then solved by FEM. In this chapter, we mainly focus on implementations of these PDEs into COMSOL Multiphysics® for finite element analyses. Step-by-step implementation routes for the first two cases are provided. Similar processes are applied to Case C and Case D with different geometries and boundary conditions. Readers are recommended to practise their modelling skills, learnt from Case A and Case B, on Case C and Case D. Using the **Postprocessing** feature provided by COMSOL®, readers can analyse the degradation behaviours, such as the number-average molecular weights, as functions of time, on the whole domain, at a specific section plane, or even at a point. Through those analyses, we find that the biodegradable device design has close relation with corresponding biodegradation rate. Different geometry parameters are identified from the four cases that are important design features. To choose an appropriate geometry parameter for a certain medical device with desired degradation rate, similar finite element analysis needs to be carried out. Please note, this chapter did not provide the simulations on mechanical behaviours of each medical device during biodegradation, and this can be a future work for readers.

Acknowledgement

COMSOL Multiphysics® software was used in all the finite element calculations presented in this chapter with a licence number 1035154.

References

1. Reed AM and Gilding DK. (1981) Biodegradable polymers for use in surgery – poly(glycolic)/poly(lactic acid) homo and copolymers: 2. *In vitro* degradation. *Polymer*, **22**, pp. 494–498.
2. Li SM, Garreau H and Vert M. (1990) Structure-property relationships in the case of the degradation of massive aliphatic poly(a-hydroxy acids) in aqueous media – Part 1: Poly(DL-lactic acid). *Journal of Materials Science: Materials in Medicine*, **1**, pp. 123–130.
3. Hurrell S and Cameron R. (2003) The effect of buffer concentration, pH and buffer ions on the degradation and drug release from polyglycolide. *Polymer International*, **52**, pp. 358–366.
4. Grizzi I, Garreau S, Li S and Vert M. (1995) Hydrolytic degradation of devices based on poly(DL-lactic acid) size-dependence. *Biomaterials*, **16**, pp. 305–311.
5. Cook RD, Malkus DS, Plesha ME and Witt RJ. (2001) *Concepts and Applications of Finite Element Analysis*. 4th edn: John Wiley & Sons, New York.

6. Huang R and Pan J. (2009) Inverse engineering of medical devices made of bioresorbable polymers. *Computer Method in Biomechanics and Biomedical Engineering*, **13**, pp. 291–303.
7. Comsol. (2012) The COMSOL Multiphysics User's Guide. COMSOL 4.3 ed: COMSOL.
8. COMSOL Multiphysics® v. 4.3b. www.comsol.com COMSOL AB, Stockholm, Sweden.
9. Hurrell S and Cameron R. (2001) Polyglycolide: degradation and drug release. Part I: Changes in morphology during degradation. *Journal of Materials Science: Materials in Medicine*, **12**, pp. 811–816.
10. Hurrell S and Cameron RE. (2002) The effect of initial polymer morphology on the degradation and drug release from polyglycolide. *Biomaterials*, **11**, pp. 2401–2409.
11. Wang Y, Han X, Pan J and Sinka C. (2010) An entropy spring model for the Young's modulus change of biodegradable polymers during biodegradation. *Journal of the Mechanical Behavior of Biomedical Materials*, **3**, pp. 14–21.
12. Schwach G and Vert M. (1999) *In vitro* and *in vivo* degradation of lactic acid-based interference screws used in cruciate ligament reconstruction. *International Journal of Biological Macromolecules*, **25**, pp. 283–291.

The effective diffusion coefficient of degrading polymers

8

X. Han
Loughborough University, Loughborough, UK

8.1 Introduction

An intensive effort has been made to use biodegradable polymers in orthopaedic fixation devices, drug delivery systems and tissue engineering scaffolds. Degraded oligomers (or dissolvable small polymer chains) produced from hydrolysis reactions are eventually removed by metabolism. The degradation of these polymers is, however, a complicated process affected by chemical composition, molecular weight, degree of crystallinity, morphology, processing details, device shape and dimensions, and even sterilisation details. A porous microstructure in a biodegradable polymer develops during its biodegradation as the hydrolysis products diffuse out. The effective diffusion coefficient of a diffusing species in the polymer changes dramatically during the process, affecting the biodegradation itself and the accompanying processes, the release of embedded drugs for example. In order to keep our general governing equations as simple as possible, and to avoid being bothered by considering details of microstructures, expressions of the effective diffusion coefficient of dissolvable small polymer chains will be introduced in this chapter.

8.1.1 Diffusion law and diffusion coefficient

Diffusion, or chemical diffusion, is a transport phenomenon that is driven by gradients of chemical potentials. Particles migrate in a system spontaneously from an initial state to a steady state with uniform chemical potential field. Based on a general relation, the average velocity for molecules of species i v_i is written as:

$$\langle v_i \rangle = -\frac{D}{RT} \cdot \nabla u_i \qquad [8.1]$$

in which the angle bracket denotes an ensemble average value. u_i is the chemical potential of species i, T is the temperature and R is the gas constant. According to the fundamental equation of chemical potential change, we have:

$$\nabla u_i = V_i \nabla p - S_i \nabla T + F_i + RT \nabla \ln a_i \qquad [8.2]$$

Modelling Degradation of Bioresorbable Polymeric Medical Devices. http://dx.doi.org/10.1533/9781782420255.2.141

where V_i and S_i are the specific molar volume and the entropy of i, respectively, F_i is the sum of external forces, p is the pressure and a_i is its activity. Substituting Equation [8.2] into Equation [8.1], we have:

$$\langle v_i \rangle = -\frac{D}{RT} \cdot \left[V_i \nabla p - S_i \nabla T + F_i + RT \nabla \ln a_i \right] \qquad [8.3]$$

where D is the diffusion coefficient. Assuming that the temperature and pressure are constants and there are no external forces, Equation [8.3] can be rewritten as:

$$\langle v_i \rangle = -D \cdot \nabla \ln a_i \qquad [8.4]$$

Now define J_i as the flux of i, and we have:

$$J_i = \langle v_i \rangle a_i = -D \cdot \nabla a_i \qquad [8.5]$$

Fick's first law is derived from Equation [8.5] if the activity a_i equals the concentration c:

$$J = -D \cdot \nabla c \qquad [8.6]$$

Diffusion coefficient D is a tensor but can be replaced by a scalar for an isotropic material.

8.2 Analytical expressions of the effective diffusion coefficient for a two-phase material

In practice, materials are heterogeneous. The diffusion coefficient of a heterogeneous material is varying and is dependent on local structures of materials. The effective diffusion coefficient, D_{eff}, is defined as a diffusion coefficient of a hypothetical homogeneous medium with the same steady-state boundary conditions applied to the heterogeneous counterpart. Crank[1] has provided compressive coverage on a set of analytical expressions for effective diffusion coefficient of two-phase materials, assuming different material structures. In this chapter, we will only introduce those expressions briefly, while the corresponding detailed derivations can be found in Crank.[1] In the last subsection, we will also introduce an expression for the effective diffusion coefficient of a solute diffusing in a cross-linked polymer obtained based on statistics.

8.2.1 Suspended array of geometries in a continuum

In the early work, Maxwell[2] published the first report stating an analytical solution of an effective diffusion coefficient in porous material:

$$\frac{D_{\text{eff}} - D_s}{D_{\text{eff}} + 2D_s} = V_f \frac{D_f - D_s}{D_f + 2D_s} \quad [8.7]$$

In the material, two phases S and f are identified, which are the continuing phase (the bulk material) and the dispersed phase (the pores), respectively. D_s,D_f denote their corresponding diffusion coefficients. V_f is the volume fraction of dispersed phase over the whole volume. A generalised Maxwell's equation developed by Fricke[3] is expressed as follows:

$$\frac{D_{\text{eff}} - D_s}{D_{\text{eff}} + xD_s} = V_f \frac{D_f - D_s}{D_f + xD_s} \quad [8.8]$$

where x is a funcion of D_s / D_f . Geometry effects are only reflected by the value of x; when f contains only spheres, x equals 2. In this case, Equation [8.8] rolls back to Maxwell's Equation [8.7]. Fricke found that when the difference of diffusion coefficients between the continuing phase and the dispersed phase is not very large, there is little geometry effect. This is true when the continuing medium has higher diffusion coefficient. Small dissolvable molecules produced from the biodegradation process, however, diffuse much faster in pores filled up with liquid media than in polymer matrix. Geometry effects thus become an important factor. An asymptotic relationship considering geometry effects was obtained by Keller.[4] He considered a dense cubic array of spheres of infinite diffusion coefficient in a continuum:

$$\frac{D_{\text{eff}}}{D_s} = -\frac{1}{2}\pi \ln\left(\left(\frac{\pi}{6}\right) - V_f\right) + \cdots \quad [8.9]$$

with $(\pi / 6) - V_f << 1$. He also concluded the relationship for a square array of cylinders. The corresponding relation is:

$$\frac{D_{\text{eff}}}{D_s} = \frac{\pi^{3/2}}{2\{\pi / 4 - V_f\}^{1/2}} + \cdots \quad [8.10]$$

$$(\pi / 4) - V_f << 1$$

8.2.2 *Series–parallel formulae*

A composite can also be considered to be composed of different components in series or parallel,[1] for example as shown in Figure 8.1. An effective diffusion coefficient

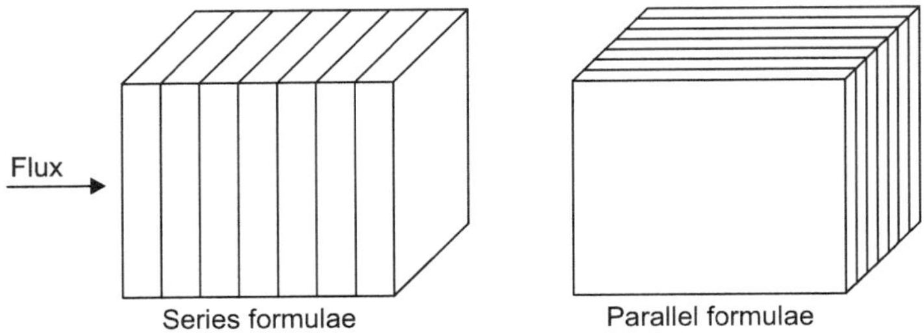

Figure 8.1 Series and parallel formulae sheets for a laminate.

along the direction of the flux (see Figure 8.1) of a laminate composed of n sheets with thicknesses $l_1, l_2, \ldots, l_n$ and diffusion coefficients $D_1, D_2, \ldots, D_n$ in series is given by:

$$\frac{l}{D_{\text{eff}}} = \frac{l_1}{D_1} + \frac{l_2}{D_2} + \cdots + \frac{l_n}{D_n} \quad [8.11]$$

and in parallel is given by:

$$lD_{\text{eff}} = l_1 D_1 + l_2 D_2 + \cdots + l_n D_n \quad [8.12]$$

in which l is the total thickness of a laminate.

8.2.3 Spheres in regular cubes

Jefferson *et al.*[5] developed a model that described a two-phase composite with small lattices. In each lattice, a sphere is suspended in the centre, which represents the dispersed phase, see Figure 8.2. They calculated the effective diffusion coefficient analytically by dividing each half cube with half suspended sphere (see Figure 8.2b) into three components *A*, *B* and *C* as shown in Figure 8.2c. A series–parallel diffusion circuit is formed by *A*, *B* and *C*. Assuming that the flux is only in the x direction, the effective diffusion coefficient is therefore given by:

$$D_{\text{eff}} = D_B \frac{A_B}{A_{\text{eff}}} + \left\{ \frac{(l_A + l_c) D_A D_C}{l_A D_C + l_C D_A} \right\} \frac{A_A}{A_{\text{eff}}} \quad [8.13]$$

in which D_A, D_B and D_C are diffusion coefficients, A_A, A_B and A_C are cross-sectional areas, l_A, l_B and l_C are the lengths of the three components *A*, *B* and *C*, respectively, and A_{eff} is the cross-sectional area of the lattice unit.

8.2.4 Randomly distributed irregular discrete phase

Analytical solutions for randomly distributed pores with irregular size and shape were derived firstly by Tsao[6] using the same idea of series–parallel formulae laminates

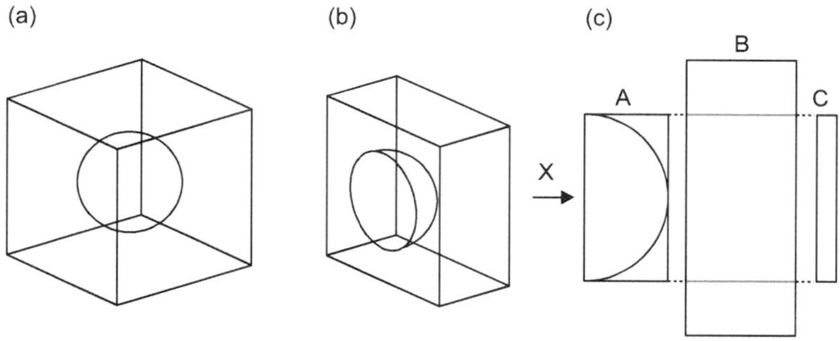

Figure 8.2 A representative unit of a two-phase composite: (a) a sphere suspends as the second phase in the centre of a lattice; (b) half a representative unit; (c) components A, B and C that compose the half unit described in (b). (*Source*: This figure is modified from References 5 and 1 with permissions.)

discussed in Section 8.2.2. He divided a laminate of a two-phase material into many parallel sheets. The dispersed phase is suspended in this laminate in a random and irregular manner. In the calculation, he assumed that diffusion occurred along only the x-axis, while the other two directions were insulated. He indicated in his calculation that the effective diffusion coefficient can be expressed in terms of not only D_s and D_f, but also P_1 and P_2, which is given by:

$$\frac{1}{D_{\text{eff}}} = \int_0^1 \frac{dP_1}{D_s + (D_f - D_s)P_2} \qquad [8.14]$$

where P_1 and P_2 are one-dimensional porosity and two-dimensional porosity, respectively. The one-dimensional porosity is defined as the fraction of the unit length occupied by the dispersed phase, while the two-dimensional porosity is defined as the fraction of area occupied by the dispersed phase. Expressions of P_1 and P_2 can be found in Crank.[1] The volume fraction V_f of the dispersed phase can be expressed using P_1 and P_2:

$$V_f = \int_0^1 P_2 dP_1 \qquad [8.15]$$

Substituting Equation [8.15] into Equation [8.14], the effective diffusion coefficient can be expressed by V_f, D_s and D_f.

Cheng and Vachon[7] developed two other expressions based on Tsao's idea:

$$\frac{1}{D_{\text{eff}}} = \frac{2}{\sqrt{EF}} \tan^{-1}\left\{\frac{B}{2}\sqrt{\frac{F}{E}}\right\} + \frac{1-B}{D_s}\left(D_s > D_f\right) \qquad [8.16]$$

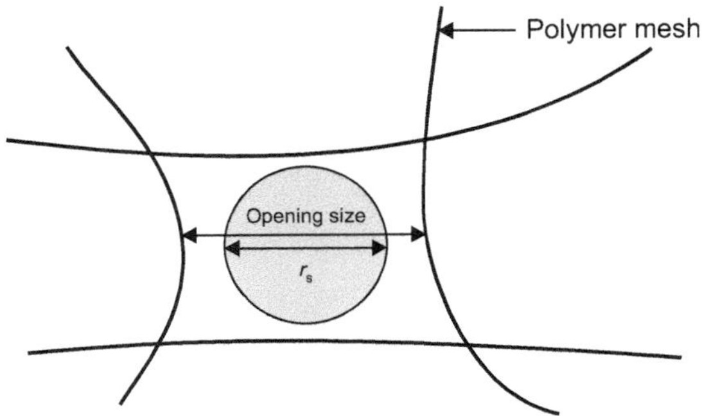

Figure 8.3 Opening size and solute radius in a cross-linked polymer mesh.

$$\frac{1}{D_{\text{eff}}} = \frac{2}{\sqrt{-EF}} \ln\left\{\frac{\sqrt{E} + \frac{1}{2}B\sqrt{-F}}{\sqrt{E} - \frac{1}{2}B\sqrt{-F}}\right\} + \frac{1-B}{D_s}\left(D_s < D_f\right) \qquad [8.17]$$

where B, E and F are functions of V_f, D_s and D_f, respectively:

$$B = \sqrt{3V_f / 2},\ E = D_s - B(D_f - D_s),\ F = -4\sqrt{2} / \left\{\sqrt{3V_f}\right\} \cdot (D_f - D_s) \qquad [8.18]$$

8.2.5 The obstruction-Scaling Model for a cross-linked polymer network

Polymer systems are of great interest in many medical applications. Due to their complicated nature, it is hard to represent their network by simple geometries. Thus probability-based techniques are widely used by researchers.[8,9] Diffusion across a cross-linked polymer network was studied by Amsden[8] using techniques in statistics, which is also known as the obstruction-scaling model. In the model, an opening is defined as a void in a polymer mesh which allows solutes to pass through once the opening size is larger than the radii of the solutes. A schematic diagram is shown in Figure 8.3, illustrating the opening size, the solute radius r_s and the polymer mesh. Polymer mesh size distribution function in his model was given by:

$$g(r) = \frac{\pi r_s}{2R^2} e^{\left(-\frac{\pi}{4}\left(\frac{r_s}{R}\right)^2\right)} \qquad [8.19]$$

in which R is the mesh size. A solute can pass a cross-linked mesh only when $R > r_s$. Thus D_{eff} / D_s becomes the probability of solute finding an opening which is large enough to pass:

$$D_{\text{eff}} / D_s = \int_{r_s}^{\infty} g(r)\,dr \qquad [8.20]$$

where D_s is the diffusion coefficient of the solute in media and D_{eff} is the effective diffusion coefficient of the solute in a cross-linked polymer.

8.3 Empirical expressions for the effective diffusion coefficient

The effective diffusion coefficient attracts large interest in the fields of controlled drug release, orthopaedic surgery and tissue engineering. An optimised drug release profile is controlled by an effective drug diffusion coefficient in drug controlled release; the diffusion of small molecules produced from the biodegradation of a medical device produces micro-voids in the medical device which will affect the comprehensive behaviour of polymer degradation; and in tissue engineering, scaffold porosity and structure of micro-channels are most important factors guaranteeing sufficient nutrient and oxygen supply for tissue cells. Empirical relations between the effective diffusion coefficient and molecular weight or degradation time for certain polymer systems have been derived by many researchers.[10–14] Faisant *et al.*[10] suggested that the effective diffusion coefficient depends on the weight-average molecular weight M_w in the following manner:

$$D_{\text{eff}}(M_w) = D_0 + \frac{k}{M_w} \qquad [8.21]$$

where D_0 is the bulk diffusion coefficient of the drug in un-degraded polymer and k is a constant. Similarly, Charlier *et al.*[12] investigated the relations between the drug release rate from a degradable polymer and the polymer degradation rate. Under the assumption that the polymer chain cleavage follows a first-order kinetics and that the effective drug diffusion coefficient is proportional to the inverse of the polymer molecular weight, they obtained:

$$D_{\text{eff}} = D_0 \exp(kt) \qquad [8.22]$$

where D_0 is the bulk diffusion coefficient of the drug prior to polymer degradation and k is the degradation rate. Joshi and Himmelstein[13] established a comprehensive reaction–diffusion–transport model and suggested that the effective diffusion coefficient is an exponential function of the polymer concentration:

$$D_{\text{eff}} = D_{\text{eff}}^0 \exp\left(\frac{\mu(C_D^0 - C_D)}{C_D^0}\right) \qquad [8.23]$$

in which D_{eff} and D_{eff}^0 are the effective diffusion coefficients of either water, acid or drug at any time and at $t = 0$, respectively, C_D^0 and C_D are the concentrations of a polymer at $t = 0$ and at any other time, respectively, and μ is a constant.

In order to calculate the drug release from poly(lactic-co-glycolic) acid-based micro-particles, Raman *et al.*[14] suggested that the effective diffusion coefficient was taken as a function of the weight-average molecular weight given by:

$$\ln D_{\text{eff}} = -0.347(\ln M_w)^3 + 10.394(\ln M_w)^2 - 104.95(\ln M_w) + 316.95 \qquad [8.24]$$

Siepmann *et al.*[11] suggested that the effective diffusion coefficient can be considered to be linearly proportional to the porosity. Empirical expressions of D_{eff} are mostly dependent on M_w or degradation time rather than real structures of polymer systems. Empirical expressions can be utilised in the same polymer system from which they were derived. They are, however, not valid for a different polymer system.

8.4 Molecular dynamics (MD) and Brownian dynamics (BD)

MD and BD are widely used numerical tools to calculate diffusion coefficients in bulk materials. Given the fact that the former is computationally expensive, MD cannot consider dispersed phase in a continuum. On the contrary, BD shows its advantages in calculating the effective diffusion coefficient of heterogeneous material. In this section, both methods are introduced in sequence in each subsection.

8.4.1 MD calculation of diffusion coefficient in bulk phase

MD is a computer-based method of simulating the motions of atoms and molecules. Forces, both external and internal, are simulated explicitly for each atom or molecule. Trajectories of atoms and molecules are obtained by solving Newton's equation of motion for a system of particles. In order to solve Newton's equation, a potential function or a force field between particles needs to be predefined. The potential function can be derived both empirically and analytically. In this chapter, we are not going to discuss the detail of selecting the potential functions. Instead, we focus on how to derive the diffusion coefficient using MD calculations. Einstein's expression related a self-diffusion coefficient with mean-squared displacement (MSD) which allows using MD directly to derive the self-diffusion coefficient.[15,16] Self-diffusion is a spontaneous mixing of molecules taking place in the absence of concentration. Its corresponding diffusion coefficient is the so-called self-diffusion coefficient. The term 'diffusion', which we discussed in previous sections and is driven by the chemical potential gradient, is also known as chemical diffusion. Chemical diffusion is a non-equilibrium process, while self-diffusion takes place under equilibrium. A relation between the chemical diffusion coefficient D_i and the self-diffusion coefficient D_i^s of a species i is given by Darken-Dehlinger relation:

$$D_i = D_i^s \left(1 + \frac{\partial \ln a_i}{\partial \ln N_i}\right) \qquad [8.25]$$

where N_i is the mole fraction of i and a_i is the thermodynamic activity coefficient of i. In a dilute solution, a_i = constant, so that $\partial \ln a_i / \partial \ln c_i = 0$, then $D_i = D_i^s$. The self-diffusion coefficient of species i can be calculated using Einstein's expression:

$$D_i^s = \lim_{t \to \infty} \frac{1}{6t} \left\langle |\mathrm{r}(t) - \mathrm{r}(0)|^2 \right\rangle \quad [8.26]$$

where $\left\langle |\mathrm{r}(t) - \mathrm{r}(0)|^2 \right\rangle = \frac{1}{N} \sum_{i=1}^{N} |\mathrm{r}_i(t) - \mathrm{r}_i(0)|^2$ which can be calculated directly using MD. Another expression of this is known as the Green-Kubo relation:

$$D^s = \frac{1}{3} \int_0^\infty dt \left\langle v(t)v(0) \right\rangle \quad [8.27]$$

where $\left\langle v(t)v(0) \right\rangle = \frac{1}{N} \sum_{i=1}^{N} \left\langle v_i(t)v_i(0) \right\rangle$. Using Equation [8.27], the self-diffusion coefficient is derived by integrating the velocity autocorrelation function. Both expressions can be used to calculate the self-diffusion coefficient. Substituting Equation [8.26] or [8.27] into Equation [8.25], the chemical diffusion coefficient is derived. For inter-diffusion in a binary system containing species i and j, its diffusion coefficient D is related to the chemical diffusion coefficients D_i and D_j for species i and j, respectively, by using the Darken equation:

$$D = N_i \bar{V}_i D_i + N_j \bar{V}_j D_j \quad [8.28]$$

where $\bar{V}_i$ and $\bar{V}_j$ are the partial molar volumes for species i and j. N_i and N_j are their respective mole fractions.

8.4.2 BD calculation for the diffusion coefficient in bulk materials

In Langevin dynamics, a stochastic differential equation is used to simulate movements of molecules. This equation is also known as the Langevin equation:

$$m \frac{d^2 r_i}{dt^2} = -\gamma \frac{dr_i}{dt} + F_i + R_i \quad [8.29]$$

The three terms on the right hand side of Equation [8.29] describe the total instantaneous forces applied on particle i. The first term denotes a friction effect on particle

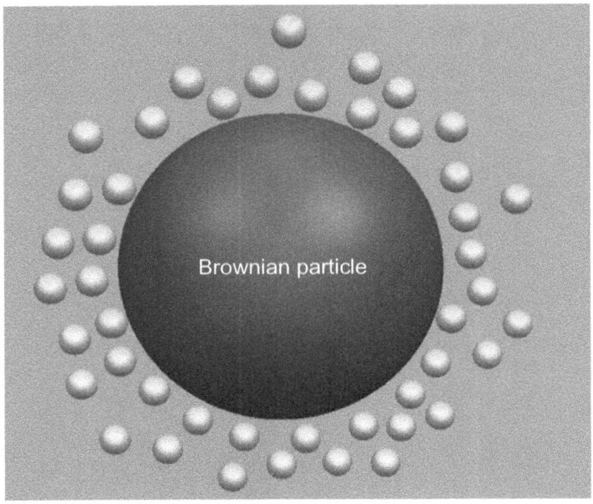

Figure 8.4 Langevin dynamics system.

i. The friction force is proportional to the particle velocity but in the opposite direction. The second term represents the explicit external forces applied on particle i. The third term on the right hand side of Equation [8.29] is a noise term representing the effect of the collisions from small molecules. A combination of the first term and the third term approximates the effect from particles that are not explicitly present in the system, solvent molecules for example. A schematic picture is shown in Figure 8.4, illustrating a typical Langevin dynamics motion system. The macroscopic particle in the centre is known as a Brownian particle, surrounded by a number of microscopic particles. These small particles, such as solvent molecules, do not enter a Langevin system explicitly. BD is a special case of Langevin dynamics where no average acceleration (in a very low Reynolds number environment) takes place in simulation. Letting the left hand side of Equation [8.29] equal zero, we obtain:

$$\gamma \frac{dr_i}{dt} = F_i + R_i \qquad [8.30]$$

Equation [8.30] is the basis of BD. Einstein showed that the noise term R_i is in accord with Gaussian distribution for an infinite time. Using Equation [8.30], one can calculate a trajectory time evolution of a Brownian particle. Einstein gave a relation between the MSD of a Brownian particle and the diffusion coefficient:

$$\langle r_i^2 \rangle = 6Dt \qquad [8.31]$$

Rearranging Equation [8.30] to obtain the MSD of particle i, the diffusion coefficient D can be derived from Equation [8.31].

A classic time step of MD is in the order of 1 fs (10^{-15} s), as a particle will undergo roughly the order of 10^{-21} collisions per second. BD, that apply a noise term and a friction term to represent small particles, have a time step that can be as large as 10^{-5} s which greatly reduces the calculation cost.

8.4.3 BD calculation for the diffusion coefficient of polymer chains in solute

Small polymer chains produced from the hydrolysis reaction during degradation are diffusible. The diffusion mechanism of small polymer chains in solute and the corresponding diffusion coefficient are of great interest in the area of polymer degradation. A BD model for simulating the diffusion of small polymer chains and calculating the diffusion coefficient is introduced in this section.

8.4.3.1 Polymer configuration

Mesoscopic polymer models simulate polymer chains by using an integrated unit to represent the detailed chemical structure of each repeat unit. They were developed from atomistic models by means of coarse-graining procedures by scientists,[17–19] in which the bead–rod and the bead–spring models are most attractive. The bead–rod model uses a rigid rod to bridge two beads and applies different bending potentials to the rod. An example of the bead–rod model is shown in Figure 8.5: a polymer chain with five repeat units is connected by four solid rods. Each bead is kept apart from each of the others by a constant distance, which is the length of its connection rod. The governing equation for the dynamics of the bead–rod chain in a solute is given as follows[17]:

$$F_i^H + F_i^C + F_i^B = 0, \qquad i = 1, 2, \cdots, N \qquad [8.32]$$

where i is bead number, and F_i^H, F_i^C and F_i^B are the hydrodynamics drag force, the constraint force and the Brownian force, respectively. The hydrodynamics drag force is also known as friction force in a viscous fluid, which is expressed by Stokes' law. The constraint force keeps two neighbouring beads apart by a certain fixed distance, which can be written in terms of the tension in the rods. The Brownian force is the noise term in Equation [8.30] which represents collisions between solvent molecules and the beads.

The bead–spring model is more popularly used in polymer kinetic simulations to represent polymer chains with different configurations: linear polymers and cross-linked polymers.[17,18] In a bead–spring model, two neighbouring beads of a polymer chain are connected by a spring. Each bead represents a repeat unit of a polymer

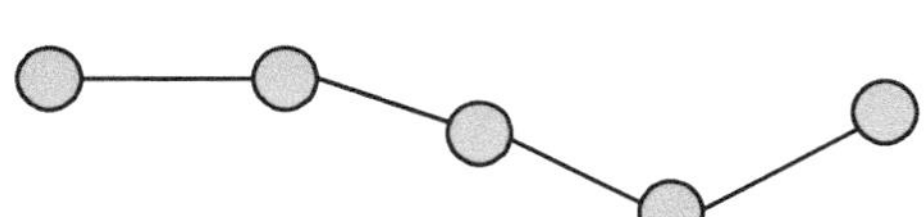

Figure 8.5 Bead–rod model.

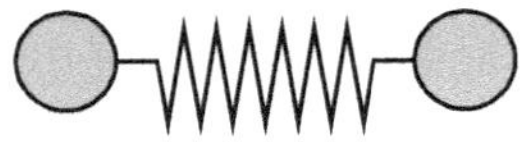

Figure 8.6 Bead–spring model.

chain. The advantage of the bead–spring model is that the gap between two beads is flexible compared to the bead–rod model. Figure 8.6 illustrates a bead–spring model: as can be seen, two beads are connected by a spring. The general governing equation is written as:

$$F_i^H + F_i^E + F_i^B = 0, \qquad i = 1, 2, \cdots, N \tag{8.33}$$

where i is the bead number, and F_i^H, F_i^E and F_i^B are the hydrodynamics drag force, the effective spring force and the Brownian force, respectively. The definitions of the hydrodynamics drag force and the Brownian force are the same as in a bead–rod model. The effective spring force can be characterised by using different spring force laws.[17–21] One of these can be written as follows:

$$F_i^E(r) = \left(\frac{k_B T}{A_{\text{eff}}}\right) \cdot \left\{\left(\frac{r}{L_0}\right) - \frac{1}{4} + \frac{1}{4\left(1 - r / L_0\right)^2}\right\} \tag{8.34}$$

Equation [8.34] is a force–extension relationship from Marko and Siggia,[21] where r is the compression or extension distance of a spring, A_{eff} is the persistence distance, L_0 is contour length, k_B is the Boltzmann constant and T is the absolute temperature.

8.4.3.2 The solvent force

The solvent molecules are not modelled explicitly in a BD model. The forces applied on each repeat unit from the solvent molecules are collisions and frictions. They can be virtually expressed by the friction term (thermodynamics drag term) and the noise term (Brownian force term) in Equation [8.32] or [8.33] for different polymer chain configuration models.

8.4.3.3 The integration scheme

Combining the polymer chain configuration models, forces from solvent molecules and using the Brownian Equation [8.30], we can develop a complete model for polymer chains diffusing in solvent. The trajectories of polymer chains over time can then be obtained. The diffusion coefficient can thus be derived from Equation [8.31]. The Velocity-Verlet method is a mathematical method used to integrate the equation of motion, which is widely applied in calculating trajectories. This method produces position and velocity for particles at each time step, which reduces memory usage significantly without storing past data. According to the Velocity-Verlet method, the formulae for calculating position and velocity are:

$$r(t+\Delta t) = r(t) + v(t)\Delta t + \frac{1}{2}F(t)\frac{\Delta t^2}{m} \quad [8.35]$$

and $$v(t+\Delta t) = v(t) + \frac{1}{2}\frac{\Delta t^2}{m}(F(t) + F(t+\Delta t)) \quad [8.36]$$

where $F(t)$ is sum of forces and Δt is the time step, r is the current position and v is the velocity. The details of this algorithm can be summarised as four steps[22]:

Step 1: Calculate $F(t)$, $v(t)$ at current time step;

Step 2: Use Equation [8.35] to derive $r(t+\Delta t)$ by substituting $F(t)$ and $v(t)$ from Step 1;

Step3: Calculate $F(t+\Delta t)$ at updated position using Equation [8.30];

Step 4: Calculate $v(t+\Delta t)$ using Equation [8.36] and go back to Step 1 for next time step.

The BD simulation discussed in this section can also be used in simulating small polymer chain diffusion in heterogeneous solute. Extra constraints, such as orientation constraints, hydrodynamic interactions and finite boundaries, can be added into Equation [8.30] in order to represent a heterogeneous solute. The effective diffusion coefficient of a non-uniform system is calculated by comparing the trajectories of small polymer chains in heterogeneous solute to a hypothetical homogeneous medium with the same boundary conditions.

8.5 The direct finite element (DFE) method for effective diffusion coefficients

A porous microstructure develops in a degrading polymer during its biodegradation due to the diffusion of diffusible polymer chains. The effective diffusion coefficient of a diffusing species in the polymer changes dramatically during the process, affecting the biodegradation itself and the accompanying processes. In order to precisely simulate small polymer chain diffusion in a degrading polymer, a DFE approach was developed. A large finite element model using very fine elements is generated by a DFE method in order to simulate the microstructure of the device. The accuracy of the effective diffusion coefficient compared to the realistic microstructure is entirely dependent on the mesh size of the model. The larger the mesh size is, the higher is the computational power. It is inefficient when this method is directly used in a reaction–diffusion degradation model. A simple formula is therefore needed to describe the relation between the effective diffusion coefficient and the porous microstructures. In this section, we will introduce a DFE model and the derivation of its corresponding formula for calculating the effective diffusion coefficient. This work was initiated by Wenguang Jiang and completed by Xiaoxiao Han. It was partially published in Reference 23.

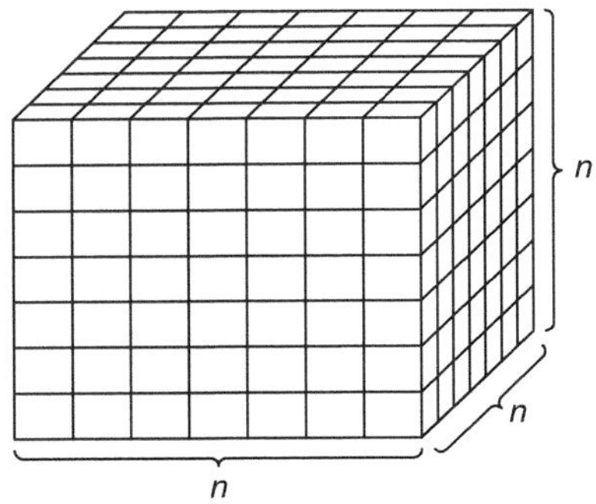

Figure 8.7 Geometry of a representative cubic volume with a total of $n \times n \times n$ sub-cubes.

Firstly, a series of random porous structures of different porosities are represented by generating a number of cubic finite elements in a representative volume. Figure 8.7 illustrates a cubic representative volume containing $n \times n \times n$ sub-cubes. n is the number of elements in each dimension. Each of the sub-cubic volumes has been assigned a material property of either a fast diffusion phase or a slow diffusion phase with different diffusion coefficients. Two phases can be either uniformly or randomly distributed in a representative unit. This is achieved by assigning different material properties uniformly or randomly on selected sub-cubes with a desired volume fraction. In this section, three geometry cases will be introduced: (1) the fast diffusion phase is randomly distributed; (2) the fast diffusion phase is distributed in parallel with the slow diffusion phase; and (3) the fast diffusion phase is located in the centre of a cubic representative unit.

8.5.1 Geometry generations of randomly distributed fast diffusion phase

A material indicator p is introduced here to separate two phases. $p = 1$ indicates a fast diffusion phase with diffusion coefficient D_f, while $p = 0$ indicates a slow diffusion phase with diffusion coefficient D_s on each sub-cube. The volume fraction V_f is defined as the ratio of volume of fast diffusion phase of material over the total volume of the composite, which can be written as:

$$V_f = \frac{V_{\text{fast}}}{V_{\text{total}}} \qquad [8.37]$$

A series of randomly distributed two-phase composites with different volume fractions from $V_f = 0.1$ to $V_f = 0.9$ are shown in Figure 8.8. Black blocks indicate a fast diffusion phase with $p = 1$, while white blocks represent a slow diffusion phase with $p = 0$.

8.5.2 Finite element procedures

To establish the finite element model, each sub-cube in a representative unit volume is further discretised into 10 × 10 × 10 8-noded linear iso-parametric brick finite

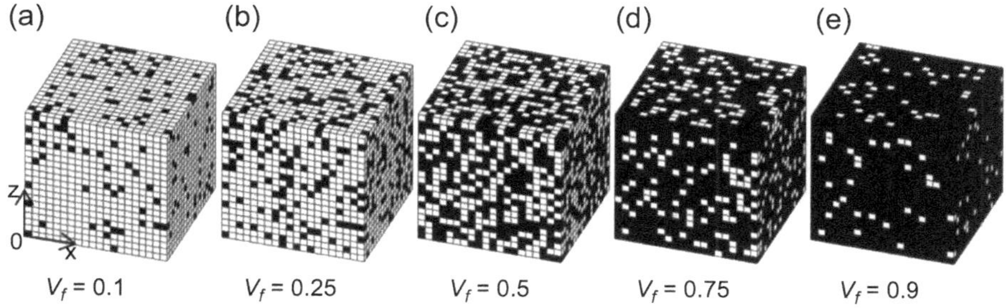

Figure 8.8 (a–e) Plots of the material phase distribution for different volume fractions – black sub-blocks represent fast diffusion phase of material. (a) $V_f = 0.1$, (b) $V_f = 0.25$, (c) $V_f = 0.5$, (d) $V_f = 0.75$, and (e) $V_f = 0.9$.

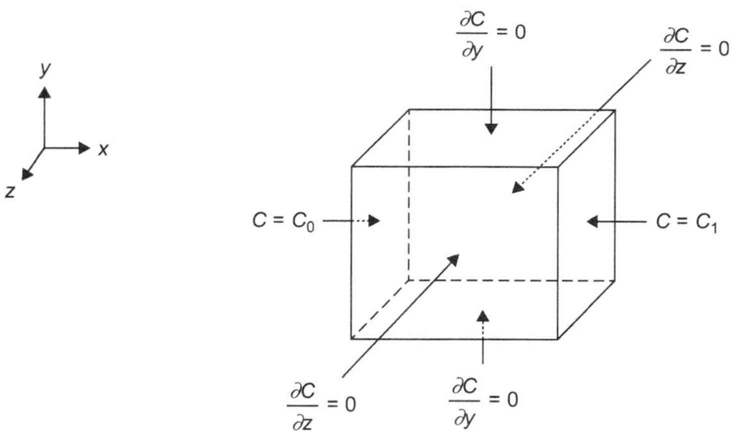

Figure 8.9 Boundary conditions of a finite element model.

elements. Thus, a typical finite element model consists of a total number of $8000n^3$ elements. Numerical analysis results show that there is no significant difference between the mesh refinement levels when $n = 3$ and $n = 4$. Therefore, for all numerical results presented in the section, the mesh refinement with $n = 4$ is used throughout, which is believed to yield converged results. Boundary conditions of a three-dimensional finite element model are shown in Figure 8.9. In Figure 8.9, the left and the right boundaries have fixed concentrations while the top, the bottom, the front and the back boundaries are insulated. Fick's first law in Equation [8.6] is applied to the DFE model. When the system reaches a steady state, the mean flux over a transverse cross-section J_{mean} can be calculated. A hypothesis homogenous representative volume is also established with the same boundary conditions shown in Figure 8.9. According to Fick's first law, the effective diffusion coefficient can be calculated:

$$D_{\text{eff}} = J_{\text{mean}} \Delta x / \Delta C \qquad [8.38]$$

where $\Delta x = x_1 - x_0$ is the distance in the x direction. $\Delta C = C_1 - C_0$ is the applied difference of concentration. Substituting J_{mean} obtained from the heterogeneous DFE model into Equation [8.38], D_{eff} is found.

8.5.2 Results and discussions

Here is introduced a normalised effective diffusion coefficient, D_N, which is defined as:

$$D_N = (D_{\text{eff}} - D_s)/(D_f - D_s) \qquad [8.39]$$

The normalised effective coefficient, as function of the volume fractions with different values of D_f/D_s, is given in Figure 8.10. A fitting curve is also illustrated in Figure 8.10, which is obtained using:

$$D_N = -0.3V_f^3 + 1.3V_f^2 \qquad [8.40]$$

It can be seen from Figure 8.10 that when the value of D_f/D_s increases, the effective coefficient tends to approach the fitting curve. So the fitting Equation [8.40] can

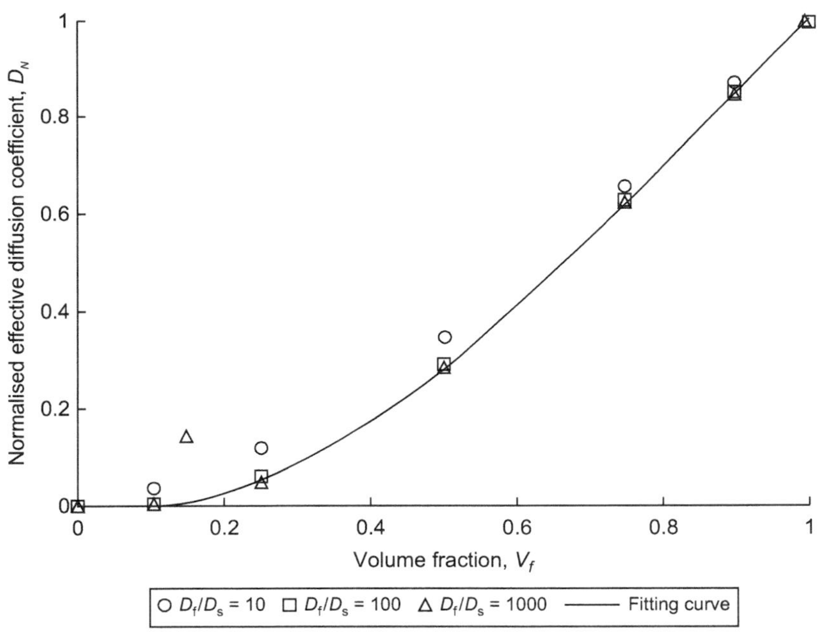

Figure 8.10 The normalised effective diffusion coefficients as functions of volume fractions for different values of D_f/D_s.

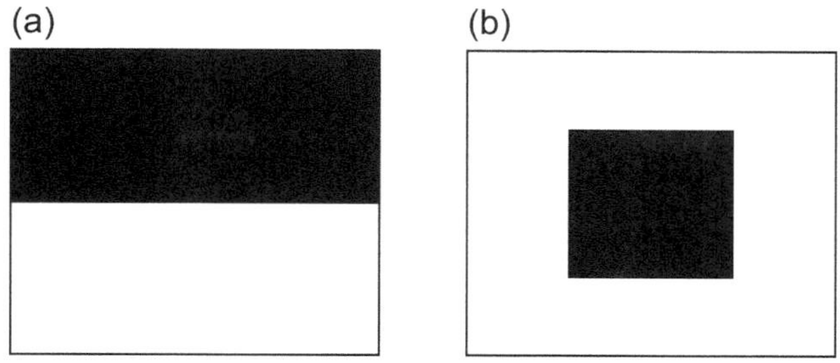

Figure 8.11 Two cross-sections of two extreme cases: (a) case one: the heterogeneous system is composed of two phases in parallel and (b) case two: the heterogeneous system is a centrally located fast diffusion phase and the surrounding slow diffusion phase.

be applied to a heterogeneous system if $D_f >> D_s$ for calculating the effective diffusion coefficient as a function of volume fraction V_f. Figure 8.10 also indicates that the effective diffusion coefficient increases gently with the volume fraction V_f in the early stage. A steep increase of the diffusion coefficient is detected when V_f is larger than a critical value. A tunnelling effect is believed to be the main reason. The percolation theory predicts that cubic pores randomly introduced in a 3D solid become interconnected at the threshold volume fraction of 31.16%.[24,25] Observing Figure 8.10, we can find that the numerical predictions agree well with the percolation theory.

Another two DFE simulations are also carried out with different distributions of the fast diffusion phase in order to discover the upper bound and lower bound of the relation between the effective coefficient and the volume fraction. Figure 8.11 describes the two cross-sections of the two cases: in the first case, the heterogeneous system is composed of two phases in parallel, while in the second case the system is composed of a centrally located fast diffusion phase and a surrounding slow diffusion phase. Figure 8.12 illustrates three relations between the normalised effective diffusion coefficients obtained from the randomly distributed, the parallel distributed and the central distributed fast diffusion phase. It can be seen clearly in Figure 8.12 that the $D_N - V_f$ relation calculated from the first case yields the upper bound while that from the second case yields the lower bound.

In amorphous polymer degradation, pores generated during degradation due to the diffusion of small polymer chains can be considered as the fast diffusion phase, while the polymer matrix is considered as the slow diffusion phase. The diffusion coefficient of pores is far greater than that of the polymer matrix, so that Equation [8.40] can be used as a general formula for calculating the effective diffusion coefficient in polymer degradation. According to Jiang *et al.* Equation [8.40] can also be written as:

$$D_{\text{eff}} = D_{\text{matrix}}\left[1+\left(1.3V_f^2 - 0.3V_f^3\right)\left(\frac{D_{\text{pore}}}{D_{\text{matrix}}} - 1\right)\right] \qquad [8.41]$$

in polymer degradation, where D_{matrix} and D_{pore} represent the diffusion coefficients of small polymer chains in the polymer matrix and pores, respectively. It is part of the

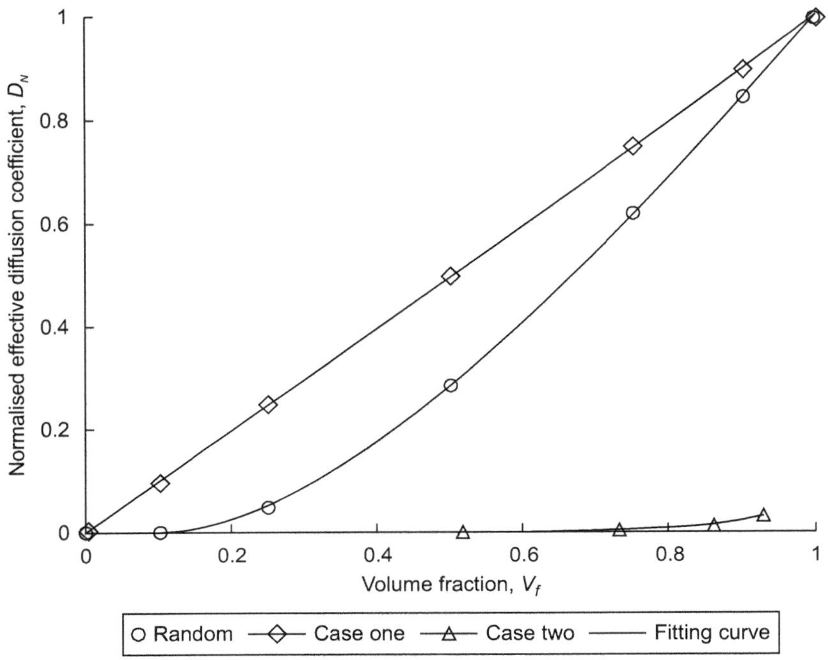

Figure 8.12 The normalised effective diffusion coefficients of the random case shown in Figure 8.8, the parallel case and the central case shown in Figure 8.12 versus the volume fraction when $D_f/D_s = 1000$.

reaction–diffusion degradation model of degradable polymers discussed in previous chapters. Using D_0 to represent the diffusion coefficient of small polymer chains in amorphous polymer, we have $D_{\text{matrix}} = D_0$ for an amorphous polymer system. For a semi-crystallised polymer system, the polymer matrix consists of an amorphous phase and a crystalline phase. It can be assumed that the diffusion of small polymer chains in a crystalline phase is zero. The effective diffusion coefficient for a semi-crystalline polymer can be still derived from Equation [8.40], but the expression of D_{matrix} is different, given by:

$$D_{\text{matrix}} = (1.3V_a^2 - 0.3V_a^3)D_0 \qquad [8.42]$$

where V_a is the volume fraction of amorphous phase over the whole polymer matrix.

8.6 Summary

Relations between D_N and V_f are discussed in this chapter. Several equations are introduced, including analytical Equations [8.7], [8.9], [8.12], [8.17] and the fitting

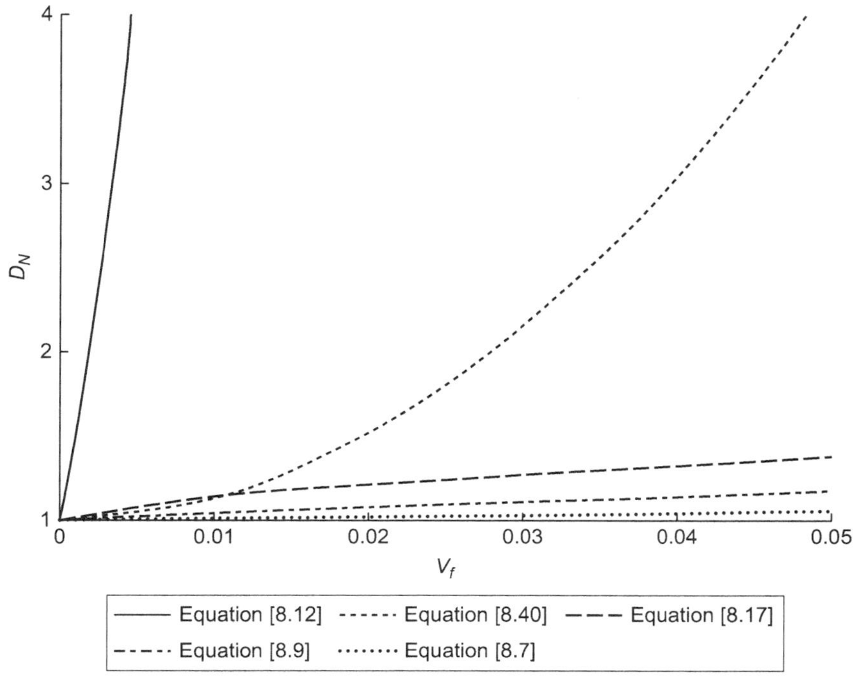

Figure 8.13 A summary of $D_N - V_f$ relations from different equations using $D_f / D_s = 1000$ excepting for Equation [8.9].

Equation [8.40]. As a summary, $D_N - V_f$ relations obtained from the above equations are all plotted in Figure 8.13. Figure 8.13 reveals that the $D_N - V_f$ relation obtained from Equation [8.7] is the lower bound, while that obtained from Equation [8.12] is the upper bound. Relations obtained from Equations [8.17] and [8.9] are very close to the lower bound. On the other hand, relations from Equations [8.12] and [8.40] give very much steeper increases of D_N as functions of V_f. This can be explained by percolation theory. In Equation [8.12], the percolation threshold value is zero while the threshold values in Equations [8.17], [8.9] and [8.7] are infinite.

8.7 Conclusions

In this chapter, analytical expressions that are used to calculate the effective diffusion coefficient of two-phase materials are firstly presented, and are followed by numerical methods. MD can be used to calculate the self-diffusion coefficient, while BD can be applied to obtain chemical diffusion coefficient for both homogenous materials and heterogeneous materials. A BD-based model is also presented in detail, which is used to calculate the diffusion coefficient of small polymer chains in solute. Subsequently, a DFE method is demonstrated. Using the DFE model, the microstructure of a degrading polymer can be considered. A fitting equation is generated based on simulation results from the DFE model that can describe the relation between the effective coefficient and the volume fraction of a second phase. This equation can calculate the effective diffusion coefficient of small polymer chains during degradation, not only in an amorphous polymer system but also in a semi-crystalline polymer system. It is part of the reaction–diffusion degradation model discussed in Part One. At last, $D_N - V_f$ relations obtained from different equation are discussed in this chapter and plotted in Figure 8.13 in summary.

Acknowledgements

The analytical expressions for calculating effective diffusion coefficients in a two-phase material presented in this chapter were firstly summarised in the reference below and are reproduced here in part with modifications with the permission of Oxford University Press.

- Crank J. *The* mathematics *of Diffusion*, 2nd edition. Oxford: Oxford University Press; 1975.

Figure 8.2 presented in this chapter was firstly produced in the reference below and is reproduced with modifications here in part with the permission of ACS publications.

- Jefferson T, Witzell O and Sibbtt W. Thermal conductivity of graphite – silicone oil and graphite-water suspensions, *Industrial and Engineering Chemistry*, 1958. pp. 1589–1592.

The author would like to acknowledge Wenguang Jiang for his contribution to the work presented in Section 8.5.

References

1. Crank J. (1975) *The Mathematics of Diffusion*. Oxford: Oxford University Press.
2. Maxwell JC. (1881) *A Treatise on Electricity and Magnetism*, second edition. Oxford: Claredon Press.
3. Fricke H. (1931) The electric conductivity and capacity of disperse systems. *Journal of Applied Physics*, **1**, pp. 106–115.
4. Keller JB. (1963) Conductivity of a medium containing a dense array of perfectly conducting spheres or cylinders or nonconducting cylinders. *Journal of Applied Physics*, **34**, pp. 991–993.
5. Jefferson T, Witzell O and Sibbtt W. (1958) Thermal conductivity of graphite – silicone oil and graphite-water suspensions. *Industrial and Engineering Chemistry*, **50**, pp. 1589–1592.
6. Tsao GT. (1961) Thermal conductivity of two-phase materials. *Industrial and Engineering Chemistry*, **53**, pp. 395–397.
7. Cheng SC and Vachon RI. (1969) The prediction of the thermal conductivity of two and three phase solid heterogeneous mixtures. *International Journal of Heat and Mass Transfer*, **12**, pp. 249–264.

8. Amsden B. (1999) An obstruction-scaling model for diffusion in homogeneous hydrogels. *Macromolecules*, **32**, pp. 874–879.
9. Brenner H. (1977) A model of surface diffusion on solids. *Journal of Colloid and Interface Science*, **62**, pp. 238–258.
10. Faisant N, Siepmann J and Benoit JP. (2002) PLGA-based microparticles: elucidation of mechanisms and a new, simple mathematical model quantifying drug release. *European Journal of Pharmaceutical Sciences*, **15**, pp. 355–366.
11. Siepmann J, Faisant N and Benoit JP. (2002) A new mathematical model quantifying drug release from bioerodible micro-particles using Monte Carlo simulations. *Pharmaceutics Research*, **19**, pp. 1885–1893.
12. Charlier A, Leclerc B and Couarraze G. (2000) Release of mifepristone from biodegradable matrices: experimental and theoretical evaluations. *International Journal of Pharmacutics*, **200**, pp. 115–120.
13. Joshi A and Himmelstein KJ. (1991) Dynamics of controlled release from bioerodible matrices. *Journal of Controlled Release*, **15**, pp. 95–104.
14. Raman C, Berkland C, Kim K and Pack DW. (2005) Modeling small-molecule release from PLG microspheres: effects of polymer degradation and nonuniform drug distribution. *Journal of Controlled Release*, **103**, pp. 149–158.
15. Li WZ, Chen C and Yang J. (2008) Molecular dynamics simulation of self-diffusion coefficient and its relation with temperature using simple Lennard-Jones potential. *Heat Transfer – Asian Research*, **37**, pp. 86–93.
16. Wang J and Hou T. (2011) Application of molecular dynamics simulations in molecular property prediction II: diffusion coefficient. *Journal of Computational Chemistry*, **32**, pp. 3505–3519.
17. Somasi M, Khomami B and Woo NJ. (2002) Brownian dynamics simulations of bad-rod and bead-spring chains: numerical algorithms and coarse-graining issues. *Journal of Non-Newtonian Fluid Mechanics*, **108**, pp. 227–255.
18. Underhill PT and Doyle PS. (2004) On the coarse-graining of polymer into bead-spring chains. *Journal of Non-Newtonian Fluid Mechanics*, **122**, pp. 3–31.
19. Underhill PT and Doyle PS. (2005) Development of bead-spring polymer models using the constant extension ensemble. *The Society of Rheology, Inc. Journal of Rheology*, **49**, pp. 963–987.
20. Underhill PT and Doyle PS. (2006) Alternative spring force law for bead-spring chain models of the worm-like chain. *Journal of Rheology*, **50**, pp. 513–529.
21. Marko JF and Siggia ED. (1995) Stretching DNA. *Macromolecules*, **28**, pp. 8759–8770.
22. Sivasubramanian A. (2003) *Molecular Dynamics Simulations of Small Molecule Diffusion in Hydrogels*. Philadelphia: Drexel University.
23. Pan J and Han X. (2011) A model for biodegradation of composite materials made of polyesters and tricalcium phosphates. *Biomaterials*, **39**, 2248–2255.
24. Stauffer D and Aharony A. (1994) *Introduction to Percolation Theory*. London: Taylor & Francis.
25. Reyes S and Jensen KF. (1985) Estimation of effective transport coefficients in porous solids based on percolation concepts. *Chemical Engineering Science*, **40**, pp. 1723–1734.

Mechanical properties of biodegradable polymers for medical applications

9

A. Gleadall
University of Nottingham, Nottingham, UK

9.1 Fundamentals of mechanical properties in polymers

Due to the complexity of the molecular structure of polymers compared to other materials, the understanding of mechanical properties with respect to molecular interaction is currently quite limited. One of the most important factors in polymer mechanical properties is the glass transition temperature (T_g), which is quite well understood. Polymers deform via different mechanisms at temperatures above and below their T_g. The polymer chains are effectively frozen in position for 'glassy' polymers below T_g and only small strains (typically <5%) can be accommodated elastically, during which the distance between polymer chains slightly increases or decreases. For 'rubbery' polymers above T_g, however, the chains can slide over one another and elongation is accommodated by chains straightening out in the direction of strain.

9.1.1 *Elastic deformation of polymers*

For a glassy polymer, elastic deformation is accommodated by small displacements between polymer chains, as shown in Figure 9.1. The average distance between adjacent polymer chains is likely to increase slightly in the direction of an applied tensile strain. This separation is expected to be aided by small deformations of the polymer chains too. It is not expected that the distance of main-chain covalent bonds changes, because these bonds are much stronger than weak interactions between chains. However, the polymer chains may be able to bend or twist to a small degree in order to assist deformation between polymer chains. The elastic deformation of glassy polymers is not well understood, so simple generally accepted theories for Young's modulus in terms of molecular interaction do not exist.

Another mechanism for elastic deformation is for polymer chains to straighten out and orientate in the direction of applied strain. This is also shown in Figure 9.1 and can facilitate large elastic deformation (>500%) but it is only possible in polymers that are above their glass transition temperature. Below T_g, the polymer chains are not able to slide over one another in order to straighten out. For this type of deformation to still be considered elastic in nature, the polymer chains must return to their original position after the stress is removed. For rubbery elasticity, the polymer chains return to their original position due to entropy. In order to consider entropy,

Modelling Degradation of Bioresorbable Polymeric Medical Devices. http://dx.doi.org/10.1533/9781782420255.2.163

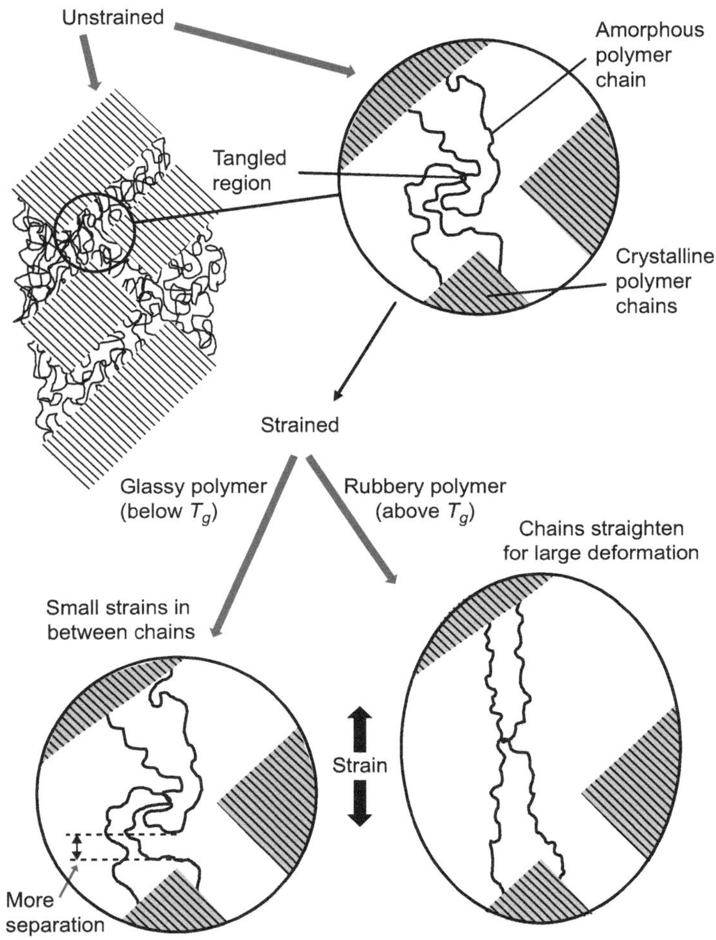

Figure 9.1 Elastic deformation occurs in the amorphous phase of polymers. Mechanisms for glassy deformation (small strains) and rubbery deformation (large strains) are shown.

the deformation of polymers is often discussed in terms of Helmholtz free energy, F, which is given as

$$F = E - TS \qquad [9.1]$$

in which the internal energy, E, is the kinetic and potential energy of all atoms and atomic interactions, S is the entropy of the system, and T is temperature. During the deformation of glassy polymers, free energy is dominated by the potential energy change that results from variation in the distance between atoms. This can be simply physically interpreted by considering strain to be resisted by bond elongation/compression. The entropy term can be considered as negligible for a polymer below T_g, since elastic deformation is limited to small strains: significant entropy changes only result from large strains, as demonstrated by rubbery polymers. In rubber elasticity the polymer chains slide over one another and rearrange with relative ease to adopt a considerably different configuration (strained) without significant change to the internal energy. The entropy of the system does change, however, so it is variation of entropy as the polymer is strained that dominates the free energy change. Entropy theory cannot be described with such an intuitive interpretation as internal energy. It is related to the total possible configurations of chains in a polymer. Consider a polymer chain whose ends are quite close to each other. The middle section of the polymer chains can occupy a large number of different configurations without the polymer ends having to change position, as shown in Figure 9.2. This means entropy is high: the structure is not highly ordered. When the overall polymer is elongated, however, the distance between the chain-ends (end-to-end distance) increases. For a longer end-to-end distance the polymer chain cannot exist in as many different configurations, as demonstrated in Figure 9.3. Entropy decreases, free energy increases, and therefore work must be applied to the system. In statistical mechanics, entropy can be defined as

$$S = k_b \ln \Omega \qquad [9.2]$$

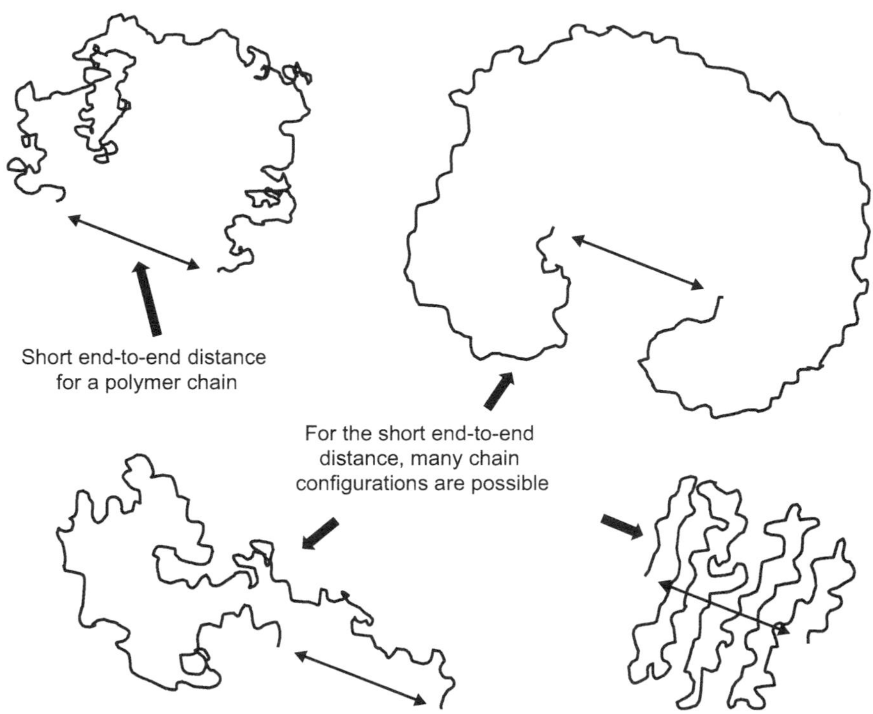

Figure 9.2 A long polymer chain can take many different configurations if it has a short end-to-end distance. The entropy of the system is therefore high.

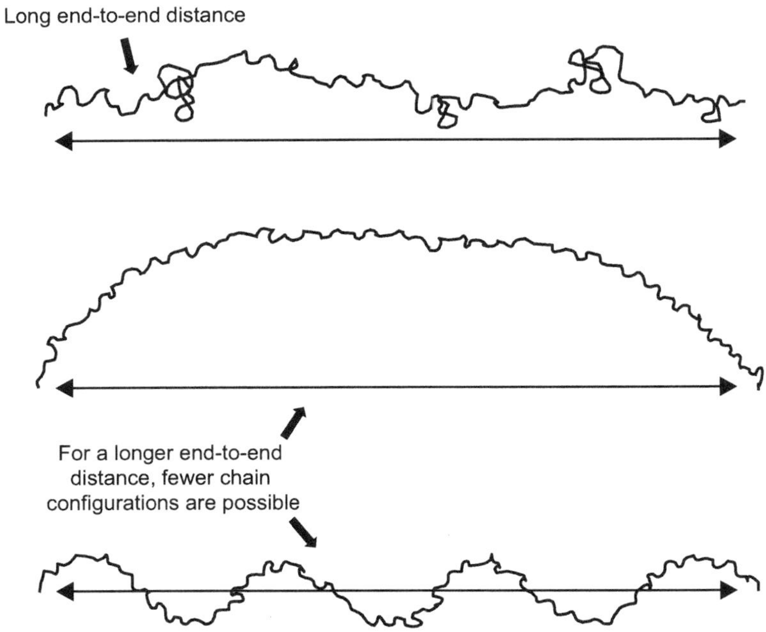

Figure 9.3 A long polymer chain can take fewer configurations if it has a longer end-to-end distance as a result of applied strain. Entropy is lower than for a short end-to-end distance.

in which k_b is Boltzmann's constant and Ω is the number of possible configurations for the polymer chains. When a polymer is elongated, the chains adopt a more aligned configuration on average than they would naturally be in. When the applied force is removed, random thermal motion means that the chains naturally return to their original un-aligned positions in a structure with minimum potential energy. Because the chains are inclined to return to their original unstrained configuration, they exert a retractive force. The sum contribution of all the polymer chains' retractive forces is equal and opposite to the external force that must be applied in order to keep the polymer in a strained state. The stiffness of the polymer is simply the rate at which this retractive force changes with elongation. The entropy change as a result of strain can be calculated in order to predict Young's modulus.[1] Wang *et al.*[2] discuss entropy change in relation to the molecular weight of a degrading polymer and present a modified theory. Since entropy is linearly related to temperature, it is expected that Young's modulus should increase when the temperature of a rubbery polymer increases; this interesting trend is known to be true experimentally.

9.1.2 Plastic deformation of polymers

In rubbery polymers, high strains of several hundred per cent are often possible without plastic deformation. Yielding occurs when the polymer chains do not return to their original positions of minimum energy. A new minimum energy configuration may result from polymer chains being broken, if crosslinks break or reposition, or if chain entanglements untangle. During plastic deformation, necking occurs and the polymer chains become highly aligned with each other. As a result, the stiffness typically increases at high strains because further deformation requires the physical stretching or breaking of bonds, as opposed to the straightening out of chains. For glassy polymers, the polymer chains do not straighten out, so yielding occurs at lower strains (typically <5%). For elastic deformation of glassy polymers, the strain is accommodated by changes in the inter-molecular distance between polymer chains but when the applied stress exceeds the limit of elasticity, plastic deformation occurs as a result of polymer segments shifting relative to one another. Plate VIII in the colour section between pages 130 and 131 shows how three segments of polymer can shift relative to one another without any deformation occurring within each segment. Once the segments have been forced into new positions, they do not return to their original position upon removal of the force; the chains are frozen in the new position unless further plastic deformation occurs.

For semi-crystalline polymers, it is different again; the amorphous phases can deform in the manner described above, depending on whether the polymer is above or below the glass transition temperature, but the crystallites also deform plastically. Figure 9.4 shows how, initially, the crystallites shear in the direction of stress to align

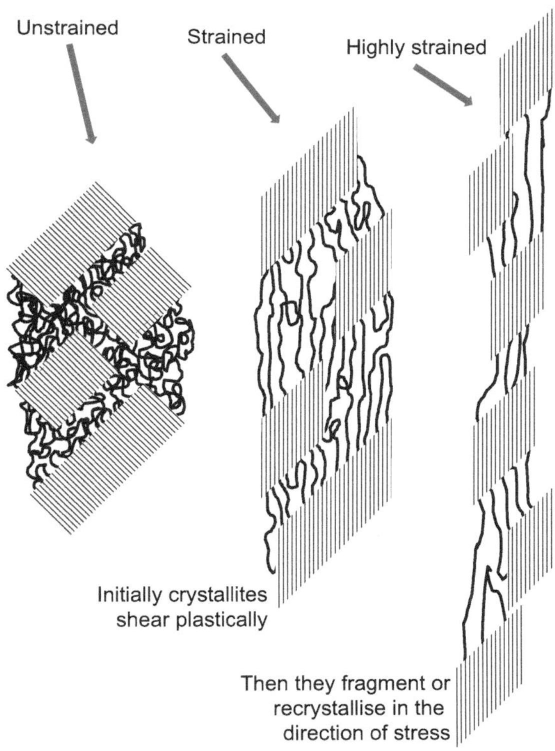

Figure 9.4 Plastic deformation of crystallites in a semi-crystalline polymer.

the chains in that direction. Upon further straining, the crystallites fragment into smaller crystallites, which allows the amorphous phase to deform more freely.

9.1.3 Strength of polymers

Strength is more complicated than stiffness, because it concerns polymers in the highly plastically strained state and is ultimately dictated by a small concentration of features in the polymer such as cross links or chain entanglements. In glassy polymers which display brittle behaviour, the strength may be dictated by the single weakest point in a polymer which initiates a crack during plastic deformation. Such weaknesses in a glassy polymer may result from features such as the local chain configuration, material imperfections (void and impurities), or surface imperfections. Increases in crystallinity may result in an increased overall strength due to the crystalline fraction having high strength but may have the opposite affect and reduce overall strength as a result of extra constraints on the amorphous phase. Rubbery polymers may only break at very high strains and the strength is affected by small concentration factors such as the frequency and distribution of crosslinks or entanglements. Crystallites may act as extra entanglements which increase strength.

9.2 Methods of measurement for mechanical properties

There are a wide range of techniques that may be used to determine mechanical properties. A well-trusted method is tensile testing, in which the two ends of a tensile sample are clamped in a tensile testing machine and pulled apart as shown in Figure 9.5. While the sample is being stretched, the forces that the machine must apply are measured. The greater the required forces, the higher is the stiffness of the sample. The Young's modulus is determined by relating stress in the sample to strain. The strength of a sample is determined from the maximum force applied at any time during a test in which the specimen is broken into two halves. Other mechanical properties may also be determined. Elongation-at-break is frequently published in experimental publications related to biodegradable polymers, and can be calculated through comparison of the initial length of the tensile sample to the final length of the sample immediately before it breaks.

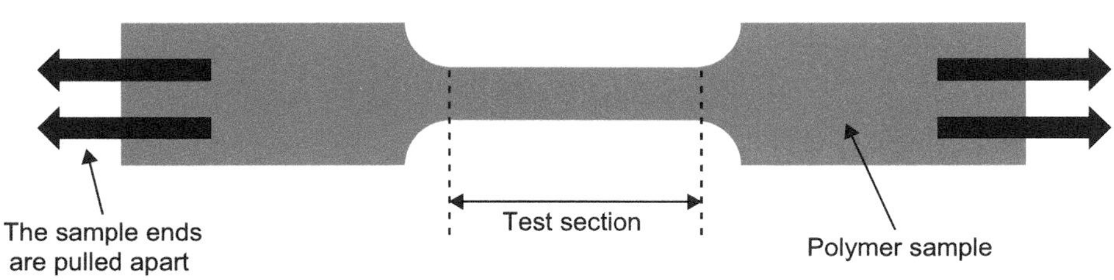

Figure 9.5 Example of a polymer specimen used in a tensile testing machine in order to analyse mechanical properties.

In addition to tensile testing, there are many other common techniques for testing mechanical properties, such as compression, bending, and shear tests. They are all similar, in that they measure the force required for deformation or failure. In compressive testing, samples are crushed. In bending tests a sample is bent, which causes the top and bottom of the sample to be subject to opposite forces of either compression or tension. In shear tests the force required to break to sample in shear can be used to determine the shear strength. As opposed to compression or tensile tests, in which two halves of a polymer may be considered to be pulled apart or crushed together, in shear tests the two halves slide over one another similar to cutting a deck of cards. A polymer reacts to the different types of deformation in different manners. For example, a polymer chain can fold up when subject to compression without stretching the strong covalent bonds in the polymer chains, whereas under tension the covalent bonds must be stretched. It is likely that the elastic moduli calculated through tensile, compressive, and bending tests degrade in different manners.

In addition to the different testing techniques, the testing set-up is also important. Temperature and strain rate have a large impact on the measurements. Nakafuku and Takehisa[3] conducted mechanical property tests at various temperatures for 80 μm amorphous films of poly(L-lactide) and poly(DL-lactide-co-glycolide) 50:50 which had glass transition temperatures of 57.7 and 30.0°C respectively. The results are shown in Figure 9.6. There is over an order of magnitude increase in Young's modulus as the polymers transition from a rubbery state to a glassy state. Interestingly, there is also a significant increase in Young's modulus as the testing temperature of the poly(L-lactide) sample decreases from 20°C to 10°C even though both temperatures are well below T_g, and there is little change in Young's modulus for temperature changes from 35°C to 20°C. These results highlight the complexity of mechanical properties in polymers.

Since biodegradable polymers are degraded in a hydrolysis solution which is absorbed by the polymer, the water molecules plasticise the polymer chains and can affect all of the mechanical properties. In most experimental publications, the testing of mechanical properties is completed using dry samples, which have been dried to ensure the results are comparable to initial tests of samples before they were introduced to the hydrolysis solution.

Due to the number of factors that affect the mechanical properties and the fact that many of these factors are not well understood, there are often large error margins on experimental data measurements. Even before degradation begins there are many factors during polymerisation and processing that can lead to large error margins ≥50%, particularly for elongation-at-break.[4–6]

9.3 Factors that influence the mechanical properties of bioresorbable polymers before degradation

The mechanical properties that are most often measured during biodegradable polymer degradation experiments are stiffness, strength, and elongation-at-break. These mechanical properties are influenced by a large number of factors, the most important

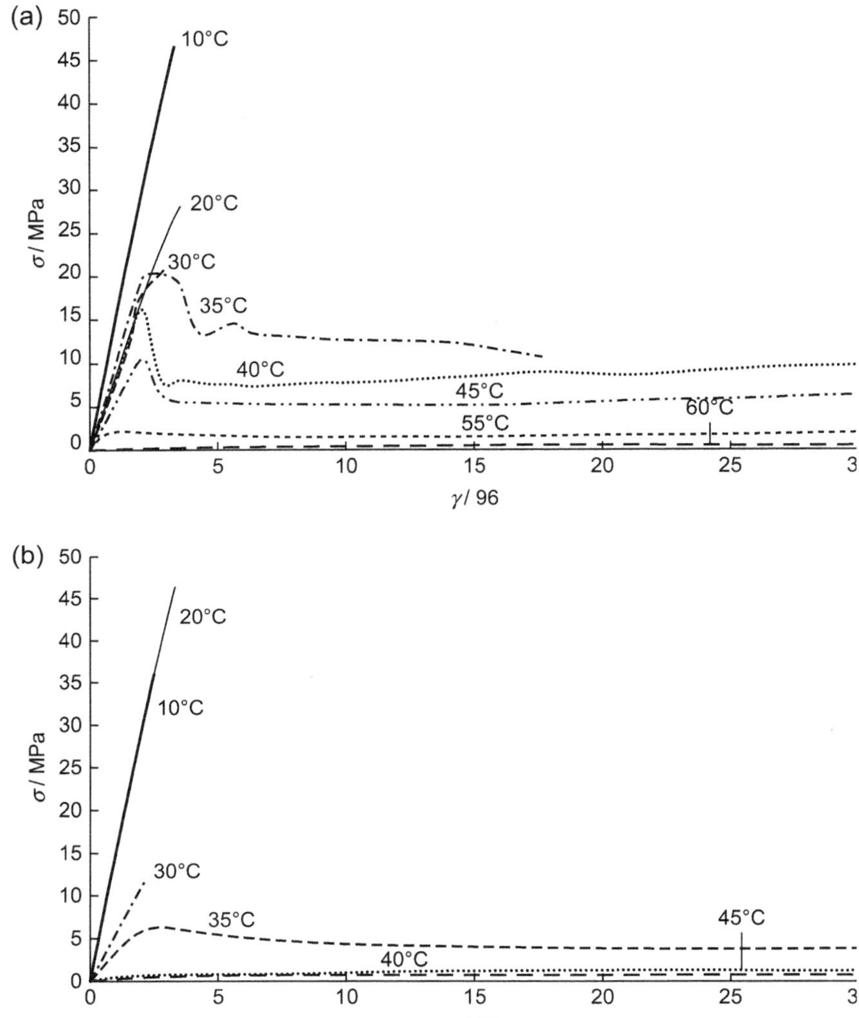

Figure 9.6 Applied stress (MPa) versus applied strain (%) at various temperatures for 80 μm amorphous films of (a) poly(L-lactide) and (b) poly(DL-lactide-co-glycolide) 50:50 reproduced from the publication of Nakafuku and Takehisa[3] with permission via the Copyright Clearance Centre.

of which may be molecular weight. As the polymer chains become longer they are likely to be more entangled. For strength, the polymer chains must either untangle from each other or physically break in order to allow a polymer sample to separate into two parts. Therefore, the more tangled a polymer, the more chains that must be broken in order for the overall polymer sample to break. Elongation-at-break increases when polymer chains are able to unravel to a greater degree without breaking so more entanglements may reduce the value of elongation-at-break. Stiffness increases with molecular weight, although as a result of the complexity of molecular interactions and the lack of comprehensive understanding there are no widely trusted theories that relate Young's modulus to molecular weight. Crystallinity affects the mechanical properties because chains that are aligned side-by-side in crystalline region are strongly bonded to each other. As a result, they become resistant to deformation, and stiffness is likely to increase significantly compared to that of the amorphous polymer phase. Strength also generally increases because the crystallites act as extra entanglements or may be considered as high-strength particles. In a similar manner to crystallinity, amorphous polymer chains may become orientated during processes such as fibre drawing or extrusion. Orientated amorphous polymer chains are aligned to a lesser degree than crystalline regions but are more closely packed than unorientated amorphous chains. The bonding between the chains is therefore stronger, so both strength and stiffness increase versus a fully unorientated amorphous polymer. Other factors that affect mechanical properties before degradation are polymer type/composition and processing techniques/conditions.

9.4 The degradation of mechanical properties

Not all of the factors discussed in the previous section vary during degradation. The rest of this chapter considers the degradation of mechanical properties and factors that affect it. The experimental data plots in Figure 9.7 are taken directly from the

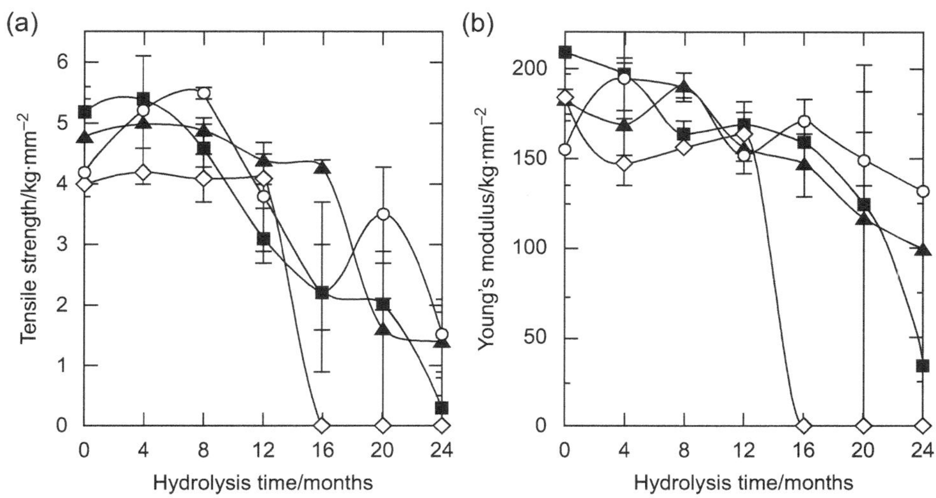

Figure 9.7 Experimental data figures reproduced from the publication of Tsuji[7] with permission via the Copyright Clearance Centre. Tensile strength (a) and Young's modulus (b) versus degradation time for various polymer compositions: poly(L-lactide) filled triangles, poly(D-lactide) ■, copolymer poly(DL-lactide) ◊, and blend polymer poly(L/D-lactide) ○.

publication of Tsuji,[7] which studies the degradation of amorphous poly(lactide) films in phosphate buffer solution (pH 7.4) at 37°C. The evolution of Young's modulus and tensile strength can be seen to be quite erratic in nature; the properties reduce and increase in value during different periods of degradation and can demonstrate a sudden drop to zero.

The erratic nature of mechanical properties degradation is a result of the high number of factors that affect them. Since the data presented in Figure 9.7 are from a single publication many of the potential factors are kept constant for all of the samples, but the trends are still temperamental and error margins are large. The standard polymer processing conditions, degradation conditions, and measuring techniques vary between institutions, which adds uncertainty when comparing data in the literature.

In many publications,[6–16] the value of Young's modulus holds or increases initially during degradation experiments, whereas in some,[5,17,18] Young's modulus reduction occurs from the outset. These trends can be linked to molecular weight degradation and changes in crystallinity, as discussed in the next few sections.

9.4.1 The effect of molecular weight degradation on Young's modulus and strength

Figure 9.8 shows the experimental data of Tsuji[12] for the Young's modulus and strength of semi-crystalline poly(lactide) films that were degraded in a phosphate buffer solution (pH 7.4) at 37°C for 30 months. The polymers used in the films were poly(D-lactide), poly(L-lactide), and a 1:1 blend of poly(D-lactide) and poly(L-lactide). The figure shows that the blended polymer retained mechanical properties for 2 years of degradation, whereas the non-blended polymers displayed a reduction in strength almost linearly from the start of hydrolysis and an initial delay of less than 1 year before the Young's modulus reduced.

The trends for the degradation of mechanical properties bear quite a resemblance to the degradation of molecular weight shown in Figure 9.9. This suggests that mechanical properties are largely dependent on molecular weight degradation. Reduction of molecular weight is generally considered to be the most important factor for long-term mechanical properties during degradation. Strength may reduce as a result of shorter polymer chains being less entangled or more able to untangle during plastic deformation. The film samples in the study[12] were tested below their glass transition temperature, but the elastic deformation of glassy polymers, and therefore Young's modulus, is not well understood.

9.4.2 A direct relationship between the degradation of Young's modulus and the degradation of molecular weight

Since molecular weight has a great impact on Young's modulus, the direct relationship between the Young's modulus and molecular weight is of interest. Mathematical models have been developed to simulate polymer chain scission and therefore the evolution of molecular weight during degradation.[19–26] By relating mechanical properties to molecular weight, the models could also be used to simulate the degradation of

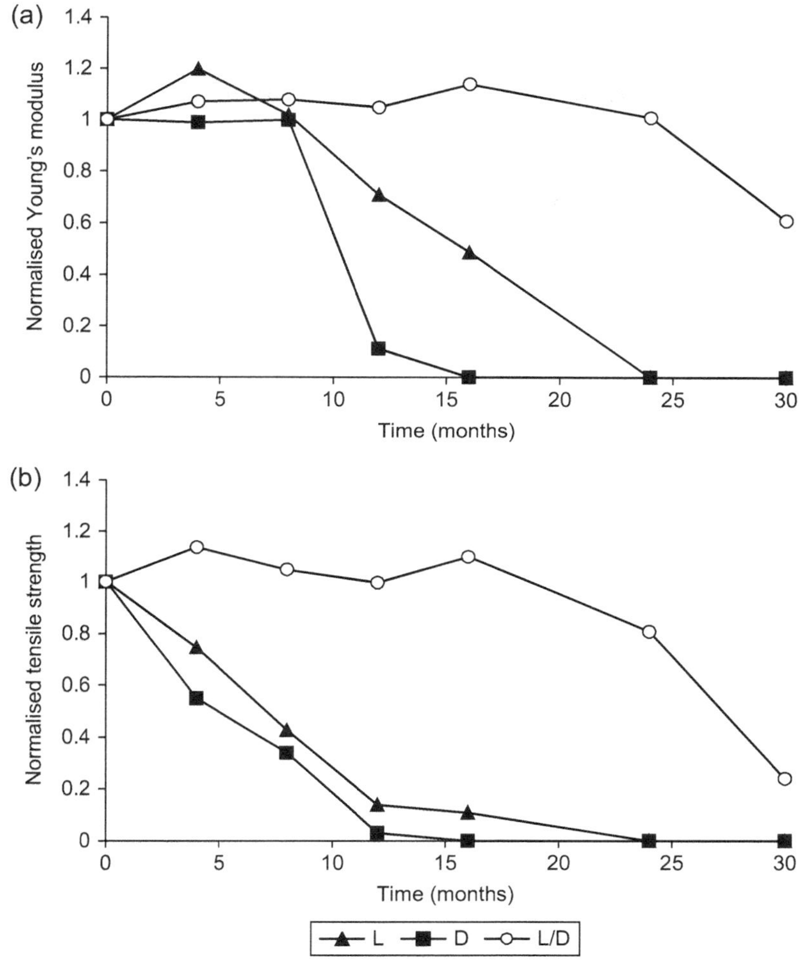

Figure 9.8 Experimental data of Tsuji[12] for the reduction of Young's modulus (a) and tensile strength (b). There is a significant difference between the degradation of mechanical properties for different polymer types: L-lactide (▲); D-lactide (■); and the polymer blend (○).

mechanical properties. It is often found experimentally that the degradation of Young's modulus occurs after molecular weight reduction, as shown in Figure 9.10.[5,7–9,11–13]

In order to determine a relationship between the Young's modulus and molecular weight, it is useful to consider a plot of the properties against one another. Figure 9.11 shows such a plot for the experimental data shown in Figures 9.8 and 9.9. Due to the loss of Young's modulus being delayed behind the loss of molecular weight, the relationship is non-linear. Molecular weight reduces by over 50% before Young's modulus begins to drop quite suddenly. The dashed line in the Figure 9.11 highlights

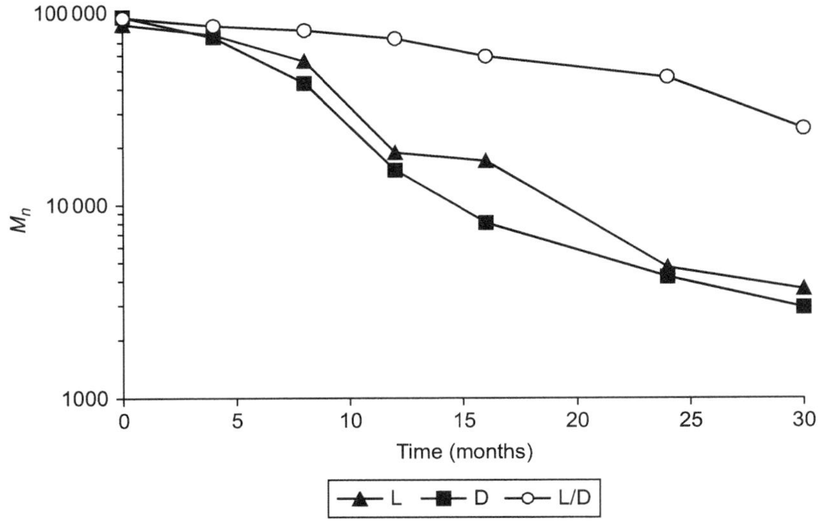

Figure 9.9 Experimental data of Tsuji[12] for the reduction number averaged molecular weight. As with mechanical properties, the rate of degradation is reduced for the blended polymer film (○) as opposed to the homopolymer films L-lactide (▲) and D-lactide (■).

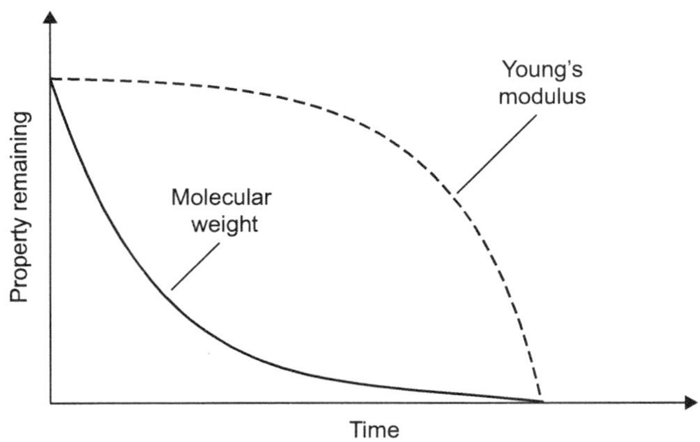

Figure 9.10 Molecular weight reduction often precedes the reduction of Young's modulus.

the typical trend that may be identified from the data to relate Young's modulus to normalised molecular weight.

The relationship between molecular weight and Young's modulus varies considerably between experimental data sets in the literature. The experimental data of Duek *et al.*[27] for Young's modulus versus molecular weight is shown in Figure 9.12. Initially, amorphous and crystalline poly(L-lactide) pins were degraded in phosphate buffer solution (pH 7.4) at 37°C for 6 months. Several of the values used

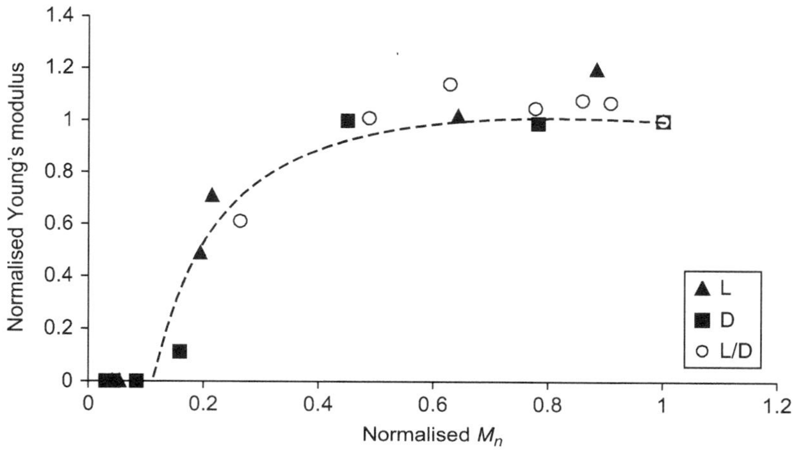

Figure 9.11 A plot of Young's modulus versus molecular weight can be used to identify a relationship between the two properties. The experimental data of Tsuji[12] (discrete symbols) are the same as used in Figures 9.8 and 9.9.

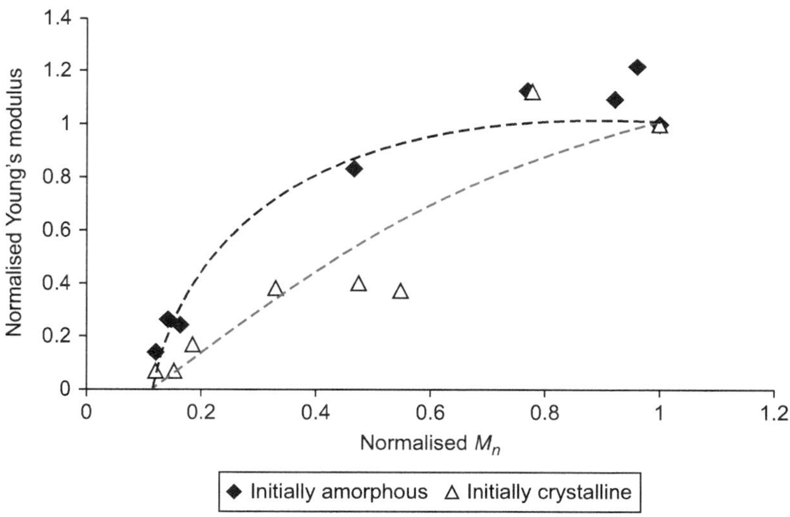

Figure 9.12 A plot of Young's modulus versus molecular weight for the experimental data of Duek *et al.*[27] for initially crystalline and initially amorphous samples during degradation.

for molecular weight in the figure are linearly interpolated (with relation to time) between measurements because molecular weight was analysed less frequently than Young's modulus and after different times of degradation. The initially amorphous sample shows a considerable initial delay in the reduction of Young's modulus compared to molecular weight, whereas the initially crystalline sample shows little delay. The effect of crystallinity on mechanical properties degradation is considered

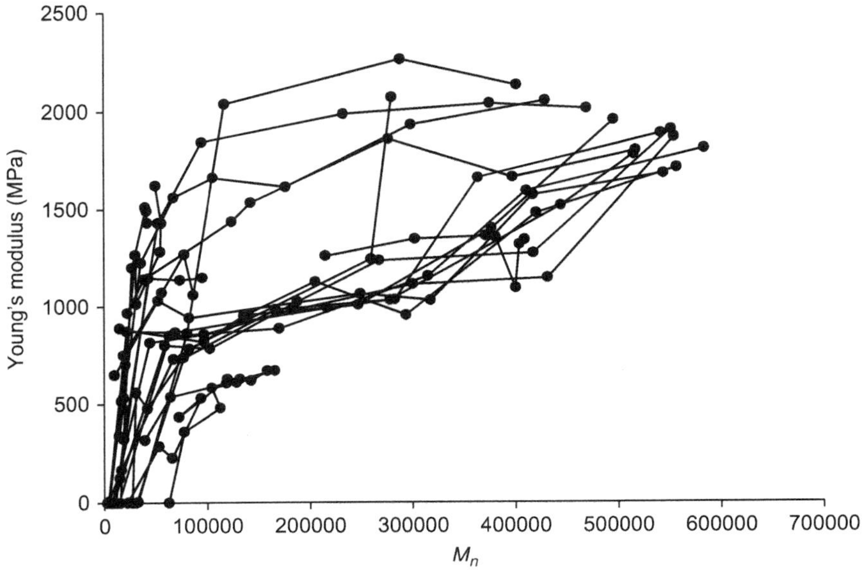

Figure 9.13 A plot of Young's modulus versus molecular weight for 21 degradation experiments of poly(lactide).[4,5,7,10,12–14,17,18,28] Each set of data points linked by lines represents a single experimental set-up.

in the next section of this chapter. The dashed black and grey curves show typical trends that may be identified from the data for the initially amorphous and crystalline samples respectively. The variation between these samples highlights how a simple relationship between Young's modulus and molecular weight is difficult to identify by considering individual samples in detail.

In order to find a simple general relationship between Young's modulus and molecular weight, 21 experimental data sets for the degradation of poly(L- or D-lactide) are analysed together[4,5,7,10,12–14,17,18,28] An overall plot of all the experimental data sets is shown in Figure 9.13. For one experimental study[18] weight-averaged molecular weight data were supplied, therefore the number-average molecular weight was calculated using a simple assumption of polydispersity = $M_w/M_n = 2$, which was the most frequent initial value measured in that study. As can be seen in the figure, almost all of the samples demonstrate a delay of Young's modulus reduction behind molecular weight reduction as previously discussed in relation to Figures 9.11 and 9.12. A single curve of best fit cannot fit the data well.

Figure 9.14 shows an alternative presentation of the data with molecular weight on a logarithmic scale. By considering $\log(M_n)$, it can be seen that the experimental data typically demonstrate a similar gradient for a linear relationship between Young's modulus degradation and the reduction of $\log(M_n)$, as highlighted by the master curves (dashed lines) which are arbitrarily offset to either side of the experimental data. For any given set of experimental data, the master curve can be shifted along the $\log(M_n)$ axis until it passes through the point of measured initial M_n and

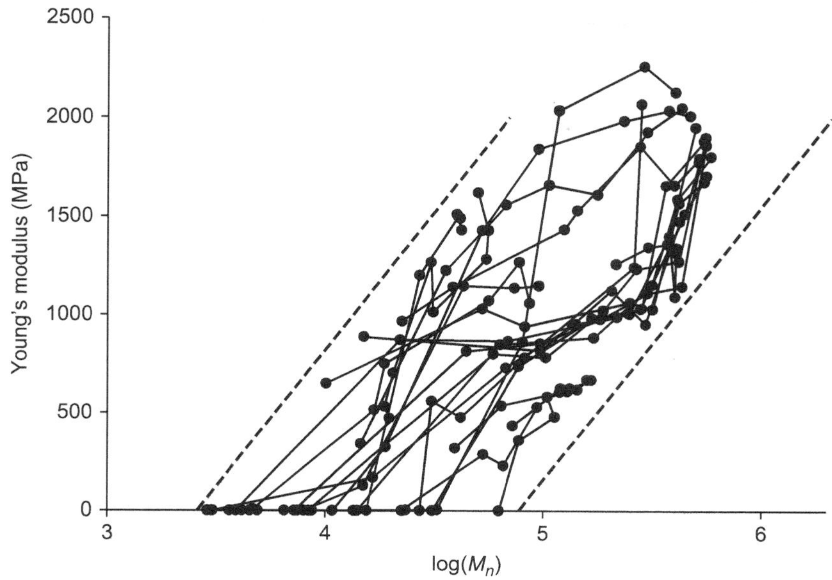

Figure 9.14 Alternative presentation of the data in Figure 9.13 with a logarithmic scale for molecular weight. The dashed lines represent a possible interpretation of the data that the Young's modulus of poly(lactide) samples during degradation is linearly related to log(M_n). The gradients of the dashed lines are 1400 MPa per order of magnitude reduction in M_n.

initial Young's modulus. The gradient of the master curves in the figure are 1400 MPa, which suggests that each time molecular weight reduces by a factor of 10, Young's modulus may reduce by ≈1400 MPa. From an alternative viewpoint, for each 500 MPa reduction in Young's modulus the molecular weight must reduce by ≈56%. This linear relationship between Young's modulus and log(M_n) can be used to predict the rate of Young's modulus degradation if M_n degradation is measured or modelled. Young's modulus can be calculated during degradation as

$$E = E_0 + k_m \log \frac{M_n}{M_{n0}} \quad [9.3]$$

in which E(GPa) and E_0 (GPa) are the instantaneous and original values of Young's modulus, respectively, k_m (GPa) is the degradation rate constant for Young's modulus, and M_n(g mol^{-1}) and M_{n0}(g mol^{-1}) are the instantaneous and original values of number averaged molecular weight, respectively. The value of k_m is 1400 GPa according to the dashed lines in Figure 9.14. It should be noted that the relationship identified here is a very general relationship, which was established from data over a broad range of experimental circumstances; initial crystallinity varies from amorphous to highly crystalline, initial molecular weight varies by over an order of magnitude, and several other factors vary, including processing conditions, degradation temperature, sample size and mechanical property measurement techniques/conditions. The master curve relating Young's modulus degradation to molecular weight degradation incorporates the uncertainties associated with these factors, including crystallinity, which is known to considerably affect Young's modulus. Equation [9.3] can be used to very simply estimate the Young's modulus of a poly(lactide) sample at any time during degradation if molecular weight is measured along with the initial value of Young's modulus.

9.4.3 The effect of increasing crystallinity during degradation on Young's modulus and strength

Crystallinity is known to increase the values of Young's modulus and strength for polymers. Figure 9.15 shows the effect of crystallinity on Young's modulus (top in figure) and strength (bottom) according to poly(L-lactide) experiments conducted by Tsuji and Ikada[29] for three different manufacturing techniques, referred to as film A, B, and C in the figure.

Crystallinity increases as a result of chain scission, so the Young's modulus and strength may be expected to increase during degradation. This effect is offset by the fact that as crystallinity increases, molecular weight reduces, which in turn reduces the values of Young's modulus and strength. Nevertheless, increases in Young's modulus or strength are often found to occur at some point during degradation experiments.[5–9,12–16,18,27,28,30] The experimental data of Duek *et al.*[27] shown in Figure 9.16 demonstrate how Young's modulus (top) and strength (bottom) can increase during degradation. These experiments were also discussed in relation to molecular weight in the previous section.

The molecular weight and crystallinity data for the same study are given in Figure 9.17. It can be seen at the top of Figure 9.17 that molecular weight drops at a greater rate for the crystalline samples than for the amorphous samples. This can explain why the mechanical properties reduce more quickly for the crystalline sample. However, consider the data after 2 weeks; the amorphous and crystalline samples demonstrate an increase in Young's modulus of 10–25% even though there is a reduction in molecular weight of up to 50%. This can be explained by the increase in crystallinity of 10–50% over the first few weeks, as shown at the bottom of Figure 9.17. Also, consider both samples after 12 weeks of degradation. The crystallinity of the initially amorphous sample has increased by ≈50%, whereas the initially crystalline sample has only increased by 10–20%. As a result, the amorphous sample retains a higher value of normalised Young's modulus even though it demonstrates a slightly greater reduction of molecular weight.

The experimental data of Saha and Tsuji[9] are shown in Figure 9.18 for crystallinity, molecular weight, Young's modulus, and strength. In the study, a sample which undergoes hydrolysis is compared to a sample which is stored at the same temperature but in the absence of water, which therefore does not undergo polymer chain scission. In the early stages of degradation, the mechanical properties are most affected by crystallinity, which increases rapidly at the start of degradation. Therefore the

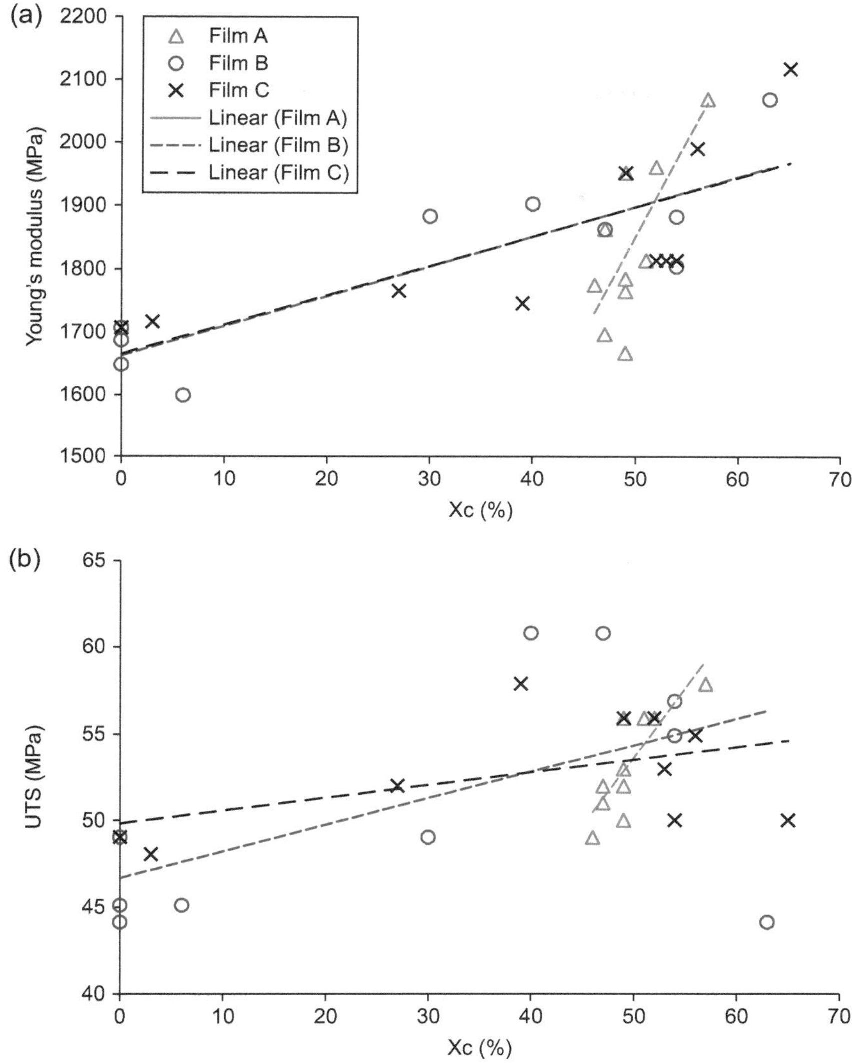

Figure 9.15 Experimental data by Tsuji and Ikada[29] for poly(L-lactide) films shows that increasing crystallinity results in an increase in polymer stiffness (a) and strength (b).

polymer becomes stiffer and stronger even though molecular weight is reducing. During the later stages of degradation, however, the reduction of molecular weight becomes the dominating factor and both Young's modulus and tensile strength properties reduce to zero. In the sample that does not degrade, crystallinity is the major factor affecting the mechanical properties throughout the experiment, so the stiffness and strength increase without subsequent reductions. The data clearly support the

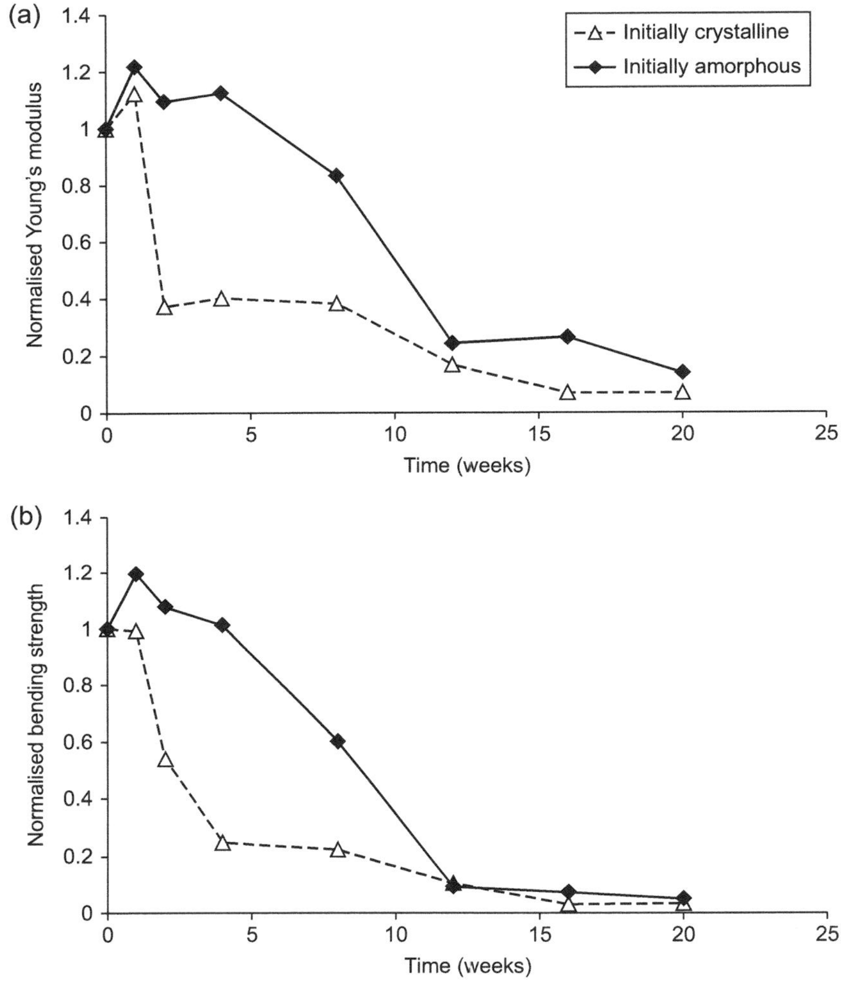

Figure 9.16 Experimental data of Duek *et al.*[27] for poly(L-lactide) pins show an increase in stiffness (a) and strength (b) during the early stages of degradation.

above discussion in regards to Figures 9.16 and 9.17 that strength and stiffness are increased by crystallinity and reduced by molecular weight.

In some experimental studies, Young's modulus increases in the early stages of degradation even if crystallinity does not.[6,7,16,3] Tsuji and Suzuyoshi[6,16,31] attributed this increase to the 'stabilized chain packing in the amorphous region in the presence of water molecules' with regards to their amorphous samples. This is similar to crystallinity increasing during annealing of the polymer; although the amorphous chains are not able to pack into a crystal form, they may reorientate into a more close-packed structure than the initial structure. If samples are stored at temperatures below 37°C before degradation, the reorientation of chains is assisted by the increased movability of

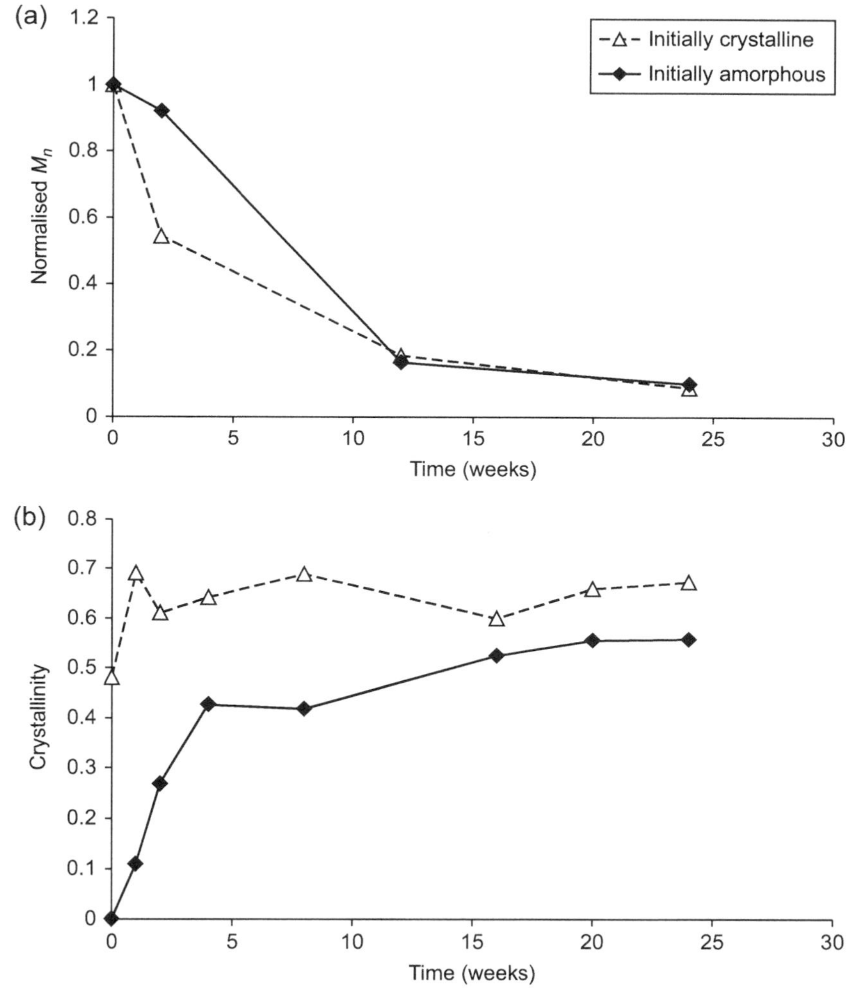

Figure 9.17 Experimental data of Duek *et al.*[27] for the molecular weight (a) and crystallinity (b) in poly(L-lactide) pins.

chains at a temperature of 37°C along with the plasticising effects of water molecules. This understanding is particularly appropriate for initially amorphous samples that are quenched from the melt, since quenching prevents the chains from relaxing into the most stable configuration. When modelling the degradation of mechanical properties, it is clearly important to consider both molecular weight and crystallinity.

9.4.4 The degradation of elongation-at-break property

Reductions in molecular weight due to chain scission during degradation generally reduce the maximum elongation sustained by the polymer before it breaks

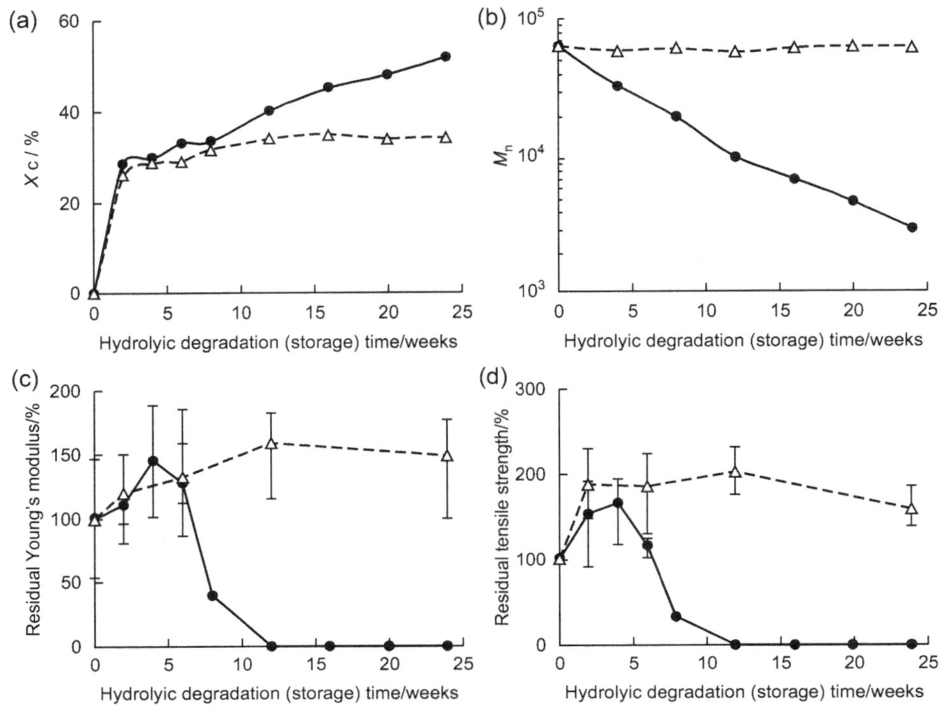

Figure 9.18 Experimental data figures reproduced from the publication of Saha and Tsuji[9] with permission via the Copyright Clearance Centre. The plots show various properties of poly(L-lactide) films during degradation: crystallinity (a); molecular weight (b); Young's modulus (c); and strength (d). Samples were either stored in the absence of water (Δ) or degraded via hydrolysis (•).

(elongation-at-break). The variation of elongation-at-break with degradation time is often more erratic than for strength and Young's modulus. The data presented in Figure 9.19. are from the study of Tsuji[12] which was discussed in relation to Figures 9.8 and 9.9. It demonstrates how elongation-at-break values can reduce and increase dramatically, and how the error margins can be large. Such large error margins may indicate that the value of elongation-at-break is not dependent on overall macroscale polymer structure, since variability in the polymer would then be expected to average out and reduce error margins. It may be the case that the elongation-at-break value is dependent on the material properties in the single weakest section of the polymer sample. This is analogous to the unpredictable strength in ceramics which is dependent on the largest flaw size.

Elongation-at-break may be expected to decrease as molecular weight degrades because shorter chains can untangle more easily, so two halves of a polymer sample can be pulled apart at a lower elongation percentage. Conversely, if chain scission results in the glass transition temperature of a polymer reducing, the deformation mechanism for the polymer may change from a glassy to rubbery deformation, in which case

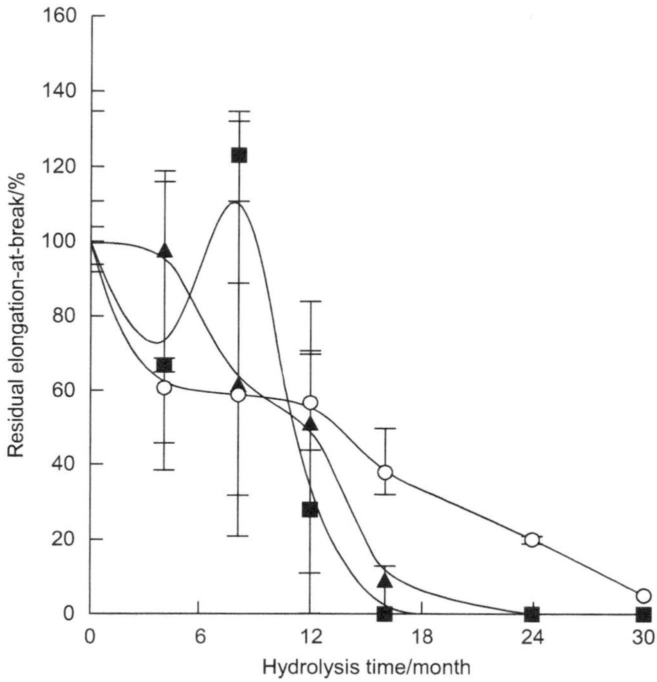

Figure 9.19 Experimental data figure reproduced from the publication of Tsuji[12] with permission via the Copyright Clearance Centre for elongation-at-break versus time. The data is quite erratic and has high error margins. Three polymers are studied: L-lactide (▲); D-lactide (■); and a 1:1 blend of L- and D-lactide (○).

elongation-at-break would significantly increase. Similarly, if chain scission reduces the chain entanglement, it is possible that elongation-at-break values could increase due to the polymer chains being more able to unravel rather than break during deformation. As mechanical properties reduce towards zero, however, the polymer approaches a state where it falls apart under its own weight, so elongation-at-break also approaches zero. The effect of chain scission is a complicated interplay between these effects, and probably many others, but in general for long-term degradation the value of elongation-at-break reduces as molecular weight reduces. This can be seen in the data presented in Figures 9.9 and 9.19, because the molecular weight reduces more quickly for the homopolymers than the polymer blend, as does long-term elongation-at-break.

In addition to changes that result from molecular weight, increases in crystallinity (as a result of chain scission) also affect elongation-at-break. In contrast to Young's modulus and strength, increasing crystallinity reduces the value of elongation-at-break because the stiff crystal particles cannot elongate like amorphous polymer chains and they may constrain the chains in a similar manner to chain entanglements. The study of Tsuji and Ikada,[29] which was discussed above in relation to Figure 9.15, also considered elongation-at-break. The effect of crystallinity on elongation-at-break

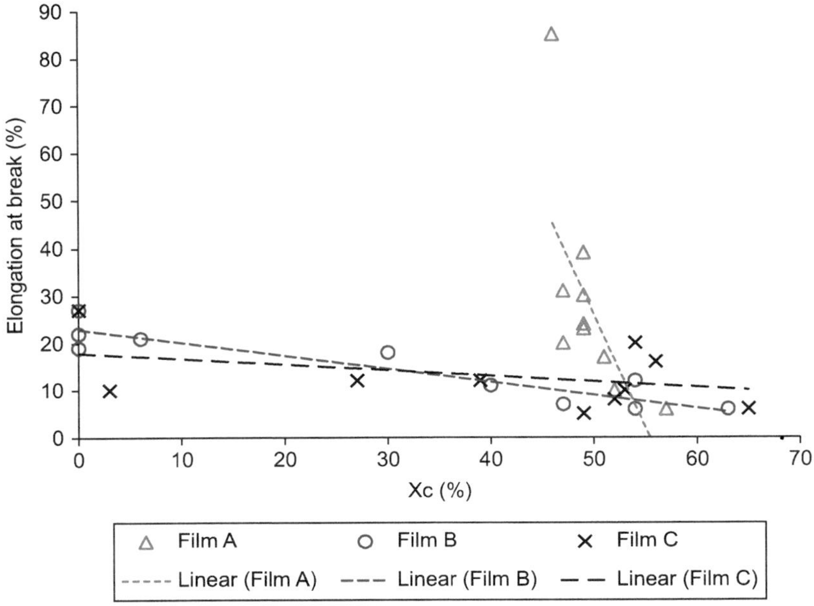

Figure 9.20 Experimental data by Tsuji and Ikada[29] for poly(L-lactide) films shows that increasing crystallinity results in a decrease in elongation-at-break.

was studied for three different manufacturing processes. The experimental data are shown in Figure 9.20 and clearly demonstrate that elongation-at-break reduces as crystallinity increases. However, the relationship is quite noisy and strongly dependent on the manufacturing process used.

The effects of both molecular weight reduction and crystallinity on elongation-at-break can be seen in the experiments of Saha and Tsuji.[9] The experimental data for elongation-at-break are shown in Figure 9.21. Molecular weight and crystallinity data are presented in Figure 9.18. Initially, amorphous samples were studied both with (solid line in the figure) and without (dashed line) hydrolytic degradation. Both samples show a sudden increase in crystallinity in the first 2 weeks and, as a result, elongation-at-break reduces sharply in that timeframe. The value of elongation-at-break for the sample which undergoes hydrolysis, and therefore experiences a reduction in molecular weight, continues to reduce and equals zero after 8 weeks of degradation, by which time Young's modulus is approximately 40% of the original value. In contrast, the sample which sees no reduction in molecular weight demonstrates a relatively constant elongation-at-break value for several weeks after the initial crystallinity-induced drop.

Although crystallinity has a considerable effect on elongation-at-break, it is reductions in molecular that ultimately reduce the value to zero. Several experimental publications[5,7,9,12,13,18,27,30] show that the samples for which molecular weight reduces most rapidly also demonstrate an earlier total loss of the elongation-at-break value. Although in many cases[5,7,12,30] the samples which degrade most rapidly in terms of molecular weight do not necessarily experience the greatest reduction

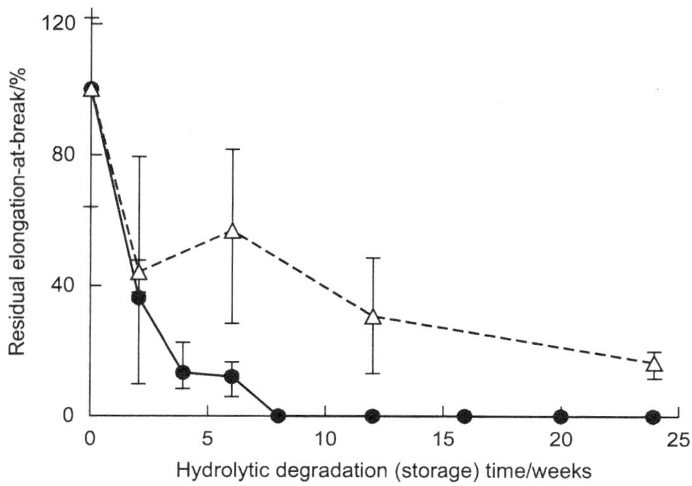

Figure 9.21 Experimental data figure reproduced from the publication of Saha and Tsuji[9] with permission via the Copyright Clearance Centre for elongation-at-break of poly(L-lactide) films. Samples were either stored in the absence of water (Δ) or degraded via hydrolysis (•).

in normalised elongation-at-break during the early stages of degradation. One important factor is that in the initial values of elongation and break can vary greatly between samples. Samples that are initially amorphous generally have a high initial value of elongation-at-break which reduces significantly in the early stages of degradation as the samples crystallise. However, these initially amorphous samples may ultimately retain non-zero values of elongation-at-break for longer because the molecular weight of initially crystalline samples tends to reduce more rapidly. This theory that less crystalline samples experience greater reduction in elongation-at-break early (due to higher initial values) but ultimately retain non-zero values longer (due to slower reduction of M_n) is the most likely situation in the experiments of Tsuji[12] and of Tsuji *et al.*[5] Other experimental studies[7,30] demonstrate significant reduction of high initial elongation-at-break values during the early stages of degradation for amorphous polymers that do not crystallise during degradation. Initially, amorphous samples are generally quenched during processing to prevent crystallisation. Therefore it may be the case that when water enters the polymer during the early stages of degradation, the amorphous polymer chains are plasticised and reorientate into a more tangled, or more orientated, configuration which does not allow high elongation-at-break.

9.4.5 *Other factors that affect the degradation of mechanical properties*

Since the reduction of molecular weight has a major effect on mechanical properties, any factors that affect the rate of molecular weight degradation in turn affect mechanical properties. In some cases, the effects may be counter-intuitive. A particular example is with regards to the structural design of fixation devices for which biodegradable polymers are being used. It has been found that the molecular weight of large polymer samples degrade more rapidly than small samples.[32] Therefore, increasing the initial strength and stiffness of a fixation device through an increase in physical size may ultimately lead to a weaker device if degradation occurs more rapidly. Factors that may affect the degradation of molecular weight include:

- Temperature, type, pH, and replacement frequency of the degradation medium along with the solution:polymer volume ratio.
- The initial molecular weight, polydispersity and residual monomer content of the polymer samples.
- Polymer micro-/nano-structure including crystallinity, orientation of amorphous chains, and spherulite size.
- Physical sample size and shape.
- Polymer, copolymer, or polymer-blend composition including any added composite particles or drug loading.
- Polymer processing conditions and techniques including polymerisation, heat treatment, shape forming, and sterilisation.
- Polymer glass transition temperature.

There are some other factors that can directly affect the degradation of mechanical properties. The initial values of mechanical properties affect the rates of their degradation, as discussed earlier in this chapter for samples with high initial values of elongation-at-break. The rate of degradation may be affected for both normalised and absolute property values. The micro-/nano-structure is mentioned in the bullet points above because it may affect the rate of chain scission. In addition to that effect, the micro-/nano-structure is likely to affect the impact that each chain scission has on mechanical properties. For example, in a drawn fibre many of the polymer chains are aligned in the fibre direction and chain scission in a fibre-orientated chain will have a different effect on mechanical properties from chain scission in a non-orientated chain. Therefore, for a given scission rate, the reduction of mechanical properties with time depends on the chain configuration in the polymer. Mass loss may be proposed to affect mechanical properties if it results in a porous structure. However, in numerous experimental publications[5,7–10,12,13,17,18,30] mass loss occurs after mechanical properties have significantly reduced or have been completely lost, so it is not expected to be an important factor for mechanical properties. The glass transition temperature (T_g) could play a significant role in the degradation of mechanical properties for polymers whose glass transition temperature is in the region of the testing temperature. During hydrolytic degradation, T_g often decreases[5,7,10,17,18,27] as a result of chain scission allowing the polymer chains to move relative to one another more easily. Although T_g may also increase, particularly in the early stages of degradation, due to an increase in crystallinity.[4,5,8,10,18] If T_g lowers to the extent that the polymer transitions from a glassy state (testing temperature below T_g) to a rubbery state (above T_g), the stiffness would dramatically reduce. This is a separate mechanism for the degradation of Young's modulus to chain scissions in a polymer which remains in a glassy state. Whether a polymer loses stiffness due to a weakening of the glassy polymer or due to a lowering of the glass transition temperature may not always be clear, particularly given that the glass transition temperature sometimes becomes poorly defined towards the later stages of degradation.[12,13] Since polymers may contain a mixture of amorphous, aligned, or crystalline polymer chains, it may be the case that some regions of the polymer are below T_g and other regions (which would facilitate the overall deformation) are above T_g.

9.5 Modelling changes in mechanical properties of degrading polymers

The master curve which relates Young's modulus to molecular weight in Figure 9.14 is simply a fitting to experimental data; the identified relationship is not a theoretical understanding of how the two material properties are related. This section reviews some models which simulate the degradation of mechanical properties based on a molecular understanding. Two models for polymer strength are considered briefly, along with more in-depth analysis of three models for Young's modulus. Flory[1] proposed that fracture strength, σ_f, could be related to initial strength, σ_∞, according to Equation [9.4] as:

$$\sigma_f = \sigma_\infty - \frac{B}{M_n} \qquad [9.4]$$

in which B is a constant. Similarly, Deng *et al.*[33] found that a fitting to their experimental data for strength retention could be described by Equation [9.5] as:

$$BSR = a + b \ln MW \qquad [9.5]$$

in which BSR is breaking-strength retention, a and b are constants to be determined from the data fitting, and MW is number or weight-average molecular weight.

The author of this chapter is only aware of three studies which relate Young's modulus to the degradation of molecular weight in bioresorbable polymers based on a theoretical understanding of how mechanical properties change during degradation: the first study was conducted by Wang *et al.*[2] and considered the entropy spring model for rubbery amorphous polymers; the second, by Ding *et al.*[34] was a molecular dynamics (MD) study of chain scission in a semi-crystalline polymer both above and below T_g; and in the third study, by Gleadall,[35] atomic-scale simulations of a glassy biodegradable polymer lead to a simple model for Young's modulus degradation.

9.5.1 *An entropy spring model for the degradation of Young's modulus by*

Wang *et al.*[2] developed a model for Young's modulus degradation based on theoretical entropy change during deformation. For polymers above their glass transition temperature,

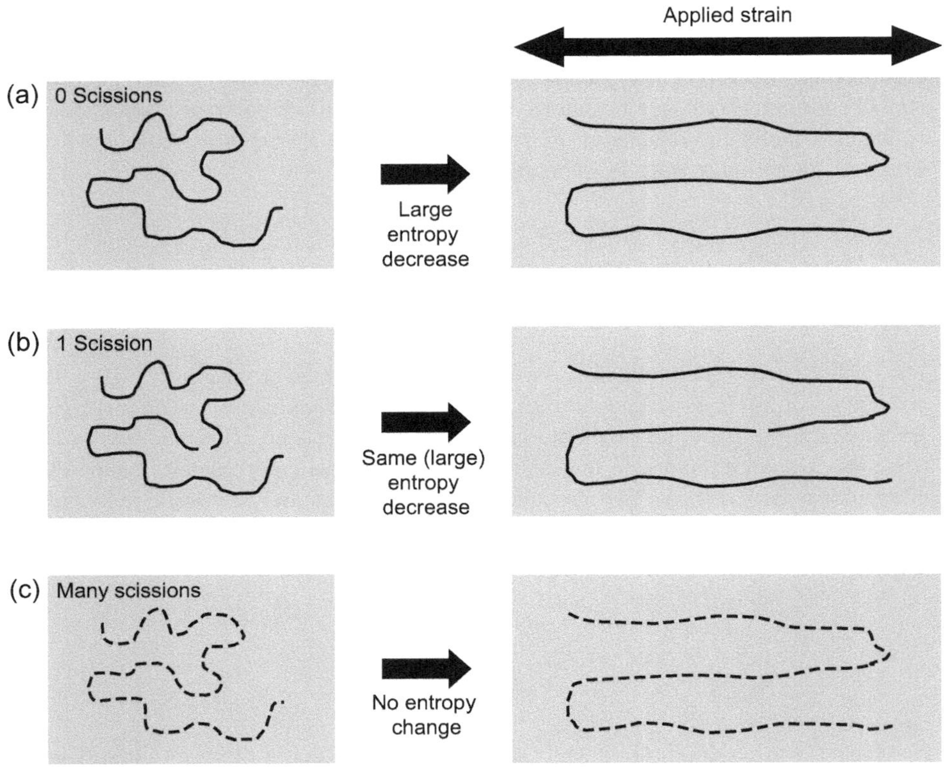

Figure 9.22 The theory presented by Wang *et al.*[2] considers how a polymer chain (black line) embedded in a matrix of other amorphous polymer chains (grey box) straightens out during elongation of the overall polymer. A chain is shown with (a) no scissions (b) a single scission, and (c) many scissions. There is little effect of a single scission on entropy change during deformation, whereas many scissions can result in entropy no longer reducing during deformation.

Young's modulus is controlled by the entropy change during degradation, as discussed at the start of this chapter. Since the polymer chains straighten out during deformation, there are fewer possible configurations for the polymer chains to occupy, which causes the entropy change. This is shown schematically in Figure 9.22a, which shows a polymer chain (black line) in a matrix of other amorphous polymer chains (grey area) before and after strain is applied. From entropy theory,[1] the Young's modulus, E, of a polymer can be related to the number of polymer chains per unit volume, N, according to

$$E = 3Nk_bT \qquad [9.6]$$

in which k_b is Boltzmann's constant and T is the absolute testing temperature. The relationship proposed in Equation [9.6] appears to indicate that Young's modulus should increase during degradation because, as chain scissions occur, the number of chains per unit volume, N, increases. However, Wang *et al.*[2] argued that (1) a fundamental assumption when deriving Equation [9.6] from entropy theory is that the end-to-end distance is much smaller than the extended chain length of a polymer chain, and (2) the end-to-end length should follow a Gaussian distribution, which is not valid for random scission. Rather than include random scission directly into entropy theory, which is a complicated task, Wang *et al.*[2] suggested an intuitive modification to Equation [9.6]. Since the individual polymer chains are highly constrained by the surrounding polymer chains, an isolated chain scission may have little effect on the overall chain configuration before and after deformation. This can be seen in Figure 9.22, by comparison of situations (a) and (b) with zero and one scissions respectively. Wang *et al.*[2] proposed that since the change in entropy is similar for both situations, isolated chain scissions can be considered to have no effect on the entropy increase during deformation, and therefore the value of N should not increase as a result of chain scission. They referred to this argument as the 'no-rise rule'. To account for the effect of chain scission, Wang *et al.*[2] suggested that once a polymer chain is cleaved to the extent that it is divided into very short chains, it no longer contributes to the overall entropy of the polymer. Figure 9.22 c shows the justification for this theory schematically because the individual chain fragments do not need to straighten out during overall polymer deformation, therefore the total entropy of all the small chains (that once made up the long chain) can be assumed not to change during deformation. Wang *et al.*[2] implemented this theory by utilising a molecular weight threshold, M_{th}. When a polymer chain undergoes chain cleavage to the extent that its molecular weight reduces below M_{th}, the chain is removed from the entropy calculation and therefore the value of N in Equation [9.6] reduces by 1.

Wang *et al.*[2] used their concepts of the 'no-rise rule' and a molecular weight threshold to relate Young's modulus to average molecular weight. They ran computer simulations of chain scissions in a discrete number of polymer chains. In the simulations, polymer chains were created numerically with random chain lengths according to an initial molecular weight distribution. Chain scissions were then numerically simulated, with consideration given to both random-scission and end-scission theories. Based on a set value of M_{th}, the value of N was calculated after each chain scission. The new value of N allowed a normalised value of Young's modulus to be calculated, according to Equation [9.6], and therefore directly related to average molecular weight which was also calculated.

Wang *et al.*[2] compared the model prediction to the experimental data of Tsuji[7] for Young's modulus and average molecular weight. In Tsuji's experiments,[7] thin films of poly(L-lactide) and poly(D-lactide) were degraded in phosphate buffer solution (pH 7.4) at 37°C. Figure 9.23 shows the experimental gel permeation chromatography (GPC) curves at four different times during degradation. A molecular weight threshold of $M_{th} = 9.36 \times 10^4$ g mol^{-1} was determined which is indicated in the figure by the shaded region. The portions of the experimental molecular weight distributions that lie within the shaded region were assumed to be too short to contribute to the entropy change during degradation. The value of N was calculated by integrating over the area to the right of the shaded region. Computer simulations were then completed to find the relationship between normalised Young's modulus and normalised average

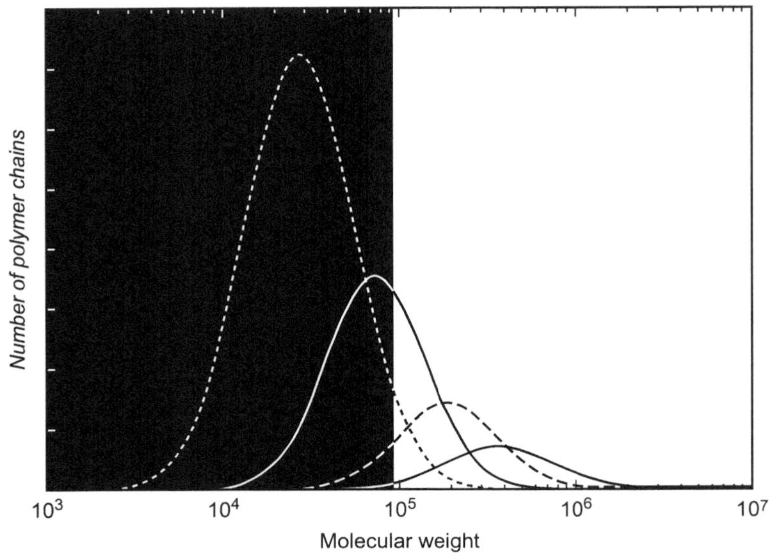

Figure 9.23 Figure reproduced with permission from the publisher Elsevier and the author Wang[2] via the Copyright Clearance Centre. Experimental GPC curves for molecular weight distributions of poly(D-lactide)[7] are shown at various times during degradation: 0, 8, 16, and 24 months from right to left. The shaded region indicates polymer chains that are below a molecular weight threshold of $M_{th} = 9.36 \times 10^4$ g mol^{-1}.

molecular weight according to Equation [9.6] utilising the 'no-rise rule' and $M_{th} = 9.36 \times 10^4$ g mol^{-1}. The relationship is shown (solid line) in Figure 9.24, along with experimental measurements of Tsuji.[7] There is clearly a very good fitting between the model and the experimental data.

Simple mathematical models exist which can simulate the degradation of average molecular weight in biodegradable polymers.[19–26] Wang *et al.*[2] combined such a model with their entropy spring model to predict the degradation of Young's modulus of a biodegradable rod using finite element analysis (FEA). Plate IX shows the results for normalised molecular weight in the rod during degradation. The rod degraded more quickly in the middle because an advanced mathematical model[19,20] was used which can consider the diffusion of short polymer chains, which accelerate the rate of chain cleavage, out of the rod near the surface. Wang *et al.*[2] completed simulations for several rod sizes, and related the predicted average molecular weight degradation to Young's modulus degradation. The results for Young's modulus versus degradation time are shown in Figure 9.25. The three different curves with non-dimensional diffusion coefficients $\bar{D}$ = 10: 0.1: 0.0001 correspond to three different normalised rod diameters of 1: 10: 100 respectively. The largest rod lost mechanical properties earliest because the short polymer chains had a further distance to diffuse before leaving the rod. The model of Wang *et al.*[2] can be used to predict the degradation of several biodegradable device designs to identify which offers the optimum mechanical properties during the degradation process.

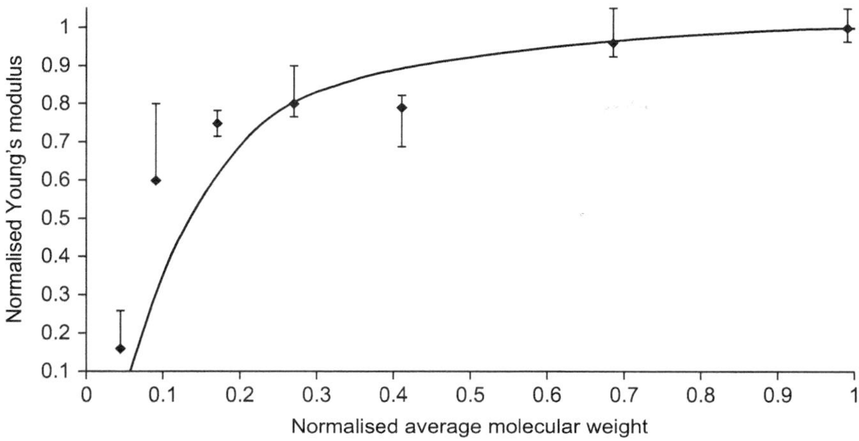

Figure 9.24 Figure reproduced with permission from the publisher Elsevier and the author Wang[2] via the Copyright Clearance Centre. Experimental data for normalised Young's modulus versus normalised average molecular weight for poly(D-lactide)[7] (discrete data points) are compared to the model prediction assuming a molecular weight threshold of $M_{th} = 9.36 \times 10^4$ g mol^{-1}.

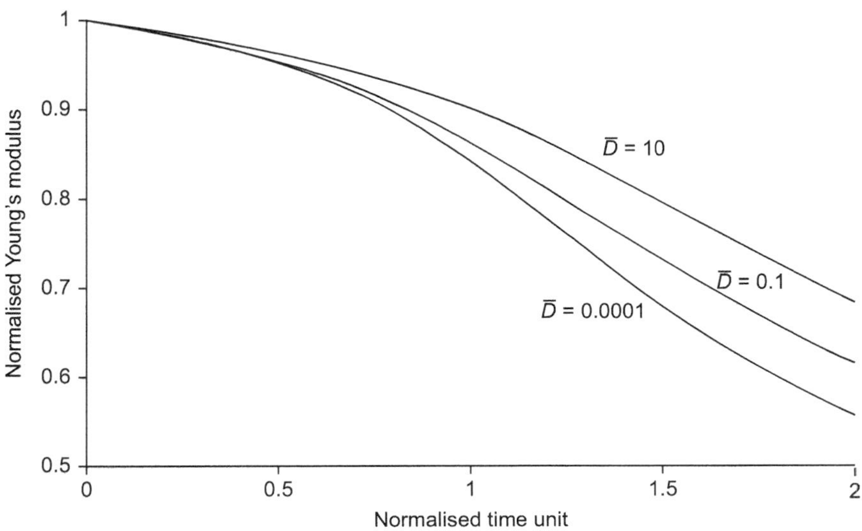

Figure 9.25 Figure reproduced with permission from the publisher Elsevier and the author Wang[2] via the Copyright Clearance Centre. The degradation of normalised Young's modulus versus time was modelled for a biodegradable rod using FEA. The non-dimensional diffusion coefficient $\bar{D}$ was varied to represent different rod diameters.

9.5.2 A molecular dynamics (MD) study of Young's modulus during degradation of bioresorbable polymers

MD is a powerful tool that can be used to simulate and understand how atoms and molecules interact in a material. Ding *et al.*[34] studied polymer chain scission with MD in order to understand the atomic effects of polymer chain scission with a particular focus on changes to Young's modulus. For MD simulations of polymers, the atoms are linked to each other by covalent bonds along with non-bonded interactions such as Lennard-Jones potentials. Plate X shows one of the semi-crystalline polymer structures that Ding *et al.*[34] produced in order to simulate the degradation of bioresorbable polymers. The structure shown in the figure is a periodic unit cell so in the simulations it was considered to repeat in all directions to infinity. Each bead represents one polymer unit. Crystalline phases exist at either end, and an amorphous phase is sandwiched in between them; this interlamellar amorphous phase represents the polymer chains that are trapped between crystal lamellae in a semi-crystalline polymer.

Chain cleavage was only simulated in the amorphous phase because the crystalline phase is known to resist hydrolysis. To calculate Young's modulus, Ding *et al.*[34] carried out the following procedure:

- Fix one crystal lamella and allow the structure to relax.
- Slowly move the other crystal lamella away from the fixed one while allowing the atoms to rearrange into a relaxed configuration during elongation.
- Sum up all the forces acting on a crystal lamella and divide by the cross-sectional area to find stress.
- Repeat this process over a range of strains up to 0.5% and then use linear regression to relate stress to strain and therefore derive the value of Young's modulus.

Temperature is considered in MD simulations based on the kinetic energy of the structure. At higher temperatures, atoms vibrate with more energy and therefore a structure can be expected to expand. In the simulations of Ding *et al.*[34] this expansion was quantified by the distance between the crystal lamellae (interlamellar spacing). Simulations were conducted at ten different temperatures, ranging from almost absolute zero to the polymer melting point. The values of interlamellar spacing and Young's modulus at the different temperatures are shown in Figure 9.26. Above a temperature of 8 (in the reduced units used in the figure) Young's modulus began to increase as temperature increased. This clearly suggested that mechanical properties at temperatures above 8 were being controlled by the entropy change during degradation rather than changes in inter-atomic potential energy, as discussed at the start of this chapter. The gradient of the slope of interlamellar spacing versus temperature becomes steeper at a temperature of 8, which also suggests the glass transition temperature was ≈8.

Figure 9.27 shows the results of the studies of Ding *et al.*[34] for the effect of chain scissions on Young's modulus both above and below the glass transition temperature. There was a considerable delay while chain scissions were applied before Young's modulus reduced for the simulations above T_g, whereas below T_g this delay may not have existed. The theory of Wang *et al.*[2] for Young's modulus degradation above T_g, discussed in the previous section of this chapter, can explain the delay in Young's

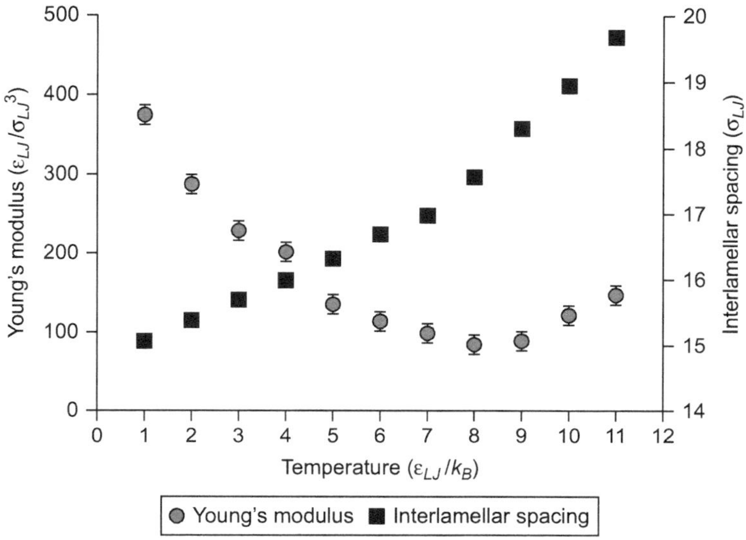

Figure 9.26 Figure reproduced with permission from the publisher Elsevier and the author Ding[34] via the Copyright Clearance Centre. The Young's modulus and distance between crystal lamellae were calculated at various temperatures. The units were based on MD parameters.

modulus versus chain scission. In that theory it was argued that scissions may have little effect on the entropy change during deformation until a polymer chain has been subjected to a significant number of scissions. For simulations both above and below T_g, the results in Figure 9.27 indicate that the average molecular weight of the structure reduced before the value of Young's modulus did which agrees with the review of experimental data in Figure 9.23.

9.5.3 The effective cavity theory for glassy polymers

Gleadall[35] have recently developed a new model for the effect of chain scission on bioresorbable polymers. The study is not yet published but a brief summary is included here because the work is very relevant to this chapter. Figure 9.28a shows the amorphous poly(lactide) structure that Gleadall[35] analysed below the glass transition temperature in atomic-scale simulations. The value of Young's modulus for the structure was found by calculating the force required for a vertically applied strain. The effect of polymer chain scission was analysed by studying the forces that individual atoms transfer vertically through the structure before and after chain cleavage. Figure 9.28b shows the same view of the polymer structure as Figure 9.28a but a chain scission had been applied and atoms are only shown if the scission caused a threshold reduction in the vertical force that they transfer through the polymer. Gleadall[35] found that there are regions of polymer above and below the scission which do not transfer as much vertical force through the polymer as a result of the chain scission.

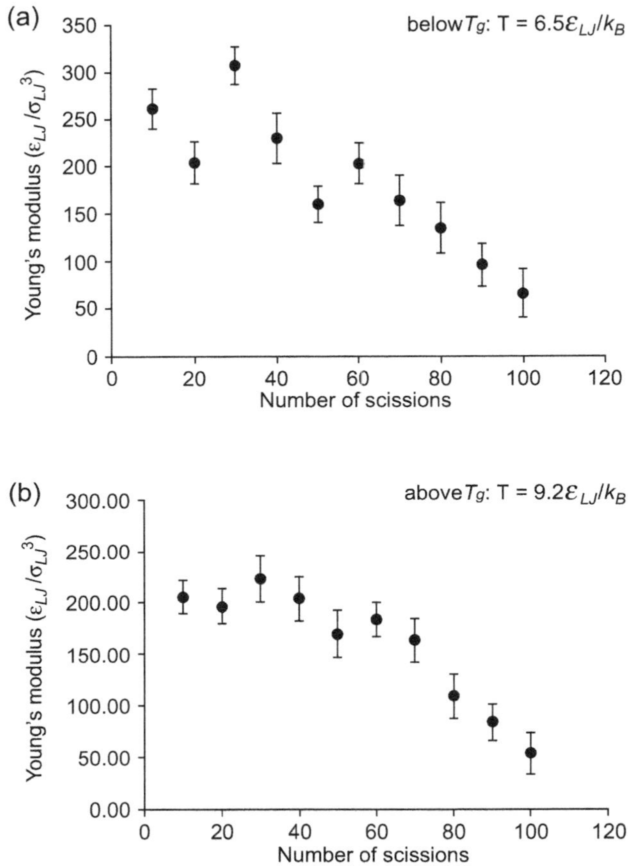

Figure 9.27 Figure reproduced with permission from the publisher Elsevier and the author Ding[34] via the Copyright Clearance Centre. Young's modulus was calculated for several numbers of chain scissions at temperatures of (a) 6.5 and (b) 9.2 which were below and above T_g respectively. The units were based on MD parameters.

Gleadall[35] proposed that chain cleavage can be represented by effective cavities around the scission. He developed the Effective Cavity Theory to model Young's modulus degradation based on this concept and also included crystallinity in the model since it is known to increase during the degradation of semi-crystalline bioresorbable polymers and affects Young's modulus. Figure 9.29 shows a representative case to demonstrate the ability of the model to fit the experimental data of Duek *et al.*[27] who studied the Young's modulus degradation of initially amorphous 3 mm poly(L-lactide) rods in phosphate buffer solution (pH 7.4) at 37°C. The volume fractions of effective cavities and crystallinity used in the model were determined directly from experimental data for molecular weight and crystallinity which are shown in Figure 9.29a. The representative fitting of the model to experimental data for the

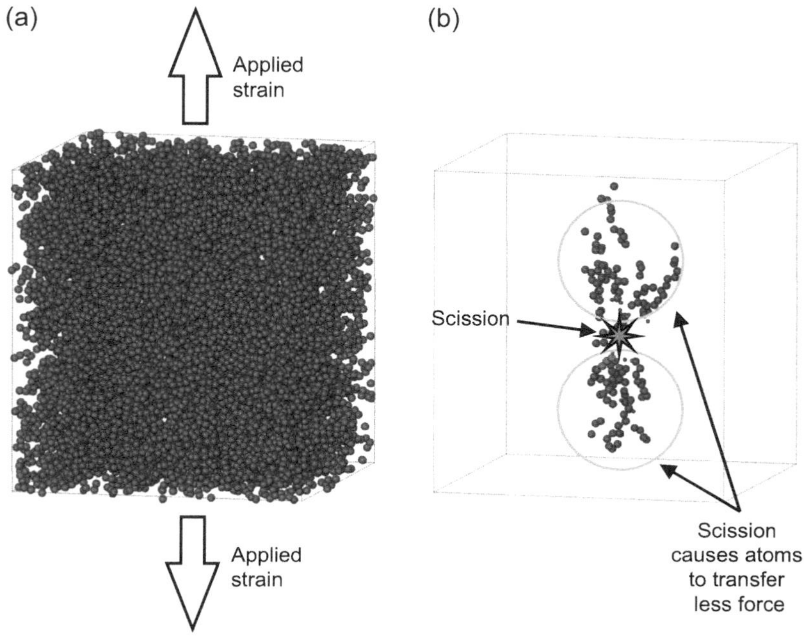

Figure 9.28 The atomic structure for poly(lactide) that was studied by Gleadall[35] is shown with (a) all atoms, and (b) only atoms for which a chain scission resulted in a threshold reduction in the force they individually transferred through the polymer.

degradation of Young's modulus is shown in Figure 9.29b. The effective cavity theory model can be seen to capture the degradation trend very accurately.

9.6 Conclusions

A literature review was carried out for both experimental and theoretical studies for the degradation of bioresorbable polymer mechanical properties. The effects of degradation of molecular weight and crystallinity were analysed in terms of changes to polymer strength, Young's modulus, and elongation-at-break values. The reduction of molecular weight during degradation was found to cause a reduction in stiffness, strength, and elongation-at-break. The experimental data for Young's modulus versus molecular weight of poly(lactide) was compared in order to identify a simple model to relate the two factors. It was found that a linear relationship exists between Young's modulus degradation and the reduction of $\log(M_n)$. This relationship was identified for polymer degradation studies over a wide range of conditions and experimental setups. It can be used to estimate Young's modulus degradation for polymer degradation studies in which mechanical properties are not measured. Increase in crystallinity, during degradation, was found to increase stiffness and strength but reduce the value of elongation-at-break. Existing models for the degradation of mechanical properties were discussed in detail.

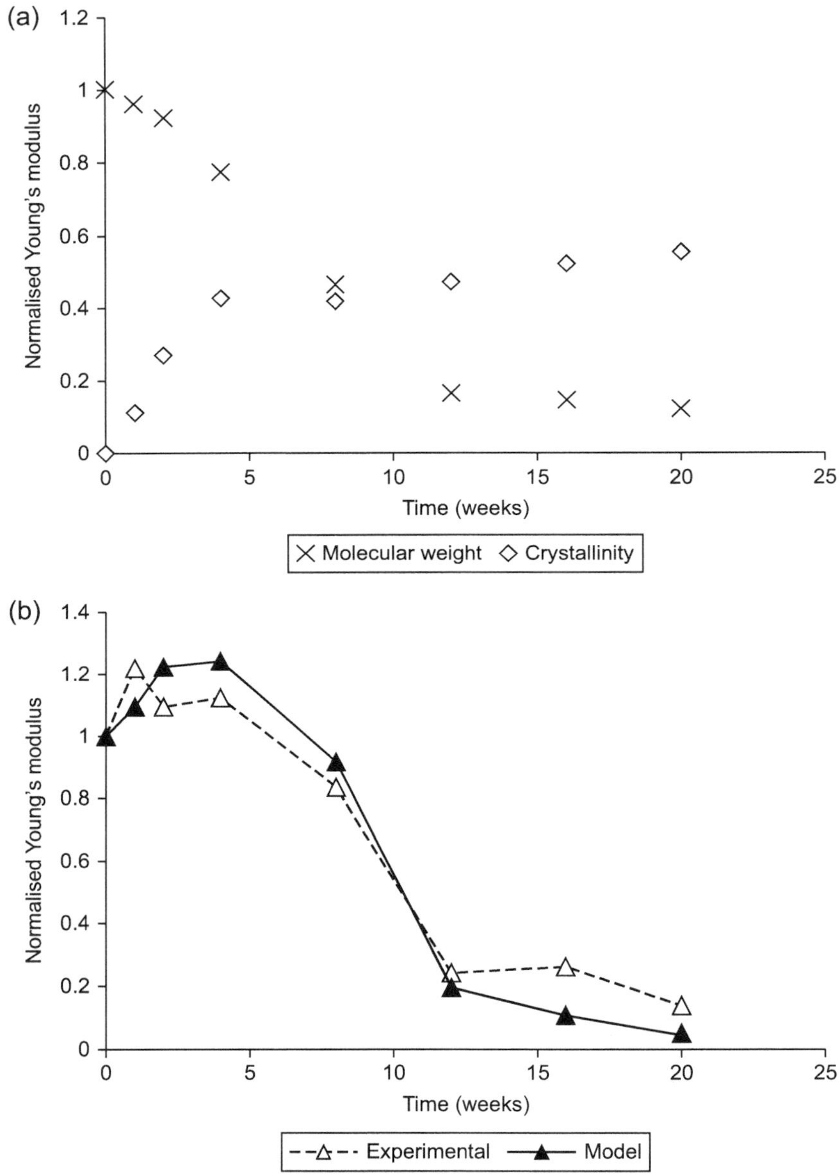

Figure 9.29 Experimental data of Duek *et al.*[27] are shown for (a) number-average molecular weight and crystallinity, and (b) Young's modulus. Also shown in (b) is a representative fitting of the effective cavity theory model of Gleadall[35] for Young's modulus degradation.

The first developed a mathematical model to relate Young's modulus to polymer chain scission and is based on entropy theory for rubber elasticity. The second was an MD study of the effect of chain scission on Young's modulus in a semi-crystalline polymer. The third study developed a model to relate Young's modulus to polymer chain scission, and is based on atomic-scale simulations for glassy polymers.

References

1. Ward IM and Hadley DW. (1993) *An Introduction to the Mechanical Properties of Solid Polymers*. Chichester, New York: Wiley-Blackwell.
2. Wang Y, Han X, Pan J and Sinka C. (2010) An entropy spring model for the Young's modulus change of biodegradable polymers during biodegradation. *Journal of the Mechanical Behavior of Biomedical Materials*, **3**:14–21.
3. Nakafuku C and Takehisa S-Y. (2004) Glass transition and mechanical properties of PLLA and PDLLA-PGA copolymer blends. *Journal of Applied Polymer Science*, **93**:2164–2173.
4. Saha SK and Tsuji H. (2006) Effects of molecular weight and small amounts of d-lactide units on hydrolytic degradation of poly(l-lactic acid)s. *Polymer Degradation and Stability*, **91**:1665–1673.
5. Tsuji H, Mizuno A and Ikada Y. (2000) Properties and morphology of poly(L-lactide). III. Effects of initial crystallinity on long-term in vitro hydrolysis of high molecular weight poly(L-lactide) film in phosphate-buffered solution. *Journal of Applied Polymer Science*, **77**:1452–1464.
6. Tsuji H and Suzuyoshi K. (2002) Environmental degradation of biodegradable polyesters 1. Poly([var epsilon]-caprolactone), poly[(R)-3-hydroxybutyrate], and poly(L-lactide) films in controlled static seawater. *Polymer Degradation and Stability*, **75**:347–355.
7. Tsuji H. (2002) Autocatalytic hydrolysis of amorphous-made polylactides: effects of L-lactide content, tacticity, and enantiomeric polymer blending. *Polymer*, **43**:1789–1796.
8. Tsuji H and Muramatsu H. (2001) Blends of aliphatic polyesters: V non-enzymatic and enzymatic hydrolysis of blends from hydrophobic poly(l-lactide) and hydrophilic poly(vinyl alcohol). *Polymer Degradation and Stability*, **71**:403–413.
9. Saha SK and Tsuji H. (2006) Effects of rapid crystallization on hydrolytic degradation and mechanical properties of poly(l-lactide-co-ε-caprolactone). *Reactive and Functional Polymers*, **66**:1362–1372.
10. Weir N, Buchanan F, Orr J and Dickson G. (2004) Degradation of poly-L-lactide. Part 1: in vitro and in vivo physiological temperature degradation. *Proceedings of the Institution of Mechanical Engineers, Part H: Journal of Engineering in Medicine,* **218**:307–319.
11. Migliaresi C, Fambri L and Cohn D. (1994) A study on the in vitro degradation of poly(lactic acid). *Journal of Biomaterials Science, Polymer Edition*, **5**:591–606.
12. Tsuji H. (2000) In vitro hydrolysis of blends from enantiomeric poly(lactide)s. Part 1. Well-stereo-complexed blend and non-blended films. *Polymer*, **41**:3621–3630.
13. Tsuji H. (2003) In vitro hydrolysis of blends from enantiomeric poly(lactide)s. Part 4: well-homo-crystallized blend and nonblended films. *Biomaterials*, **24**:537–547.
14. Lam KH, Nieuwenhuis P, Molenaar I, Esselbrugge H, Feijen J, Dijkstra PJ, Lam KH, Nieuwenhuis P, Molenaar I, Esselbrugge H, Feijen, J, Dijkstra PJ and Schakenraad JM. (1994) Biodegradation of porous versus non-porous poly(L-lactic acid) films. *Journal of Materials Science: Materials in Medicine*, **5**:181–189.

15. Yuan X, Mak AFT and Yao K. (2002) In vitro degradation of poly(L- lactic acid) fibers in phosphate buffered saline. *Journal of Applied Polymer Science*, **85**:936–943.
16. Tsuji H and Suzuyoshi K. (2002) Environmental degradation of biodegradable polyesters 2. Poly([var epsilon]-caprolactone), poly[(R)-3-hydroxybutyrate], and poly(L-lactide) films in natural dynamic seawater. *Polymer Degradation and Stability*, **75**:357–365.
17. Weir N, Buchanan F, Orr J, Farrar D and Dickson G. (2004) Degradation of poly-L-lactide. Part 2: increased temperature accelerated degradation. *Proceedings of the Institution of Mechanical Engineers, Part H: Journal of Engineering in Medicine*, **218**:321–330.
18. Tsuji H and Ikada Y. (2000) Properties and morphology of poly(L-lactide) 4. Effects of structural parameters on long-term hydrolysis of poly(L-lactide) in phosphate-buffered solution. *Polymer Degradation and Stability*, **67**:179–189.
19. Wang Y, Pan J, Han X, Sinka C and Ding L. (2008) A phenomenological model for the degradation of biodegradable polymers. *Biomaterials*, **29**:3393–3401.
20. Han X and Pan J. (2009) A model for simultaneous crystallisation and biodegradation of biodegradable polymers. *Biomaterials,* **30**:423–430.
21. Han X, Pan J, Buchanan F, Weir N and Farrar D. (2010) Analysis of degradation data of poly(l-lactide-co-l,d-lactide) and poly(l-lactide) obtained at elevated and physiological temperatures using mathematical models. *Acta Biomaterialia*, **6**:3882–3889.
22. Han X and Pan J. (2011) Polymer chain scission, oligomer production and diffusion: a two-scale model for degradation of bioresorbable polyesters. *Acta Biomaterialia*, **7**:538–547.
23. Gleadall A, Pan J and Atkinson H. (2012) A simplified theory of crystallisation induced by polymer chain scissions for biodegradable polyesters. *Polymer Degradation and Stability*, **97**:1616–1620.
24. Gleadall A, Pan J, Kruft M-A and Kellomäki M. (2013) Degradation mechanisms of bioresorbable polyesters, part 1: effects of random scission, end scission and autocatalysis. *Acta Biomaterialia,* **10**(5):2223–2232.
25. Gleadall A, Pan J, Kruft M-A and Kellomäki M. (2013) Degradation mechanisms of bioresorbable polyesters, part 2: effects of initial molecular weight and residual monomer. *Acta Biomaterialia,* **10**(5):2233–2240.
26. Gleadall A and Pan J. (2013) Computer simulation of polymer chain scission in biodegradable polymers. *Journal of Biotechnology & Biomaterials*, **3**:1–5.
27. Duek EAR, Zavaglia CAC and Belangero WD. (1999) In vitro study of poly(lactic acid) pin degradation. *Polymer*, **40**:6465–6473.
28. Karjalainen T, Hiljanen-Vainio M, Malin M and Seppälä J. (1996) Biodegradable lactone copolymers. III. Mechanical properties of ε-caprolactone and lactide copolymers after hydrolysis in vitro. *Journal of Applied Polymer Science,* **59**:1299–1304.
29. Tsuji H and Ikada Y. (1995) Properties and morphologies of poly(L-lactide): 1. Annealing condition effects on properties and morphologies of poly(L-lactide). *Polymer*, **36**:2709–2716.
30. Tsuji H and Del Carpio CA. (2002) In vitro hydrolysis of blends from enantiomeric poly(lactide)s. 3. Homocrystallized and amorphous blend films. *Biomacromolecules*, **4**:7–11.
31. Tsuji H and Ikada Y. (1998) Blends of aliphatic polyesters. II. Hydrolysis of solution-cast blends from poly(L-lactide) and poly(E-caprolactone) in phosphate-buffered solution. *Journal of Applied Polymer Science*, **67**:405–415.
32. Grizzi I, Garreau H, Li S and Vert M. (1995) Hydrolytic degradation of devices based on poly(dl-lactic acid) size-dependence. *Biomaterials,* **16**:305–311.
33. Deng M, Zhou J, Chen G, Burkley D, Xu Y, Jamiolkowski D, Deng M, Zhou J, Chen G, Burkley D, Xu Y, Jamiolkowski D and Barbolt, T. (2005) Effect of load and temperature

on in vitro degradation of poly(glycolide-co-l-lactide) multifilament braids. *Biomaterials*, **26**:4327–4336.

34. Ding L, Davidchack R and Pan J. (2011) A molecular dynamics study of Young's modulus change of semi-crystalline polymers during degradation by chain scissions. *Journal of the Mechanical Behavior of Biomedical Materials*, **5**:224–230.
35. Gleadall A. (2014) *Modelling the Degradation of Biodegradable Polymers and Their Mechanical Properties*. United Kingdom: The University of Leicester.

Molecular and multi-scale modelling methods of polymer device degradation

10

X. Han
Loughborough University, Loughborough, UK

10.1 Introduction

Degradable polymers that are applied in medical applications usually undergo chemical degradation via hydrolysis and enzyme-catalysed hydrolysis. There are three main steps during biodegradation: (a) water molecules penetrate into polymer chains, driven by the diffusion mechanism; (b) water molecules attack the ester bonds of polymer chains, causing cleavages of the chains; and (c) small molecules (oligomers/monomers) release from the device to the medium. It has been generally believed that chain scissions randomly occur at ester bonds of polymer chains. It has, however, also been reported that the chain scissions occur dominantly at the chain ends[1] with dramatically different chain scission rates for polylactic acid (PLA), polyglycolic acid (PGA) and poly(lactic-*co*-glycolic) (PLGA). Most mathematical models use the effective degradation rates for both non-catalysed hydrolysis and enzyme-catalysed hydrolysis, ignoring the kinetic rate difference between mid chain scissions and end chain scissions of certain polymer systems. Different degradable polymers are believed to experience random chain scission, end chain scissions or their combinations, depending on their chemical structure and the hydrolysis environment.[1] Definitions of random chain scission and end chain scission hydrolysis are as follows:

Random chain scission hydrolysis: the probability of a chain scission, which occurs at middle ester bonds, is the same as the probability of a chain scission happened at the end chain ester bonds: denoted by $p_{\mathrm{mid}} = p_{\mathrm{end}}$, where p_{mid} and p_{end} are probability of a chain scission in the middle and a chain scission at the end ester bonds, respectively.

End chain scission hydrolysis: probability of a chain scission occurring at the middle ester bonds is far less than that at the end chain ester bonds: denoted by $p_{\mathrm{mid}} << p_{\mathrm{end}}$, in which the chain scissions at the middle ester bonds are eliminated.

Chain ends of a polymer system have a very different electronic environment from the middle ester bonds, due to the effects of their adjacent functional groups. An example of degradable polymers is shown in Figure 10.1, giving an illustration of how chemical structures affect the rates of both hydrolysis for middle ester bonds and end ester bonds. Figure 10.1 illustrates the chemical formula of PLA. Two functional groups, the hydroxyl group and the carboxyl group, are identified at the two ends of a PLA polymer chain. The hydrogen atom in the carboxylic group is unstable that it is able to ionize, which results in a rather acidic local environment at the left end while

Modelling Degradation of Bioresorbable Polymeric Medical Devices. http://dx.doi.org/10.1533/9781782420255.2.201

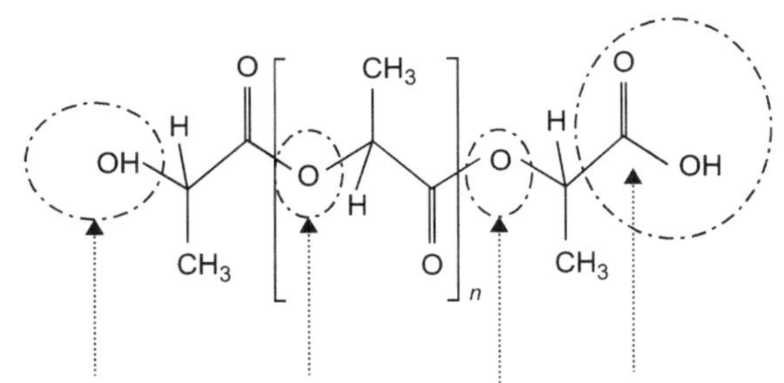

Figure 10.1 Chemical formula of PLA and its functional groups: hydroxyl group, alkoxy group and carboxyl group.

the hydroxyl group at the other end induces local alkalinity. Their areas of effect are limited to local areas. If ester bonds connected with any alkoxy group are within the effect areas, hydrolysis reaction rates increase. In a PLA polymer chain, local areas of effect are very close to the chain end ester bonds, so that hydrolysis reaction rates at the chain ends are greater than those in mid-chains. On the contrary, due to a very different chemical formula, the distance between the functional groups in the chain ends of a polycaprolactone (PCL) chain is large enough to eliminate the hydrolysis rate difference between end groups and middle ester bonds. Degradation differences between random chain scission and end chain scission are therefore very small.

Molecular weight distribution (MWD), which was not possible to be considered in the previous phenomenological model, changes during degradation due to polymer chain scissions. Polymer systems with different initial MWDs behave differently during degradation, even if they have the same initial number/weight-average molecular weight. Additionally, random chain scissions and end chain scissions have different influences on MWD changes during degradation. End chain scissions, by definition, reduces the molecular weight of a long polymer chain by yielding monomers. Monomers are diffused out of the device, so that this cleavage only changes the coordinates of an MWD, whereas the shape of an MWD remains the same. Random chain scissions lower the molecular weight by producing shorter polymers and oligomers, or even monomers in a later stage. An MWD therefore transforms to a different shape after a random chain scission dominated degradation. Figure 10.2 illustrates two examples of MWD time evolutions before and after degradation based on (a) pure end chain scission degradation, and (b) pure random chain scission degradation, respectively. Figure 10.2a clearly shows that the shape of an MWD stays the same when end chain scission is the sole mechanism of hydrolysis. Coordinate position is the only difference between the dashed plot and the initial MWD plot in Figure 10.2a due to the unchanged number of polymer chains (this shape will eventually change at a very late stage of degradation). In Figure 10.2b, hydrolysis is dominated by random scission, and thus the dashed MWD changes its mean value and shape from the initial MWD, producing a larger number of polymer chains.

Modelling chemical reactions naturally falls into a field of molecular dynamics, such as the reactive models presented by Buehler.[2,3] However, the typical time scale

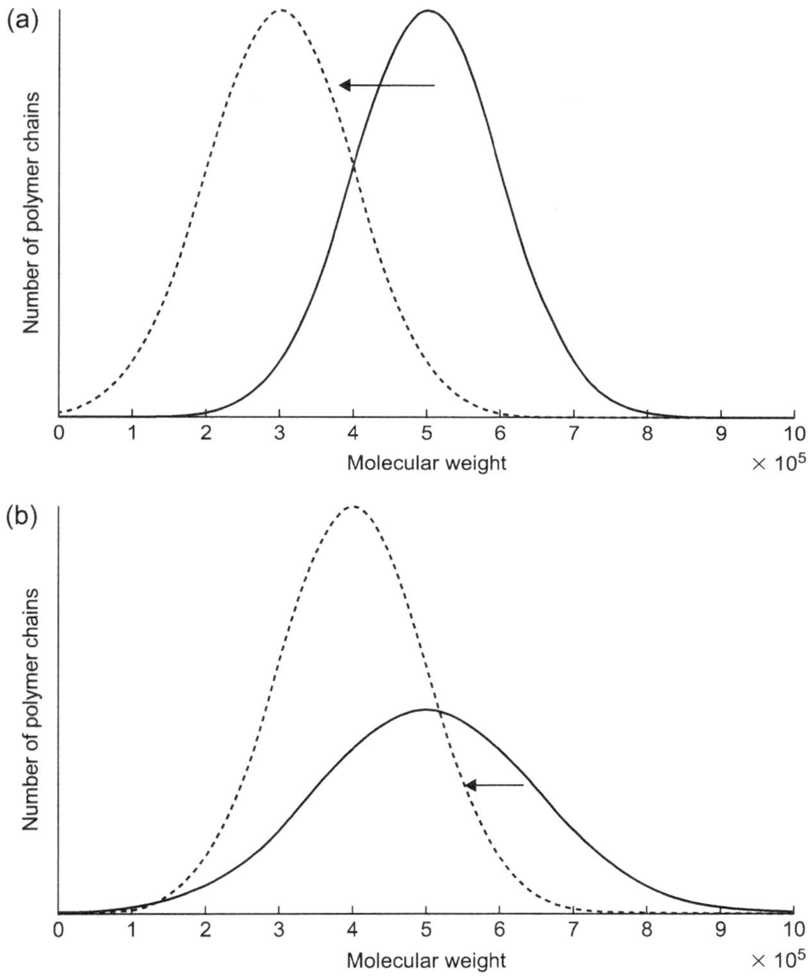

Figure 10.2 MWDs change during degradation for end sole chain scission hydrolysis (a) and random chain scission hydrolysis (b), respectively. Solid lines are MWDs before degradation, while the dashed lines are MWDs after degradation.

of hydrolysis reactions is over several weeks, which is far beyond the time scale that a molecular dynamics simulation can reach. The molecular models discussed in this chapter consider a larger scale that takes repeated units of a long polymer chain as the minimum unit in the model. Chemical structure details of a repeat unit are ignored, so that we use an integrated lumped unit instead. Plate XI in the colour section pages 130 and 131 shows that a blue bead is used to represent the repeat unit ($C_3H_4O_2$) of PLA (a) and a red bead is used to represent the repeat unit of ($C_2H_2O_2$) of PGA (b), respectively. Different colours of beads indicate a different polymer chain repeat unit with its corresponding hydrolysis rate.

Desired degradation rates for copolymers can be achieved by simply choosing different copolymer ratios for different homopolymers, PLA and PGA for example. The copolymer degradation rate and copolymer ratio follows some complicated relations.[4] In the molecular models, highly complex chemical structures of copolymers can be represented by carefully distributing different coloured beads with corresponding hydrolysis rates on one polymer chain based a certain copolymer ratio. Polymer characteristics, such as the initial MWD, degree of crystallinity and copolymer ratio, are all considered as input data in a molecular model. The model is then used to study the effect of every mechanism for both homopolymer systems and copolymer systems.

10.2 Mathematical models for polymer chain scission

An initial polymer system is characterized by (a) an initial weight distribution of polymer chains (b) an initial size distribution of polymer crystals, and (c) copolymer distributions. Implementations for each input will be discussed one by one in the succeeding sections.

10.2.1 Polymer chain seeding in molecular model

The polymer chain seeding process aims to generate a set of polymer chains with a predetermined weight distribution. Different types of polymer weight distributions can be adopted to generate polymer chains, among which the Flory-Schulz distribution and the log-normal distribution are the most used. The Flory-Schulz distribution is based on a model of chain polymerization from Paul Flory and G. V. Schulz.[5] Thus, the Flory-Schulz distribution is believed to be the most probable one.[5]

$$y_j = (1-p)p^{j-1} \quad [10.1]$$

In Equation [10.1], y_j is the Flory-Schulz mole fraction distribution for linear polymer systems. j is chain length, also known as degree of polymerization, and p is an adjustable empirical parameter. The number-average molecular weight is then calculated using Equation [10.2]:

$$\bar{M}_n = \sum_{j=1}^{\infty} y_j M_j \quad [10.2]$$

in which M_j is the molecular weight of the polymer chains with j degrees of polymerization. The weight distribution is expressed in Equation [10.3] and the weight-average molecular weight is derived by Equation [10.4].

$$w_j = j(1-p)^2 p^{j-1} \quad [10.3]$$

$$\bar{M}_w = \sum_{j=1}^{\infty} w_j M_j \qquad [10.4]$$

The polydispersity index (PDI), which is known as a ratio of weight-average molecular weight and number-average molecular weight, is given by:

$$\text{PDI} = \frac{\bar{M}_w}{\bar{M}_n} \qquad [10.5]$$

The log-normal polymer chain distribution has larger fraction of very high molecular weight polymer chains compared to the Flory-Schulz distribution and is expressed by:

$$w(M) = \frac{1}{\sigma_w \sqrt{2\pi}} \frac{M^A}{B\bar{M}_m^{A+1}} e^{\left[\frac{-(\ln M - \ln \bar{M}_m)^2}{2\sigma_w^2}\right]} \qquad [10.6]$$

in which

$$B = e^{\left[\frac{\sigma_w^2}{2}(A+1)^2\right]} \qquad [10.7]$$

where σ_w is the deviation of the log-normal distribution, $\bar{M}_m$ is the median value and A is a constant. Values of σ_w and A can be selected empirically by comparing the distribution with detected polymer chain weight distributions. Number-average molecular weight and weight-average molecular weight based on the log-normal polymer chain distribution are calculated by Equations [10.8] and [10.9]:

$$\bar{M}_n = \bar{M}_m e^{\left[\frac{\sigma_w^2}{2}(2A+1)\right]} \qquad [10.8]$$

$$\text{and } \bar{M}_w = \bar{M}_m e^{\left[\frac{\sigma_w^2}{2}(2A+3)\right]} \qquad [10.9]$$

PDI is calculated by Equation [10.10]

$$\text{PDI} = \frac{\bar{M}_w}{\bar{M}_n} = e^{\sigma_w^2} \qquad [10.10]$$

Practically, most initial MWDs are able to be detected experimentally by using the size-exclusion chromatography (SEC) method for polymers. MWDs of some polymer systems are very difficult to obtain though. Thus, two seeding processes are introduced here: (a) the polymer seeding process for a polymer system with a known MWD: apply to a selected mathematical distribution expression specific parameters which are obtained by fitting the known MWD; and (b) the seeding process for a polymer system with an unknown MWD can be achieved by comparing system values $\bar{M}_n$, $\bar{M}_w$ and PDI together from physical polymer systems with mathematical systems to obtain the unknown variables: p for the Flory-Schulz distribution and σ_w and $\bar{M}_m$ for the log-normal distribution. Mathematically, a homopolymer chain is *de facto* represented by a positive integer P whose value equals the degree of polymerization of a polymer chain. A polymer system is therefore a set of positive integers: $(P_1, P_2, \ldots, P_i)$ which follows a selected MWD.

Representing one copolymer chain needs additional information apart from a positive integer. This information depends on the types of copolymers: different types of constituent units contribute differently in a copolymer chain, and this can be classified as the following types of linear copolymers:

1. Alternating copolymer with regular alternating A and B units: -A-B-A-B-A-B-
2. Periodic copolymer: -(A-B-A-A-B-B-A-A-A-B-B-B)$_n$-
3. Random copolymer: -A-B-A-A-B-A-B-B-
4. Block copolymer: -B-B-B-B-A-A-A-A-

The mathematical representation of a copolymer chain is therefore characterized by an integer and a distribution representative based on these types of copolymers.

In a molecular model, a small simulation volume of a polymer system is taken into account and a total of n_0 polymer chains are seeded into this simulation volume. The simulation volume is related to the number of chains seeded by:

$$V_0 = \frac{n_{e0}}{C_{e0} \times N_A} \qquad [10.11]$$

where n_{e0} and C_{e0} are the total mole numbers of ester bonds in the model and the mole concentrations of the ester bonds, respectively, and N_A is the Avogadro constant which equals 6.02×10^{23} mol^{-1}.

10.2.2 Chain scission implementation methods in molecular models

In this section, we choose homopolymer chains for simplicity. Random chain scissions and end chain scissions are executed mathematically simply by dividing a positive integer into two smaller integers. Plate XII illustrates examples of random chain scission implementation and end chain scission implementation of a polymer chain in (a) and (b), respectively. Red rods and red beads represent end chain ester bonds and end chain units, respectively. In Plate XII (a), a polymer chain with five repeat units is chopped by a water molecule randomly: by the definition of random chain scission, each rod regardless of its colour has the same probability of being chopped. In Plate XII (b), a polymer chain with five repeat units undergoes an end chain scission: only the red rods can be chopped. A combination of case (a) and (b) is able to describe all types of chain scissions in hydrolysis reactions. Mathematically, an integer of a polymer chain in case (a) is divided into two shorter chains: 2 and 3, while in case (b), integer 5 changes to 4 + 1. If the value of an integer equals 1, this means it has reduced to a monomer. Chain scissions implement methods for a polymer system can be described in the two flow charts shown in Figures 10.3a and 10.3b. Integers n_i,m_i,n_e, n_{ol}, n_{H^+} and n in Figure 10.3 are the numbers of ester bonds for polymer chain i, the number of ester bonds of a daughter polymer chain produced from a parent polymer chain i, the total ester bond number of the polymers, the total

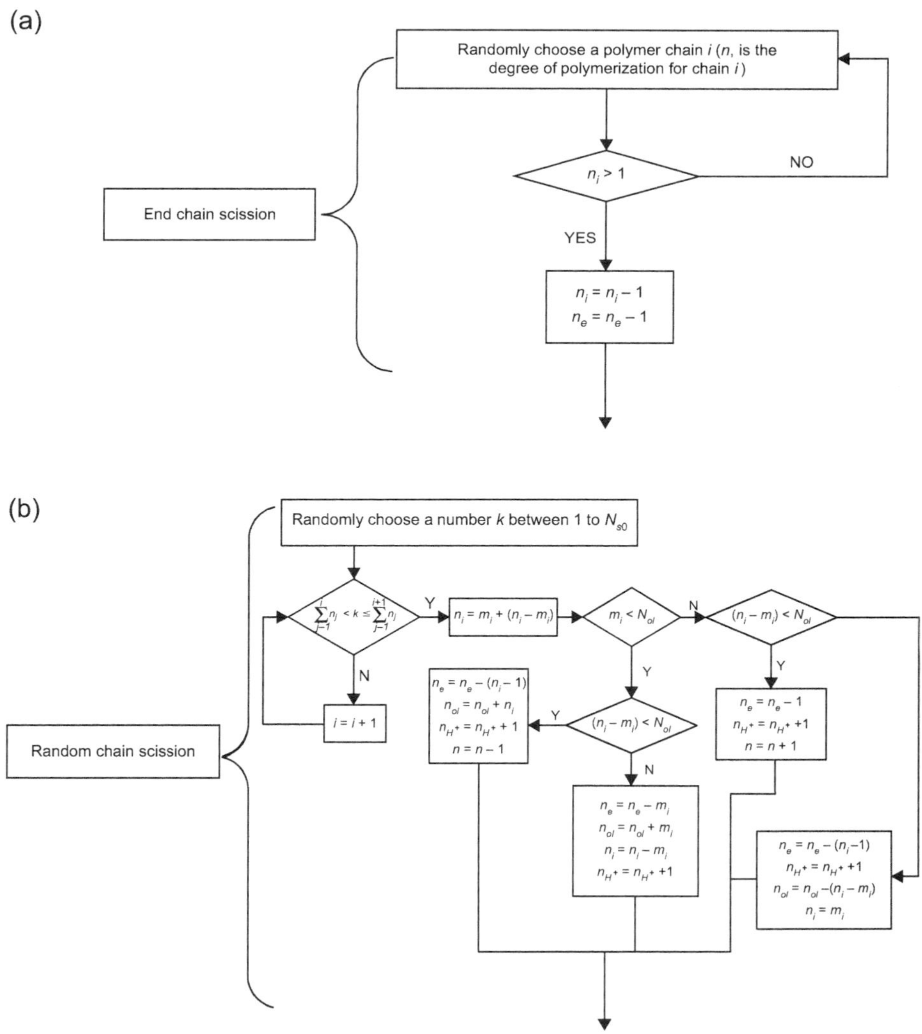

Figure 10.3 Flow charts of implementation methods for end chain scission (a) and random chain scission (b).

ester bonds of the oligomers and the number of carboxylic acids, respectively. In this chapter, an oligomer is defined by its degree of polymerization that is less than or equal to 8 (≤ 8). The flow chart in Figure 10.3a describes end chain scission procedures mathematically: firstly, randomly select a polymer chain i in the polymer system – if the degree of polymerization of this chain is greater than 1 (not a monomer), chain scission occurs at its end. The total number of ester bonds and the degree of polymerization of the current polymer chain are updated by $n_i = n_i - 1$ and $n_e = n_e - 1$, respectively. Implementing random chain scissions is relatively complicated. Refer to Figure 10.3b – as each ester bond has the same probability to react with a water molecule, a random integer k is generated between 1 and n_e. A succeeding comparison is carried out, as shown in Equation [10.12], in order to determine which polymer chain will be chopped:

$$\sum_{j=1}^{i} n_j < k \leq \sum_{j=1}^{i+1} n_j \qquad [10.12]$$

Relative binary selections and corresponding changes of variables are illustrated in Figure 10.3b. N_{ol} is the oligomer threshold of the degree of polymerization: if the degree of polymerization for a polymer chain is less than or equal to N_{ol}, it is a dissolvable oligomer. As mentioned before, $N_{ol} = 8$ is used throughout this chapter. Three possible selection cases can be summarized from Figure 10.3b:

1. Both degrees of polymerization for two daughter chains produced by a random chain scission are greater than or equal to N_{ol};
2. Either degrees of polymerization for two daughter chains produced by a random chain scission are greater than or equal to N_{ol};
3. Both degrees of polymerization for two daughter chains produced by a random chain scission are less than N_{ol}.

The third case can be discovered only at a very late stage of degradation, while the first two are the main cases during degradation. Oligomers produced from chain scissions are dissolvable in liquid media. The diffusion behaviour will be discussed in the following sections. They are still available for chain scissions until they eventually turn to a monomer. Figure 10.4 illustrates the monomer number as a function of the chain scission number for a sole end chain scission case. Chain scissions in this case only happen at the chain ends. In fact, this case, which does not occur in reality, can be used in understanding the detailed mechanism of end chain scissions. A strict linear relationship is shown in Figure 10.4, in that one monomer is produced from one end chain scission. On the other hand, Figure 10.5 illustrates a non-linear relationship for the ester bond number of oligomers as a function of the chain scission number for a pure random scission. In Figure 10.5, the gradient of the curve increases with the increasing chain scission number. This phenomenon can be explained in terms of the probability that a daughter chain, produced by a random chain scission from a parent polymer chain, falls into the oligomer group increases as the parent polymer chains became shorter. Three oligomer production stages can be identified from Figure 10.5 for random chain scission dominated degradation:

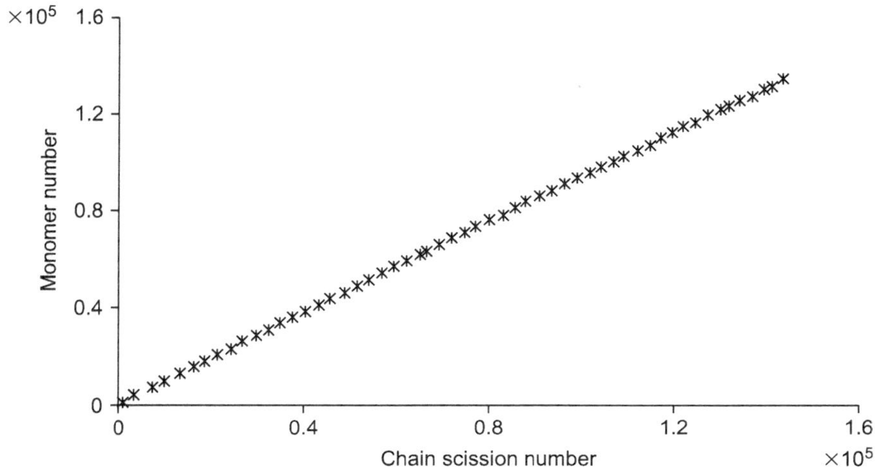

Figure 10.4 Monomer number as a function of chain scission number of sole end chain scissions.

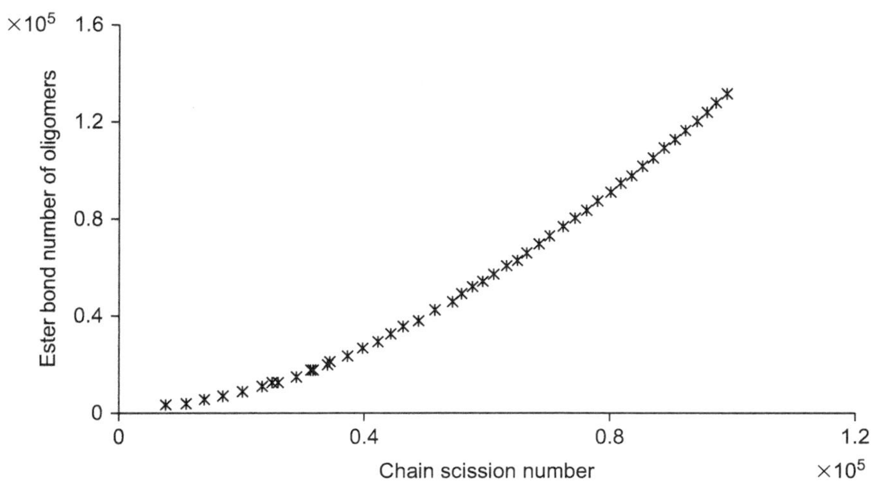

Figure 10.5 Ester bonds number of oligomers as a function of chain scission number for pure random scissions.

Stage 1: the chain scission number ranges from 0 to 0.1 $\times 10^5$. This is the stage in which most parent chains and daughter chains are larger than oligomers. In this stage, the number of polymer chains increases greatly while very small number of oligomers can be found. The molecular weight of this polymer system largely decreases as a consequence.

Stage 2: the chain scission number ranges from 0.1×10^5 to 0.7×10^5. In this stage, the rate of oligomer production increases as more and more polymer chains are chopped into oligomers. The molecular weight thus decreases more slowly.

Stage 3: the chain scission number is greater than 0.7×10^5. Oligomer production is almost proportional to the chain scission number in this stage, which indicates that most of the chains after chain scission fall into oligomers.

R_{ol} and R_s are defined as the mole concentration of oligomers generated from polymer cleavages and the mole concentration of polymer chain cleavages per unit volume, respectively. They can be counted directly from ester bonds, number of oligomers and chain scission number by considering the representative volume. A relationship of dR_{ol}/dt and dR_s/dt for sole end scission is obvious:

$$\frac{dR_{ol}}{dt} = \frac{dR_s}{dt} \qquad [10.13]$$

Flory[6] reported a most probable distribution for the number of polymer chain units of all the x-mers, R_x, under random chain scissions:

$$\frac{R_x}{C_{e0}} = x\left(\frac{R_s}{C_{e0}}\right)^2\left(1-\frac{R_s}{C_{e0}}\right)^{x-1} \qquad [10.14]$$

where C_{e0} is the initial mole concentration of ester bonds. Equation [10.14] can be rewritten for the total number of units of all the oligomers shorter or equal to m units:

$$\frac{R_{ol}}{C_{e0}} = \sum_{x=1}^{m} x\left(\frac{R_s}{C_{e0}}\right)^2\left(1-\frac{R_s}{C_{e0}}\right)^{x-1} \approx \frac{1}{2}\left(m+m^2\right)\left(\frac{R_s}{C_{e0}}\right)^2 \qquad [10.15]$$

On the right hand side, this term was derived by using series expansion, omitting the higher order terms if $R_s/C_{e0} << 1$.

From Figure 10.5, we found that this non-linear relation can be fit perfectly by a second order polynomial equation. In general, although the reaction rate of end chain scissions is faster than the rate of random chain scissions, oligomer production is, however, still dominated by random chain scissions for most cases. We apply a general polynomial form with flexible orders to express the relation between chain scission number and oligomer production number:

$$\frac{R_{ol}}{C_{e0}} = \sigma\left(\frac{R_s}{C_{e0}}\right)^{\beta} \qquad [10.16]$$

in which α and β are empirical fitting constants. We then have

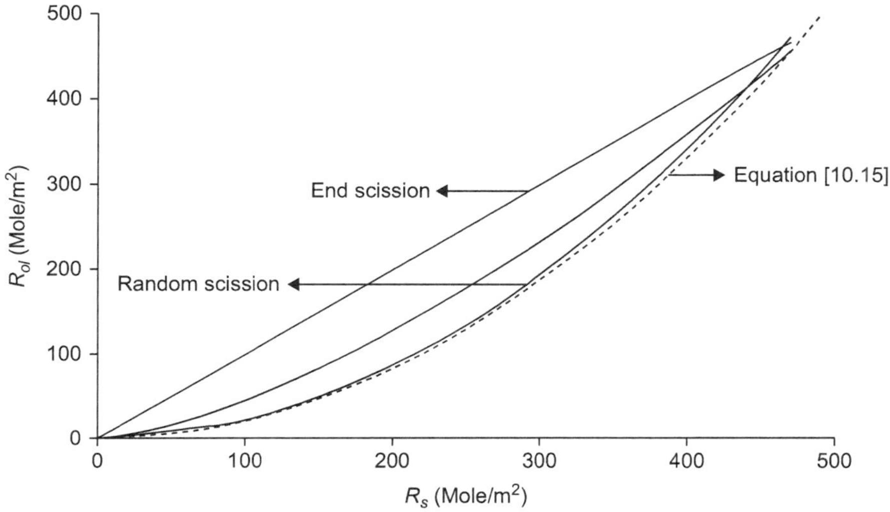

Figure 10.6 The mole concentration of oligomers as a function of mole concentration of chain scissions: predictions from molecular models of chain scissions (solid lines) and plot from Equation [10.15] (dashed lines). (*Source*: Reproduced from Reference 6 with permission.)

$$\frac{dR_{ol}}{dt} = \alpha\beta\left(\frac{R_s}{C_{e0}}\right)^{\beta-1}\frac{dR_s}{dt} \quad [10.17]$$

R_{ol} and R_s can be obtained directly by counting the numbers in chain scission implemental procedures. α and β are two empirical parameters which are obtained by fitting Equation [10.16] with values of R_{ol} and R_s. Figure 10.6 shows the relationships of R_{ol} and R_s both from Equation [10.15] (dashed line) and molecular models (solid line) for random chain scission and end scission degradation, respectively. Predictions from molecular models agree well with Equation [10.15], which validates the statistical models. The chain scission mechanism which contains both random chain scissions and end chain scissions can also be predicted using molecular models. The prediction is shown in Figure 10.6 as a middle solid plot. Using empirical Equation [10.16], three plots in Figure 10.6 can be fitted using different pairs of α and β: $\alpha = 1$ and $\beta = 1$ are used for sole end chain scissions; $\alpha = 36$ and $\beta = 2$ are used for sole random scissions. Equation [10.16] was used in the phenomenological model in previous chapters.

10.3 The Kinetic Monte Carlo (KMC) simulation of hydrolysis reactions

In this section, two chain scission methods discussed in Section 10.2 is combined together into a KMC model to represent general polymer degradations. KMC models can simulate not only amorphous polymer systems but also semi-crystallized polymer and copolymer systems simulations will be also discussed in this section. Polymer characteristics, the initial MWD, degree of crystallinity and copolymer ratio, are considered as the input data in a KMC model. After a number of KMC steps, the oligomers produced are counted according to a threshold degree of polymerization.

10.3.1 The reproduced hydrolysis reaction equations

A polymer system is characterized by (a) the weight distribution of polymer chains, (b) the size distribution of polymer crystals, and (c) the distributions of its constituent polymers for copolymers. Weight distributions of polymer chains, degree of crystallinity and copolymer ratio are available for most polymer systems. A KMC computational simulation can therefore be established using the above information as inputs for a certain polymer system. There are different types of ester bonds in a polymer system, which may have different hydrolysis rates. For example, in a PLGA copolymer system, PGA degrades much faster than PLA[7]; in a semi-crystalline polymer system, crystallized polymer chains degrade much more slowly than amorphous polymer chains[8]; ester bonds at chain ends often degrade faster than those in the middle of polymer chains[1]. All types of ester bonds can be considered in a single KMC model, and the scission rate of the i-th type of ester bond can be written as:[9]

$$\frac{dR_i}{dt} = k_i\, C_i + k_i^a C_i C_{ol}^{0.5} \qquad [10.18]$$

in which R_i represents the mole number of total chain scissions of the i-th type of ester bonds per unit volume, C_i is the mole concentration of the i-th type of ester bonds, C_{ol} is the mole concentration of the oligomers, and k_i and k_i^a are the kinetic reaction rates for the non-catalytic and auto-catalytic hydrolysis reactions.

10.3.2 The KMC scheme

The KMC method is a random sampling method to simulate the time evolution of physical or chemical processes using known kinetic rates. These rates are served as inputs to a KMC algorithm. An algorithm of a general KMC simulating a system with a set of possible processes occurring at known rates r_i is discussed in Figure 10.7.

At the current step, when $t = t_0$, system is at its **initial state**. The current system can transfer to three possible final states, with three known possibilities (kinetic rates) r_1, r_2 and r_3. The KMC method requires a random integer valued between 0 and $r_{\text{total}} = r_1 + r_2 + r_3$; if this integer falls into the region of r_i, which is clarified in Figure 10.7, the system transforms from the initial state to a final state i. The time interval Δt can then be calculated based on these kinetic rates r_i. Steps of this algorithm can be written as:

1. The KMC simulation starts, $t = 0$.
2. Input all kinetic rates into a set $\{r_1, r_2, \ldots, r_n\}$.

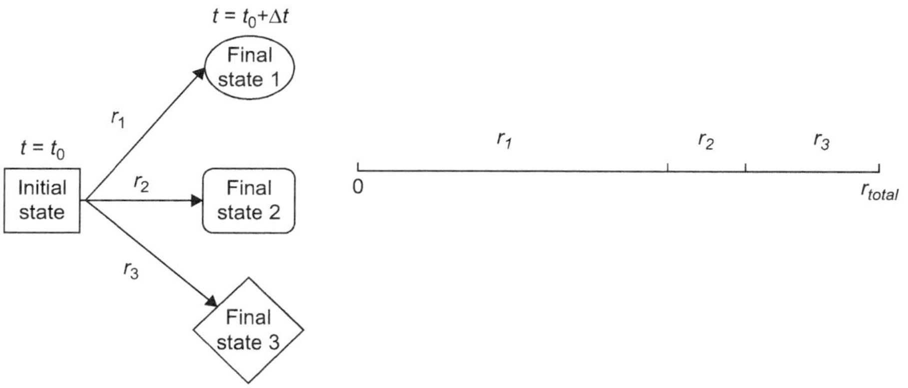

Figure 10.7 A general physical/chemical system undergoing three possible processes with three possibilities (kinetic rates):r_1, r_2 and r_3.

3. Calculate total system transform possibility using $r_{\text{total}} = \sum_{i=1}^{n} r_i$.
4. Generate a uniform random number ξ in $(0,1]$.
5. If $\sum_{i=1}^{j} r_i < \xi \times r_{\text{total}} < \sum_{i=1}^{j+1} r_i$, then carry out process j.
6. Generate another uniform random number $\xi_1 \in (0,1]$.
7. Calculate time interval Δt: $\Delta t = -\ln(\xi_1)/r_{\text{total}}$ and update $t = t + \Delta t$.
8. Recalculate all r_i for a new state, update all variables accordingly.
9. Return to step 2.

Following the KMC scheme above,[10] a chain cleavage of the i-th type of ester bonds occurs if

$$\sum_{j=1}^{i} \frac{dR_j}{dt} < \xi_2 \times \sum_{j=1}^{N} \frac{dR_j}{dt} < \sum_{j=1}^{i+1} \frac{dR_j}{dt} \qquad [10.19]$$

in which $\xi_2 \in (0,1]$ is a uniform random number and N is the total number of different types of ester bonds. The corresponding time step length of a chain cleavage is calculated by

$$\Delta t = -\frac{\ln(\xi_3)}{\sum_{j=1}^{N} \left(dR_j/dt\right)} \qquad [10.20]$$

in which ξ_3 is another uniform random number. Recalculate all kinetic rates which may change due to changes of C_i and C_{ol}. For a homogeneous polymer system, two types of ester bonds are identified: ester bonds beside the chain ends, and ester bonds in the middle. Thus Equation [10.18] for a homopolymer system can be rewritten as Equations [10.21] and [10.22]:

$$r_1 = \frac{dR_{\text{random}}}{dt} = k_{\text{random}} C_{\text{est}} + k^a_{\text{random}} C_{\text{est}} (C_{ol}^{0.5}) \qquad [10.21]$$

$$r_2 = \frac{dR_{\text{end}}}{dt} = k_{\text{end}} C_{\text{end}} + k^a_{\text{end}} C_{\text{end}} C_{ol}^{0.5} \qquad [10.22]$$

where k_{random}, k^a_{random}, k_{end} and k^a_{end} are phenomenological kinetic reaction rates for non-catalysed random chain scission, auto-catalysed random chain scission, non-catalysed end chain scission, and auto-catalysed end scission, respectively. C_{est} and C_{end} are mole concentrations of middle ester bonds and end ester bonds per unit volume, respectively. A KMC simulation flow chart of a homopolymer system experiencing both end and random scission are shown in Figure 10.8.

10.3.3 A coarse grain KMC method

The KMC scheme executes one chain cleavage at each time step, which is computationally inefficient. Therefore a number of coarse grained KMCs have been proposed by researchers.[10,11] Chatterjee *et al.*[11] showed that the following coarse grained KMC scheme can reduce computing time by a factor of 10^4:

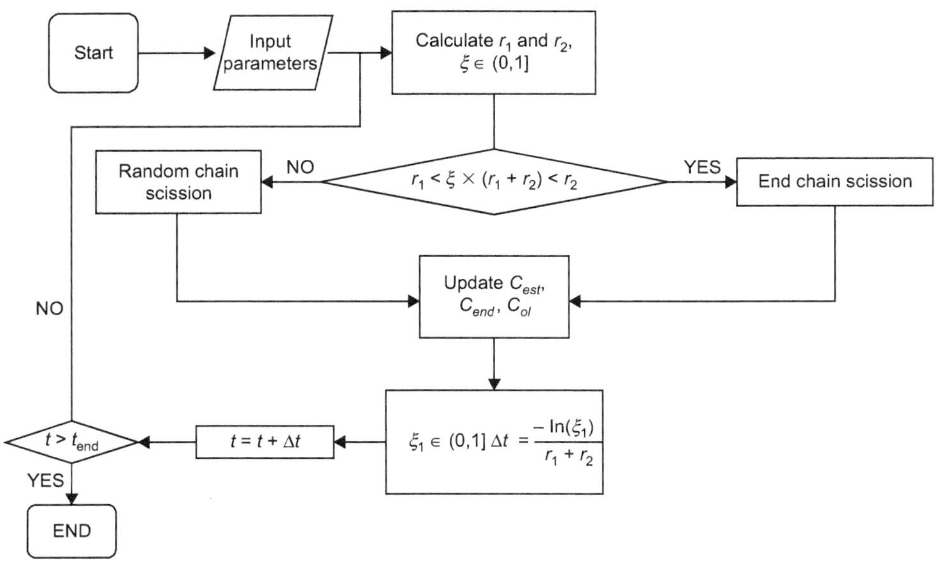

Figure 10.8 Flow chart of a KMC simulation for a homopolymer system undergoing both random chain scission and end chain scission with different rates.

Set a time step length using

$$\Delta t = \varepsilon \min_{i=1}^{N} \left(\frac{C_i}{\sum_{j=1}^{N} (dR_j / dt)} \right) \quad [10.23]$$

where ε is an empirical number, N is the total number of ester bond types.

Calculate

$$P_i = \frac{(dR_i/dt)\Delta t}{\min_{i=1}^{N}(C_i)} \quad \text{and} \quad \Delta R^{\max} = \min_{i=1}^{N}(C_i) \quad [10.24]$$

Sample the number of chain cleavages, ΔR_i, from the binomial distribution of

$$f(\Delta R_i; P_i, \Delta R^{\max}) = \frac{\Delta R^{\max}!}{\Delta R_i!(\Delta R^{\max} - \Delta R_i)!} P_i^{\Delta R_i} (1 - P_i)^{\Delta R^{\max} - \Delta R_i} \quad [10.25]$$

Update $t = t + \Delta t$ and then return to the first step. In this coarse grained KMC method, parameter ε contributes the main uncertainty of dynamics for a system when compared to a KMC method. An appropriate ε therefore needs to be selected in order to satisfy convergence conditions.

Figure 10.9 shows an example of calculated average molecular weights as functions of time for a homopolymer system using the KMC and coarse grained KMC schemes respectively. Number-average molecular weight can be calculated using its definition in Chapter 1. The initial MWD is assumed to follow a log-normal distribution. The kinetic rates used in this simulation were arbitrarily taken as $k_{\text{random}} = k_{\text{end}} = 0.003 / \text{week}$ and $k^a_{\text{random}} = k^a_{\text{end}} = 0.002\sqrt{(\text{m}^3/\text{mol})} / \text{week}$ to ensure a sole random chain scission mechanism. Asterisks in Figure 10.9 are predictions from the KMC simulation. It can be observed from this figure that when the value of ε reduces from 0.0068 to 0.0029, the coarse grained KMC converges to the KMC method.

10.3.4 Degradation behaviours of various chain scissions

In Section 10.2.2, $R_{ol} - R_s$ curves for random chain scission and end chain scission were studied. Different behaviours were clarified and distinguishing degradation stages were classified. Now using KMC (or coarse grained KMC) methods, number-average molecular weights as functions of degradation time for sole random chain scission and sole end chain scission can be obtained separately, which are illustrated in Figure 10.10. Sole random chain scissions can be achieved in the molecular model

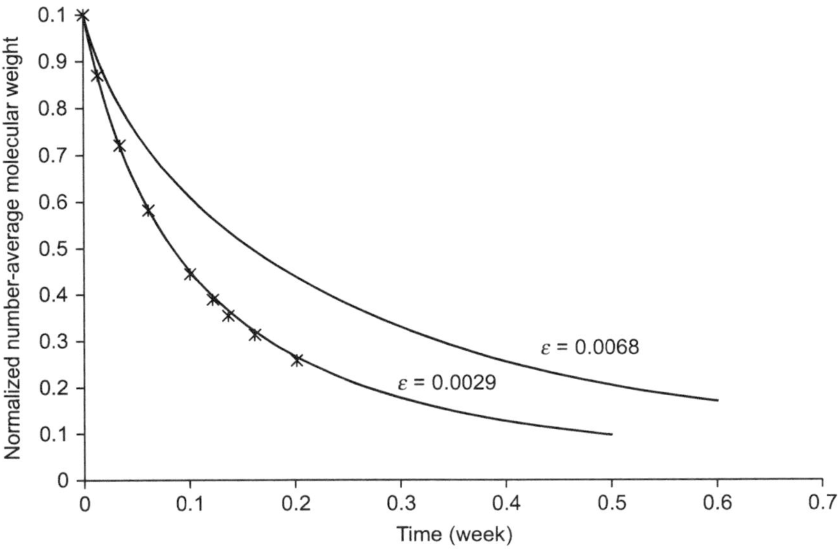

Figure 10.9 Normalized number-average molecular weight as a function of time calculated using the KMC scheme (asterisks) and coarse grained KMC scheme with different values of ε (solid lines), showing the convergence of the coarse grained KMC scheme. (*Source*: Reproduced from Reference 6 with permission.)

by setting the same chain cleavage probabilities for both middle ester bonds and end ester bonds; reaction constants therefore were taken as $k_{\text{random}} = k_{\text{end}} = 0.05\,/\,\text{week}$ and $k^a_{\text{random}} = k^a_{\text{end}} = 0.5\sqrt{(\text{m}^3\,/\,\text{mol})}\,/\text{week}$. In a KMC model, chain scissions in middle ester bonds can be switched off, by the setting k_{random} and k^a_{random} to zero, in order to give the system a sole end chain scission degradation.

Two very different degradation profiles are identified in Figures 10.10a and 10.10b. Degradation rates (number-average molecular weight decreasing rate) in Figure 10.10a decreases continually, while that of Figure 10.10b increases at the beginning and decreases thereafter. On the one hand, probability for a long polymer chain shortening into two shorter polymer chains of a random chain scission dominated degradation decreases from the very beginning, because more and more oligomer chains are produced from shorter polymer chains. On the other hand, in an end chain scission dominated degradation, a large amount of carboxylic acids result in auto-catalysed reactions, which increase the degradation rate until it reaches a turnover point when the degradation rate starts to decrease. This is because some polymer chains are eliminated to oligomers to which part of chain scissions contribute. This number of chain scissions is not counted when calculating polymer molecular weight thus decreasing the degradation rate. Furthermore, oligomer diffusion will also influence the degradation rate, which has not been considered in the examples but will be discussed.

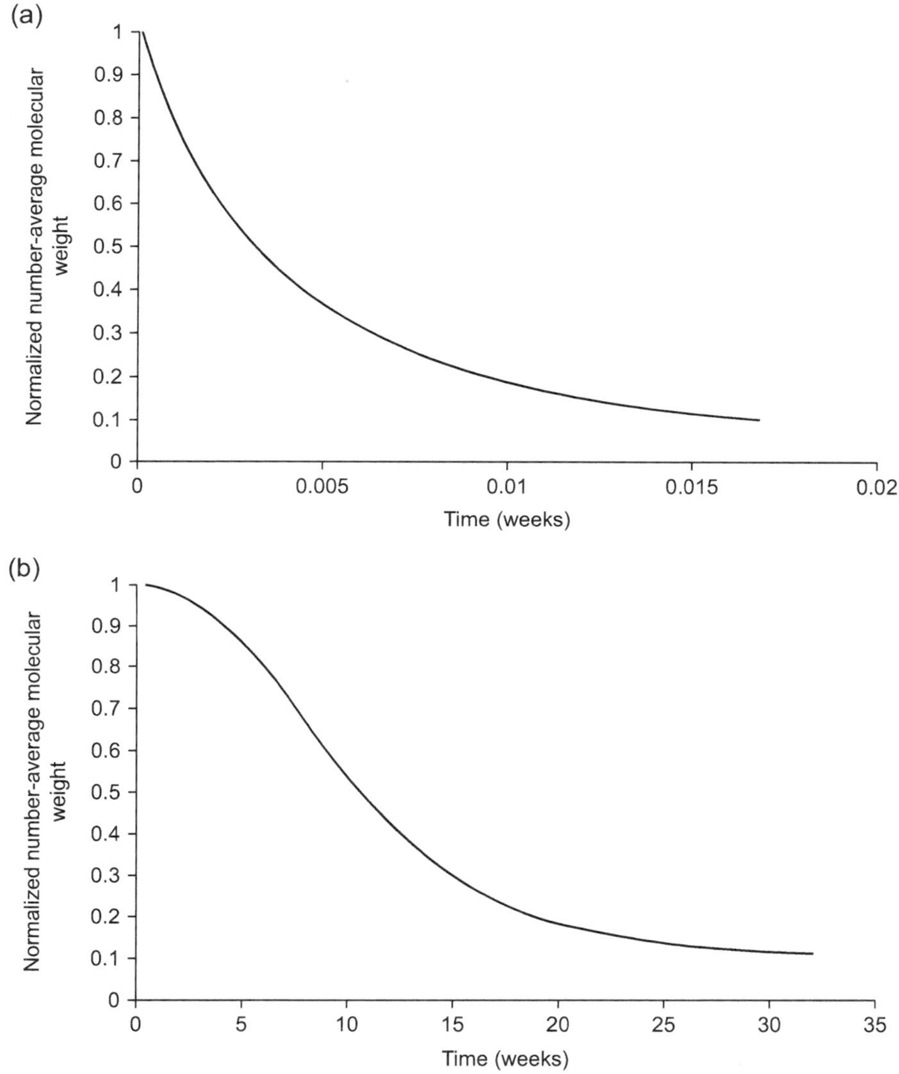

Figure 10.10 Normalized number-average molecular weights as functions of time for random chain cleavages (a) and end chain cleavages (b).

10.3.5 A KMC degradation model for copolymers

The copolymer ratio of a polymer system greatly alters its degradation rates.[8,6,12,13] Poly(DL-lactic acid) (PDLA) and PGA are the most used linear polymers, due to well-established biocompatibilities. It is possible to achieve a desired degradation rate by using different copolymer ratio of PGA and PDLA. In this section, we use a KMC degradation model for a PLGA copolymer system in order to study its innate

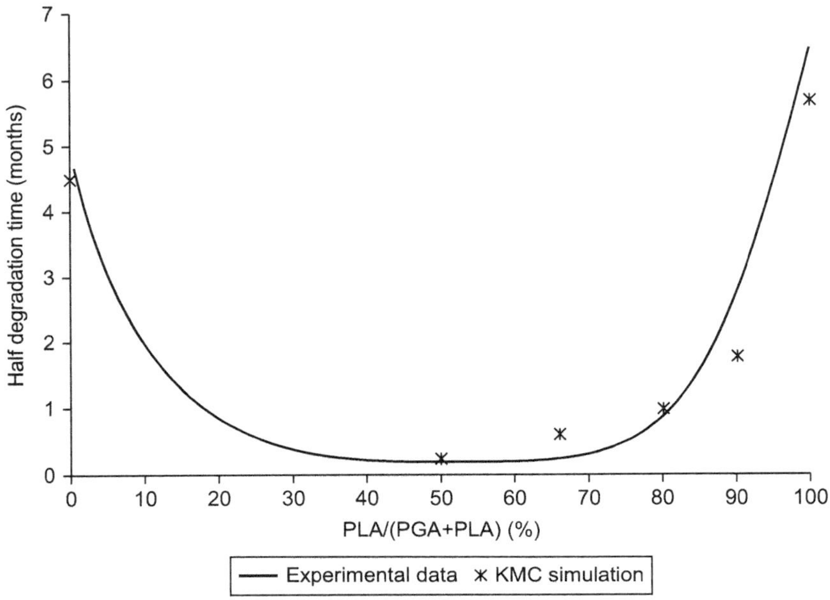

Figure 10.11 Half-life of PDLA and PGA homopolymers and copolymers from *in vivo* experiments (the solid line)[7] and the KMC simulation (asterisks). (*Source*: Reproduced from Reference 6 with permission.)

properties. PDLA is usually an amorphous polymer, while PGA is semi-crystalline. PGA has an approximately 50% initial crystallinity, which may increase to 80% during degradation.[14] In a copolymer system consisting of amorphous PDLA and semi-crystalline PGA, five types of ester bonds are identified: end ester bonds of PDLA, middle ester bonds of PDLA, end ester bonds for PGA, middle ester bonds of PGA and ester bonds in the polymer crystals. The first four kinetic rates are input parameters, while the last rate constant is set to zero (i.e. assuming that all crystals are non-degradable). It is assumed that the PGA has a constant degree of crystallinity of 70% (an average value of crystallinity during degradation: 60% at the beginning and 80% after degradation) during degradation, for simplicity. PGA monomers are uniformly distributed in polymer chains (type 1 copolymer is assumed). A half-degradation time of a polymer system is defined as the time taken for the polymer to halve its average molecular weight. Figure 10.11 shows the half-degradation time of PLGA, as a function of the copolymer ratio obtained experimentally (the solid line)[4] and by the KMC simulations (discrete symbols). Figure 10.12 presents the average molecular weights of PDLA, PGA and their copolymers as functions of time, calculated by KMC models. All the parameter values used in the KMC simulation are shown in Table 10.1. The reaction rates for PGA and PDLA are determined by fitting half-degradation times for pure PGA and PDLA respectively, which are also provided in Table 10.1. They are kept consistent in the KMC models predicting half-degradation times for copolymer PLGA of four different copolymer ratios. Experimental data in Figure 10.11 show that the

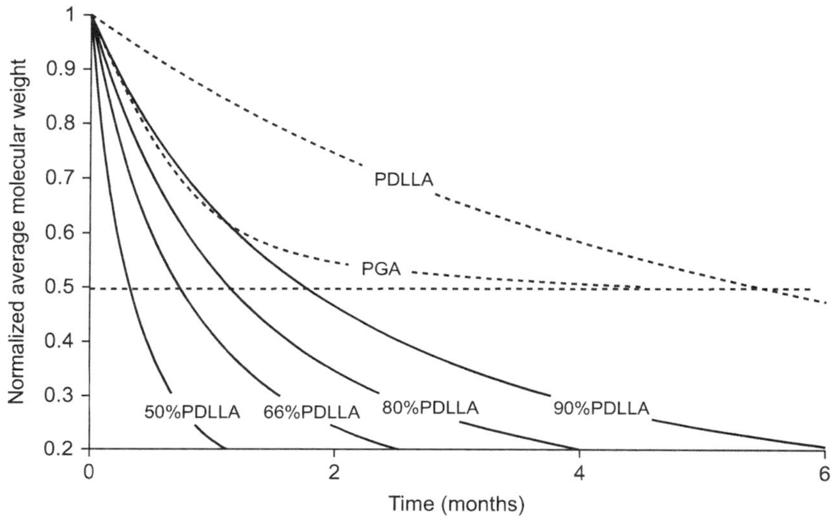

Figure 10.12 Normalized number-average molecular weight as a function of time for PDLA, PGA (solid lines) and their copolymers of different copolymer ratios (dashed lines) from the KMC simulation. (*Source*: Reproduced from Reference 6 with permission.)

half-degradation time of the copolymer reduces sharply as PDLA is introduced into the copolymer system. This is because the copolymer has a reduced degree of crystallinity in comparison to that of the pure PGA. Copolymers that contain a higher percentage of PDLA are regarded as amorphous polymers. A higher percentage of PDLA increases half-degradation time, because of a slower degradation rate for PDLA than PGA. The KMC model predictions of half times, shown as asterisks in Figure 10.11, were obtained from Figure 10.12 by finding the corresponding time when the normalized average molecular weight equals 0.5. Figure 10.13 shows calculated MWDs at three different times for the six cases. It can be observed that the distribution remains log-normal except for the pure PGA case, which developed a bimodal distribution because of the non-degradable crystalline phase.

Figure 10.14 shows the PDIs as functions of time for six cases. Calculated PDIs vary during degradation time from 1.5 to 2, except for pure PGA, which is in consistency with experimental observations[15,16] due to the exited crystal phase.

10.4 A multi-scale model for device degradations

A multi-scale model is introduced in this section, using KMC simulation for polymer chain scissions which occur in a microscopic stage while applying a diffusion equation for the macroscopic oligomer diffusion. In this section, the development of the multi-scale model is discussed, providing details of models in each scale and especially focusing on the combination of these two scales. An application is also provided in this section to demonstrate advantages that this model can deliver.

Table 10.1 Model parameters used in the case studies

Parameters Cases in	D_0 (m^2/week)	k_{random} (1/week)	k^a_{random} $\left(\sqrt{(m^3/mol)}\ /\ week\right)$	k_{end} (1/week)	k^a_{end} $\left(\sqrt{(m^3/mol)}\ /\ week\right)$	Polymers
Figures 10.10–10.13	Diffusion not considered	7×10^{-6}	7×10^{-6}	2.3×10^{-5}	2.3×10^{-5}	PDLA
	Diffusion not considered	1.9×10^{-4}	1.9×10^{-4}	1.2×10^{-3}	1.2×10^{-3}	PGA
Figures 10.15,10.16	2×10^{-9}	$k = 0.042$/week		$k^a = 0.001\left(\sqrt{(m^3/mol)}/week\right)$		PLA
Figures 10.18–10.21	2×10^{-9}	5×10^{-5}	2.5×10^{-5}	0.1	0.1	PLA

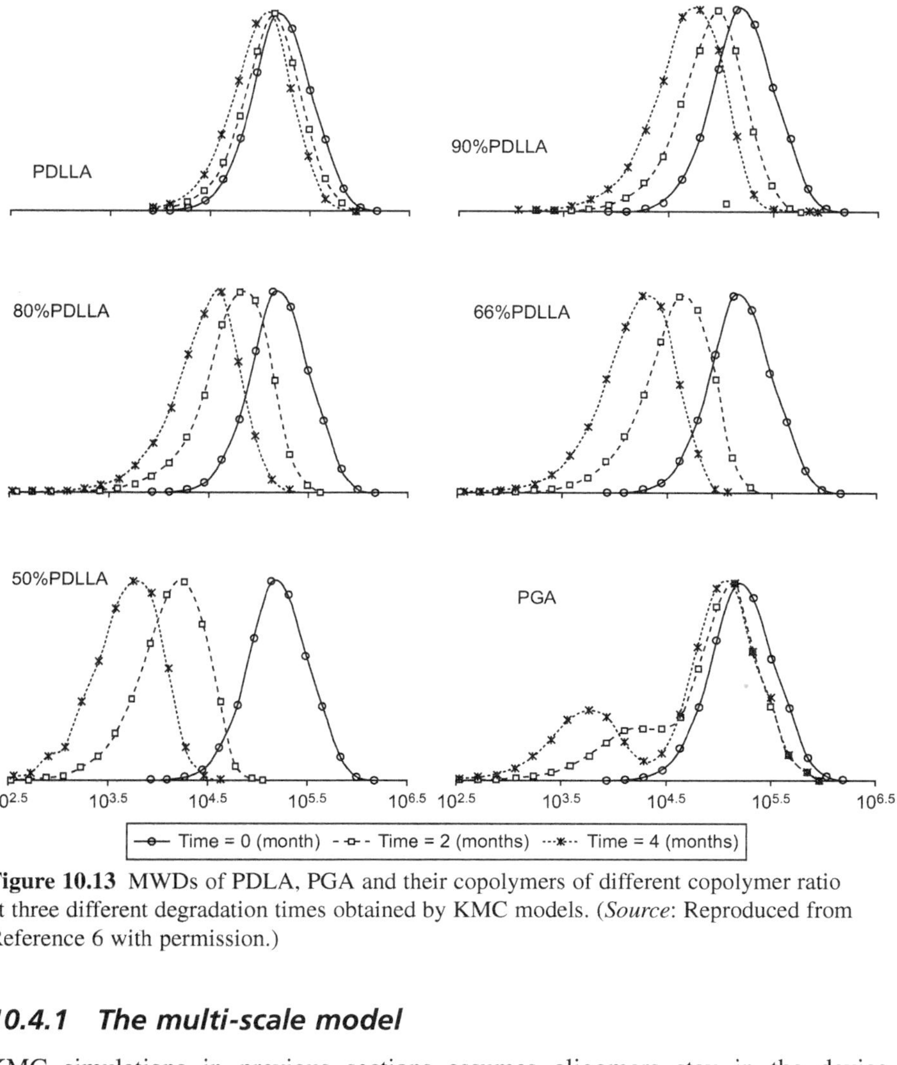

Figure 10.13 MWDs of PDLA, PGA and their copolymers of different copolymer ratio at three different degradation times obtained by KMC models. (*Source*: Reproduced from Reference 6 with permission.)

10.4.1 The multi-scale model

KMC simulations in previous sections assumes oligomers stay in the device. Oligomers are small molecules which are water soluble and will diffuse out of the device during degradation. The non-uniform diffusion profile of oligomers will cause a heterogeneous degradation due to auto-catalysed chain scissions. In the phenomenological model, the following governing equation was used to describe the change in the oligomer concentration due to oligomer diffusion:

$$\frac{dC_{ol}}{dt} = \frac{dR_{ol}}{dt} + \underset{x_i}{\text{div}}\left(\text{D}\,\underset{x_i}{\text{grad}}\left(C_{ol}\right)\right) \quad [10.26]$$

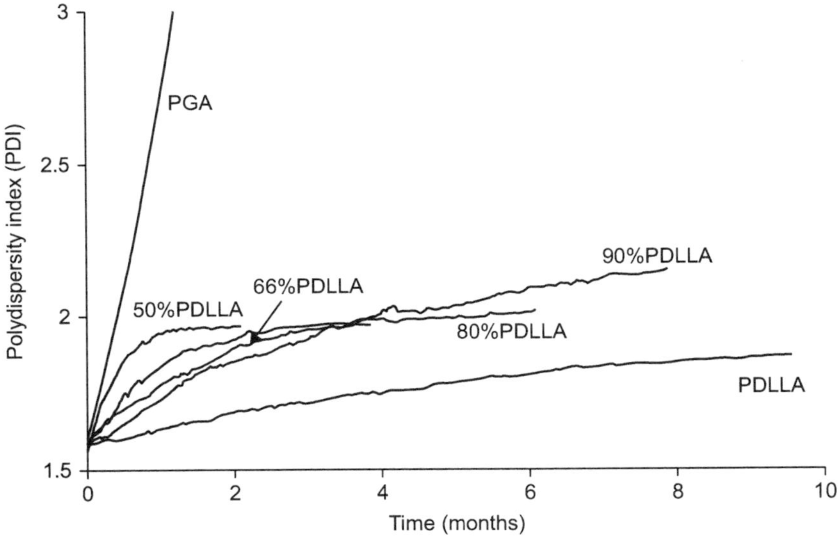

Figure 10.14 Polydispersity index (PDI) as a function of time for PDLA, PGA and their copolymers of different copolymer ratio obtained from the KMC simulations. (*Source*: Reproduced from Reference 6 with permission.)

where C_{ol} is the mole concentration of oligomers, D is the effective diffusion coefficient of the oligomers that depends on the porosity of the polymer:

$$D = D_0 + \left(1.3p^2 - 0.3p^3\right)\left(D_1 - D_0\right) \qquad [10.27]$$

where p is porosity, which is given by:

$$p = 1 - \left(\frac{C_e}{C_{e0}}\right) - \frac{C_{ol}}{C_{e0}} \qquad [10.28]$$

In equation [10.27] D_0 is the diffusion coefficient of oligomers in non-degraded amorphous polymer, D_1 is the diffusion coefficient of oligomers in micro-pores and C_e is the mole concentration of the ester bonds of all the polymer chains. Equation [10.26] can be solved numerically using either the finite element method or the finite difference method for a device. At each integration point of either the finite element method or the finite difference node, the first term on the right hand side in Equation [10.26] can be calculated from KMC simulation at that local point by counting the number of chains shorter than N_{ol} at each time step. Oligomers produced from the KMC model diffuse over the entire device globally, which is described by the second term on the right hand side in Equation [10.26]. These two terms combine a molecular KMC model and a global diffusion model. Figure 10.15 illustrates the two-scale model for the degradation of a plate schematically. In Figure 10.15, we consider an

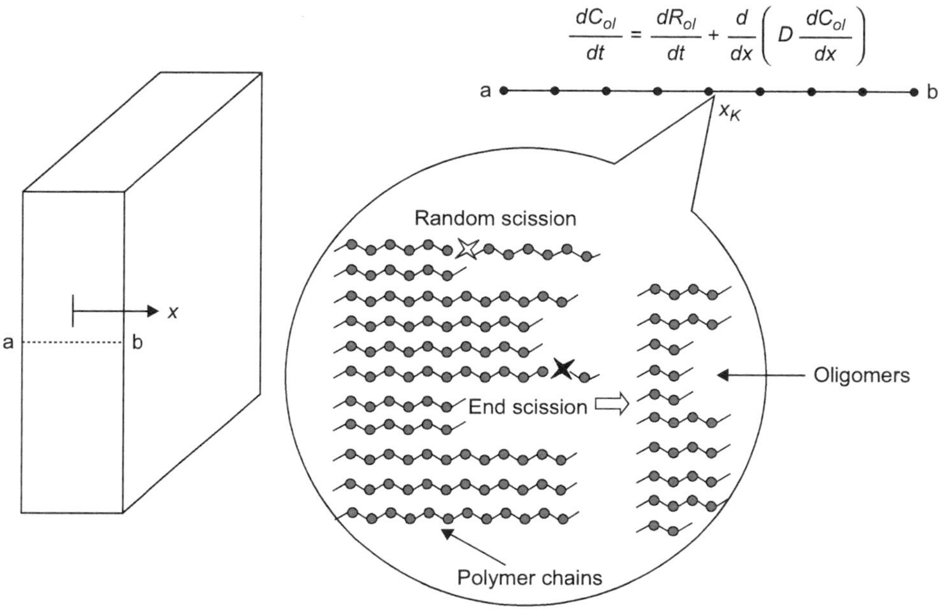

Figure 10.15 Schematic diagram of the two-scale model for the biodegradation of a plate in which the diffusion of oligomers occurs only in the thickness direction (a–b) of the plate. (*Source*: Reproduced from Reference 6 with permission.)

infinitively large plate in which the oligomer diffusion occurs only in the x direction (marked as a–b). A finite difference scheme is utilized to discretize the spatial differentiation in Equation [10.26] with respect to x. At each finite difference node x_K, N_e of the polymer chains are generated according to the initial MWD seeding process of the polymer system. Chain scissions are executed using the KMC scheme at each node based on kinetic rates on this node, which provides concentrations of oligomers and the different types of ester bonds on the polymer chains. The change in oligomer concentration due to global diffusion is calculated using a finite difference representation of the second term of Equation [10.26]. Direct Euler scheme is used for the time integration. The time step length required by the KMC scheme is typically much smaller than that needed by the global diffusion. Therefore, two different time steps are used for oligomer diffusion and chain scissions, respectively. After a number of local time steps, the local concentrations of different quantities are passed to the global calculation for oligomer diffusion. Oligomer concentrations after the diffusion at all nodes are then fed back to the local KMC scheme. Thus, a two-scale model is perfectly combined. The detailed algorithm can be found in Reference 17.

10.4.2 An application of multi-scale molecular model

Li *et al.*[8,6,13] reported the finding in their experiments that the degradation of their disc samples made of PLA and PLGA is highly heterogeneous. The centres of the samples degrade much faster than the device surface. Shell-like samples were found at a very late stage of degradation. Grizzi *et al.*[18] later showed that a thinner film of 0.3 mm in thickness degrades slower than a thicker plate of 2 mm made of the same PLA. They explained that the heterogeneous[13] degradation and size effect phenomenon result from the autocatalytic nature of the hydrolysis reaction of polyesters. Heterogeneous shorter chains' diffusion profile thus plays a key role in controlling the overall degradation rate. A thicker plate degrades faster than a thinner one, as the short chains with acid end groups in a thick plate cannot diffuse out quickly enough and an acidic environment is built up at the core of the plate. The core of a thick plate also degrades faster than the surface of the plate. However, the size effect and heterogeneous degradation were observed during an early stage of the degradation test when very little weight loss, L-lactic acid release and pH change were measured.[8,6,13,18] This is interesting, in that the obvious size effect and heterogeneous degradation would require significant smaller chains to diffuse out of the samples. To demonstrate this point, the conceptional analysis by Grizzi *et al.*[18] is carried through quantitatively using a diffusion–reaction model. The multi-scale model in this chapter assumes the polymer device remains a solid during biodegradation. In the biodegradation tests by Grizzi, Li and their co-worker, the core of the polymer discs became viscous in the later stage of the degradation. We therefore limit the numerical analysis to the first 11 weeks of the tests. The parameters in the model were obtained by fitting the molecular weight data of the thin film and the thick plate and fitting the weight loss data of the thick plate simultaneously. This procedure gives $k = 0.042/\text{week}$, $k^a = 0.001\sqrt{(\text{m}^3/\text{mol})}/\text{week}$ and $D_0 = 2\times10^{-9}\,\text{m}^2/\text{week}$. These parameters are then used to calculate the weight loss of the thin film. Figures 10.16 and 10.17 show the fit between the model prediction and the experimental data for average molecular weight and weight loss as functions of time. Figure 10.17 indicates that significantly more weight loss in the thin film is required by the model to achieve the observed size effect than the experimental measurement.

10.4.3 A thin layer of the multi-scale model

The observed size effect without significant weight loss reported by Grizzi *et al.*[18] can be achieved in the multi-scale model by introducing a thin surface layer in which the hydrolysis is not autocatalytic ($k^a = 0$) as shown in Figure 10.18. The different hydrolysis kinetics in the surface layer can be due to either the neutralization of the carboxylic end groups at the surface or the instant dissolution of the oligomers into the liquid media. Hundreds of finite difference nodes are generated along the thickness of the plate. At each node, 20 000 polymer chains are generated following the SEC data provided by Grizzi *et al.*[18] A log-normal MWD is generated based on fitting SEC data. Material parameters are found by fitting the experimental data of MWDs and weight loss at various degradation times which are: $k_{\text{random}} = 5\times10^{-5}/\text{week}$, $k^a_{\text{random}} = 2.5\times10^{-5}\sqrt{(\text{m}^3/\text{mol})}/\text{week}$, $k_{\text{end}} = 0.1/\text{week}$, $k^a_{\text{random}} = 0.1\sqrt{(\text{m}^3/\text{mol})}/\text{week}$ and $D_0 = 2\times10^{-9}\,\text{m}^2/\text{week}$. For the finite difference nodes within the surface layer,

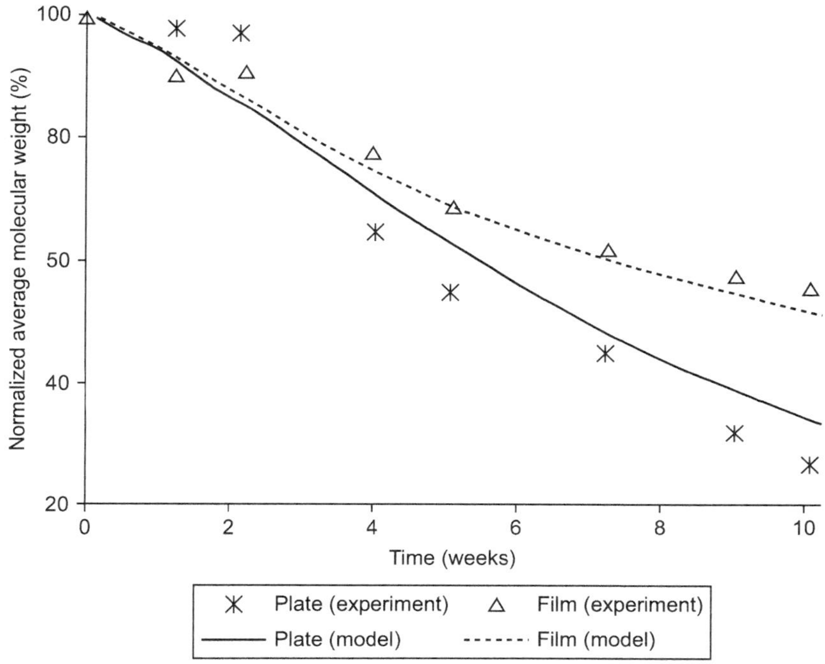

Figure 10.16 Normalized weight-averaged molecular weight as a function of time for a PLA plate of 2 mm and a film of 0.3 mm made of the same PLA. The discrete symbols are experimental data[13] and the lines are fit using a reaction–diffusion model[9]. (*Source*: Reproduced from Reference 6 with permission.)

k^a_{random} and k^a_{end} are set as zero. The thickness of the surface layer is set as 100 μm for both plate and film according to Grizzi *et al.*[18] The model parameters are summarized in Table 10.1. Figures 10.19–10.21 show the comparison between the calculated predictions and experimental molecular weight-averaged over the thickness of sample, weight loss of the sample and MWD averaged over the thickness of the sample as functions of time, respectively. It can be observed from the figures that the two-scale reaction–diffusion model with surface layer can fit all the experimental data by Grizzi *et al.*[18] very well. In particular, the size effect is obtained even when the weight losses of the thick plate and thin film are very similar, as shown in Figure 10.20. Figure 10.21 shows that the model is able to capture the transition from the initial monomodal MWD to a bimodal distribution by week 11 in the thick plate, while predicting a monomodal MWD in the thin film throughout the degradation process. Figure 10.22 shows the calculated MWDs of the central and surface points for the thick and thin samples respectively at 0 and 11 weeks. It can be observed that the thick plate shows much more differentiated degradation than the thin one, entirely due to the slower diffusion of the oligomers out of the thick plate, as suggested by Grizzi *et al.*[18]

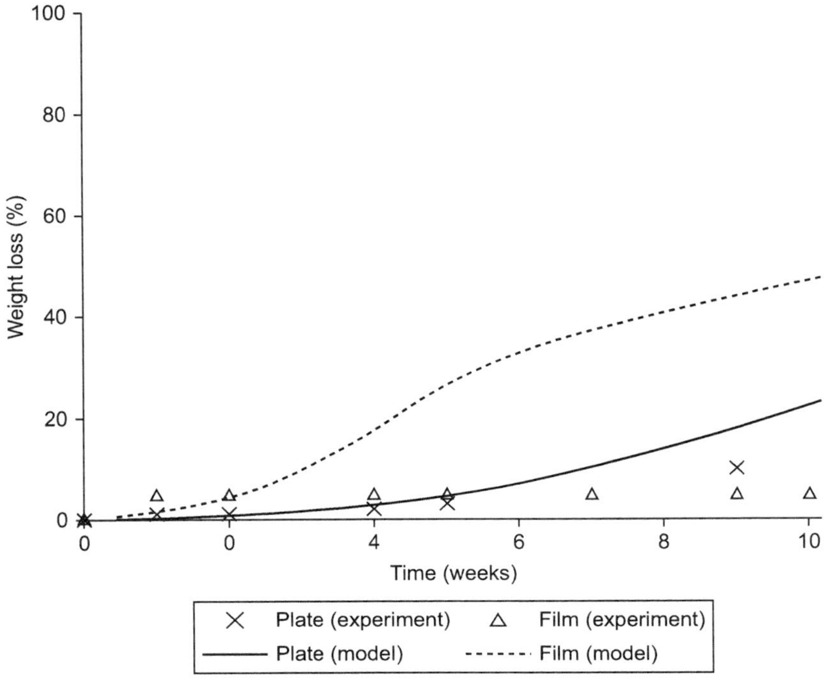

Figure 10.17 Weight loss as a function of time for a PLA plate of 2 mm and a film of 0.3 mm made of the same PLA. The discrete symbols are experimental data[8,13] and lines are fit using a reaction–diffusion model.[9] (*Source*: Reproduced from Reference 6 with permission.)

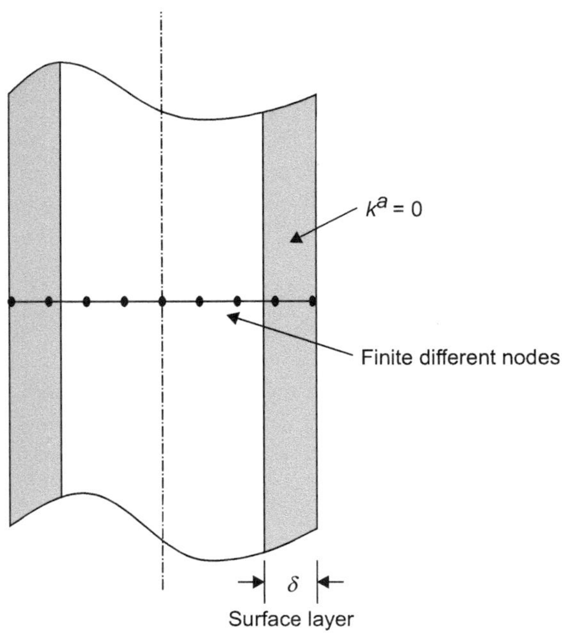

Figure 10.18 A schematic diagram of a plate with a surface layer in which the carboxylic end groups are neutralized. (*Source*: Reproduced from Reference 6 with permission.)

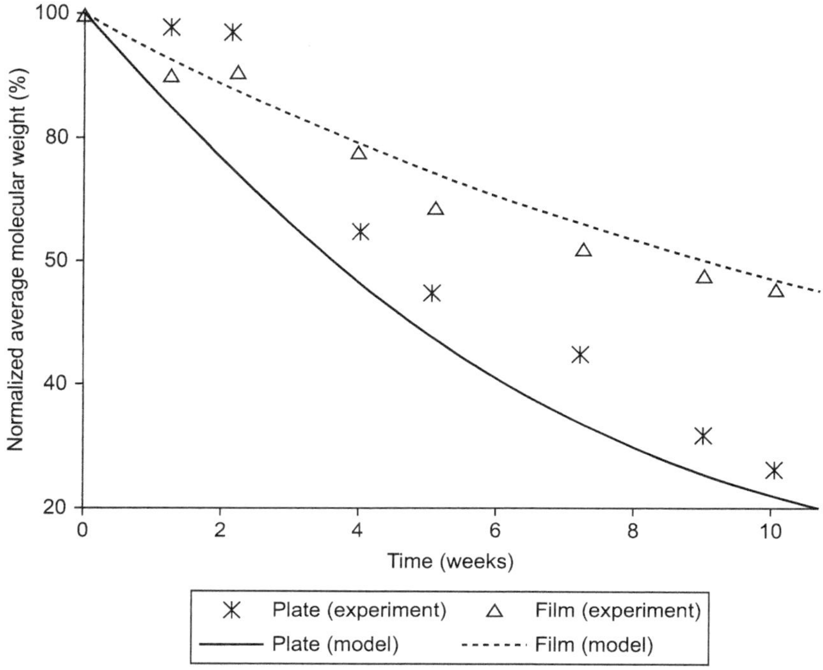

Figure 10.19 Refitting of the data shown in Figure 10.16 using the two-scale model with a surface layer. (*Source*: Reproduced from Reference 6 with permission.)

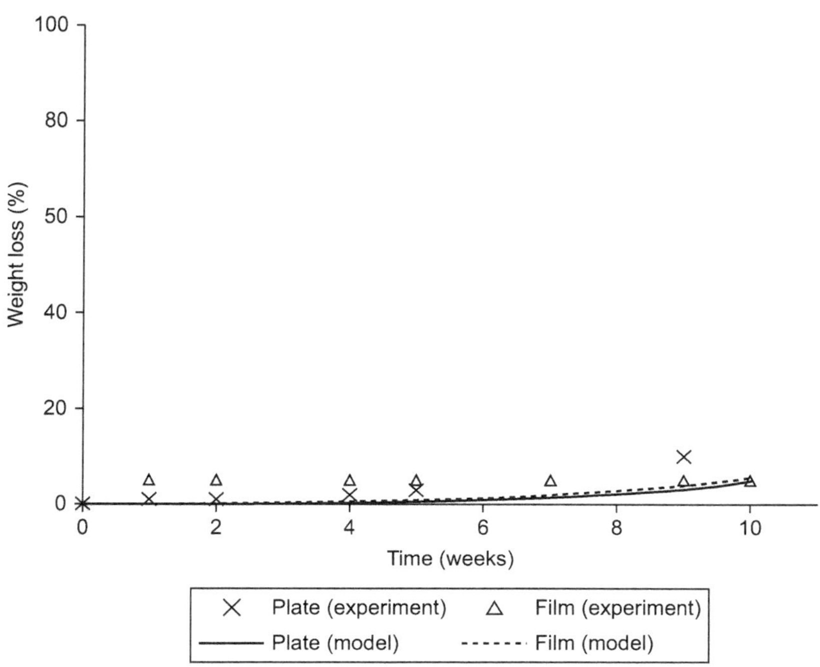

Figure 10.20 Refitting of the data shown in Figure 10.17 using the two-scale model with a surface layer. (*Source*: Reproduced from Reference 6 with permission.)

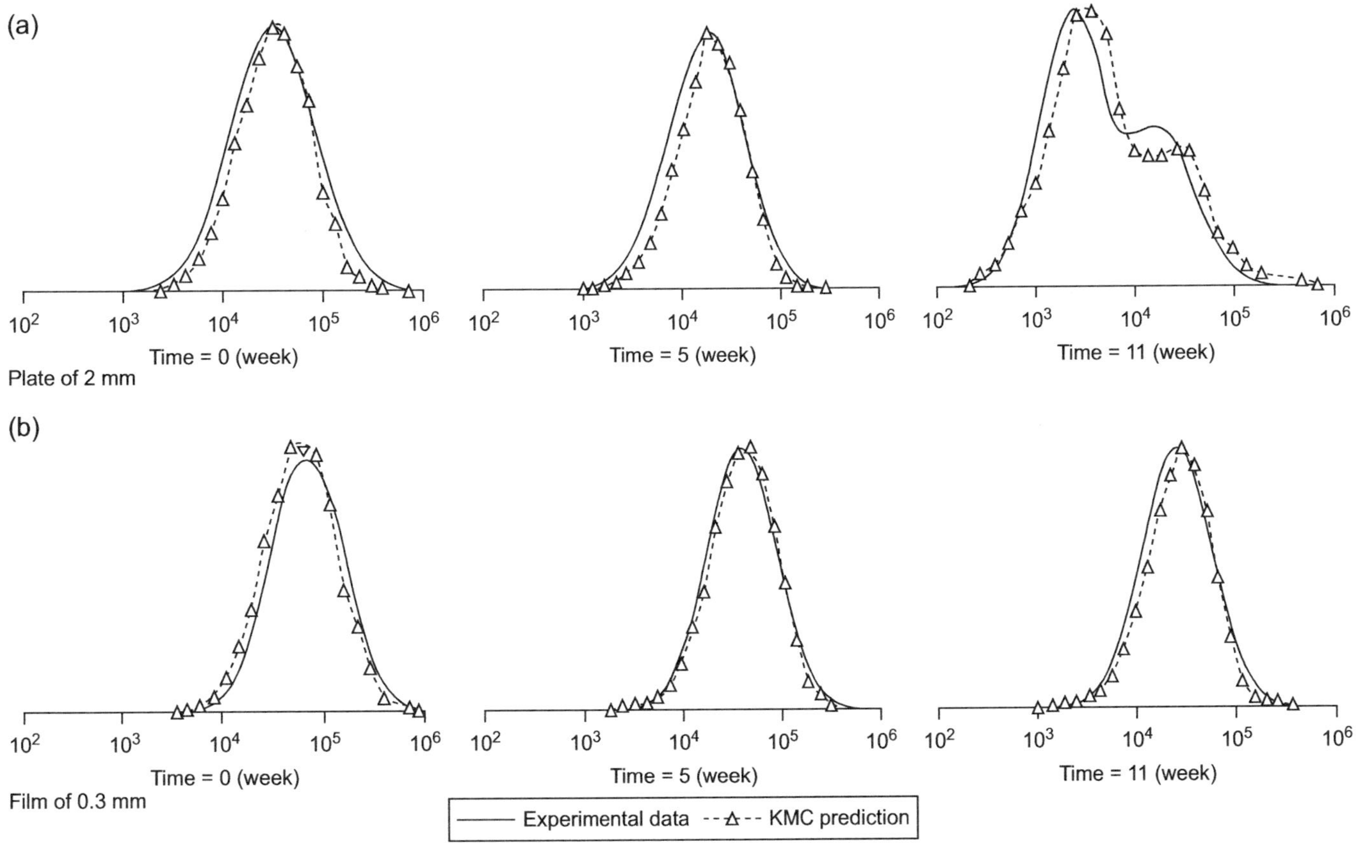

Figure 10.21 MWDs averaged over the sample thickness for (a) the plate and (b) the film at different times from the experimental data[13] and the two-scale model. (*Source*: Reproduced from Reference 6 with permission.)

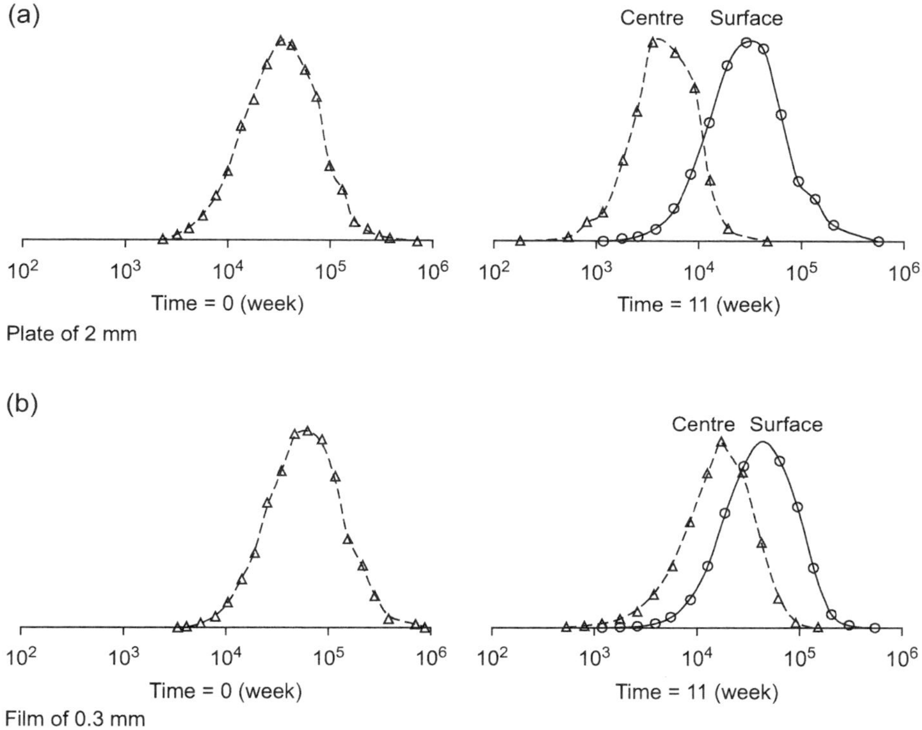

Figure 10.22 Calculated MWDs of a centre and surface nodes in the finite difference model at the beginning and after 11 weeks of the degradation for (a) plate of 2 mm and (b) film of 0.3 mm. (*Source*: Reproduced from Reference 6 with permission.)

10.5 Conclusions

In this chapter, we introduce molecular and multi-scale modelling methods of polymer device degradation. Molecular models can consider the detailed information about the polymer system, such as the initial MWD, copolymer ratio, degree of crystallinity, end chain scission and random chain scission rates. Using the KMC scheme, molecular models of polymer chain scission can be predicted for both homopolymers and copolymers. It is also shown that the KMC scheme can accurately predict the effect of copolymer ratio between PGA and PDLA on the degradation rate of the copolymer. A multi-scale model is used to simulate polymer degradation considering both chain scissions and the small molecule diffusion. The numerical study shows that the conceptional reaction–diffusion model suggested by Grizzi *et al.*[18] needs to be extended in order to fully explain the size effect and heterogonous degradation observed in the experiment. A possible extension is to introduce a surface layer in which the carboxylic end groups are neutralized. It is shown that such a model can capture all the experimental data well. However, the exact cause of the neutralization is unclear and remains to be explored in future studies. For devices of sophisticated shapes, such as an internal fixation screw, the finite element method can be used to perform the global diffusion analysis. The local KMC analysis can be connected with the finite element analysis at the integration points of the finite element mesh.

Acknowledgement

The molecular models and the multi-scale model described in this chapter were first reported in the reference below and the figures are reproduced here in part or in full with the permission of Elsevier Science & Technology Journals.

X. Han and J. Pan (2010), Polymer chain scission, oligomer production and diffusion: A two-scale model for degradation of bioresorbable polyesters. *Acta Biomaterialia*, **7**: 538–547.

References

1. Shih C. (1995) Chain-end scission in acid catalyzed hydrolysis of poly(D,L-lactide) in solution. *Journal of Controlled Release*, **34**:9–15.
2. Buehler MJ. (2007) Hierarchical chemo-nanomechanics of proteins: entropic elasticity, protein unfolding and molecular fracture. *Journal of Mechanics of Materials and Structures*, **2**:1019–1057.
3. Ackbarow T and Buehler MJ. (2007) Superelasticity, energy dissipation and strain hardening of vimentin coiled-coil intermediate filaments: atomistic and continuum studies. *Journal of Material Science*, **42**:8771–8887.
4. Miller R, Brady J and Cutright DE. (1977) Degradation rates of oral resorbable implants (polylactates and polyglycolates): rate modification with changes in PLA/PGA copolymer ratios. *Journal of Biomedical Materials Research*, **11**:711–719.
5. Flory PJ. (1953) *Principles of Polymer Chemistry*, New York, Cornell University Press.
6. Li SM, H.Garreau and Vert M. (1990) Structure-property relationships in the case of the degradation of massive poly(a-hydroxy acids) in aqueous media-Part 2 Degradation of lactide-glycolide copolymers: PLA37.5GA25 and PLA75GA25. *Journal of Materials Science: Materials in Medicine*. **1**:131–139.
7. Cameron RE and Kamvari-Moghaddam A. (2008) Synthetic bioresorbable polymers. In: Fraser Buchanan (ed.). *Degradation Rate of Bioresorbable Materials Prediction and Evaluation* Boca Raton, CRC Press, 3-43-66.
8. Li SM, Garreau H and Vert M. (1990) Structure-property relationships in the case of the degradation of massive poly(a-hydroxy acids) in aqueous media- Part 3 Influence of the morphology of poly(L-lactic acid). *Journal of Materials Science: Materials in Medicine*. **1**:198–206.
9. Han X, Pan J, Buchanan F, Weir N and Farrar D. (2010) Analysis of degradation data of poly(l-lactide–co-l,d-lactide) and poly(l-lactide) obtained at elevated and physiological temperatures using mathematical models. *Acta Biomaterialia*, **6**:3882–3889.
10. Gillespie DT. (1976) A general method for numerically simulating the stochastic time evolution of coupled chemical reactions. *Journal of Computational Physics*, **22**:403–434.

11. Chatterjee A and Vlachos DG. (2005) Binomial distribution based t-leap accelerated stochastic simulation. *The Journal of Chemical Physics*. **122**:024112.
12. Zong, X-H, Wang Z-G, Hsiao BS and Chu B. (1999) Structure and morphology changes in absorbable poly(glycolide) and poly(glycolide-co-lactide) during *in vitro* degradation. *Macromolecules*, **32**:8107–8114.
13. Li SM, Garreau H and Vert M. (1990) Structure-property relationships in the case of the degradation of massive aliphatic poly(a-hydroxy acids) in aqueous media – Part 1: Poly(DL-lactic acid). *Journal of Materials Science: Materials in Medicine*, **1**:123–130.
14. Lee JW and Gardella JA. (2001) *In vitro* hydrolytic surface degradation of poly(glycolic acid): role of the surface segregated amorphous region in the induction period of bulk erosion. *Macromolecules*, 3928–3937.
15. Saha S and Tsuji H. (2006) Effects of molecular weight and small amounts of D-lactide units on hydrolytic degradation of poly(l-lactic acid)s. *Polymer Degradation and Stability*, **34**,1665–1673.
16. Grayson A, Cima M and Langer R. (2005) Size and temperature effects on poly(lactic-co-glycolic acid) degradation and microreservoir device performance. *Biomaterials*, **36**, 2137–2145.
17. Han X and Pan J. (2011) Polymer chain scission, oligomer production and diffusion: A two-scale model for degradation of bioresorbable polyesters. *Acta Biomaterialia*, **7**, 538–547.
18. Grizzi I, Garreau S, Li S and Vert M. (1995) Hydrolytic degradation of devices based on poly(DL-lactic acid) size-dependence. *Biomaterials*, **16**, 305–311.

Index

FSC
www.fsc.org
MIX
Papier | Fördert
gute Waldnutzung
FSC® C083411

Kolibri 360 GmbH
Ferdinand-Jühlke-Straße 7
99095 Erfurt, Deutschland
produktsicherheit@kolibri360.de